HEADACHE AND
Facial Pain
MEDICINE

T0289910

HEADACHE AND
Facial Pain
MEDICINE

Editor

Sait Ashina, MD

Assistant Professor of Neurology and Anesthesia
BIDMC Comprehensive Headache Center
Department of Neurology and Department of Anesthesia
Critical Care and Pain Medicine
Harvard Medical School
Beth Israel Deaconess Medical Center
Boston, Massachusetts

Headache and Facial Pain Medicine

Copyright © 2025 by McGraw Hill LLC. All rights reserved. Printed in China. Except as permitted under the United States Copyright Act of 1976, no part of this publication may be reproduced or distributed in any form or by any means, or stored in a database or retrieval system, without the prior written permission of the publisher.

1 2 3 4 5 6 7 8 9 DSS 29 28 27 26 25 24

ISBN 978-1-264-80312-5
MHID 1-264-80312-5

This book was set in Minion Pro by MPS Limited.
The editors were Timothy Y. Hiscock and Kim J. Davis.
The production supervisor was Richard Ruzycka.
Project management was provided by Poonam Bisht of MPS Limited.
The cover designer was W2 Design.
This book is printed on acid-free paper.

Library of Congress Cataloging-in-Publication Data

Names: Ashina, Sait, editor.
Title: Headache and facial pain medicine / editor, Sait Ashina.
Description: New York : McGraw Hill, [2024] | Includes bibliographical
   references and index. | Summary: "The book covers epidemiology,
   pathophysiology, diagnosis and treatment of primary and secondary
   headache disorders and facial pain disorders described in the third and
   latest edition of the International Classification of Headache Disorders
   (ICHD-3)"—Provided by publisher.
Identifiers: LCCN 2023052564 (print) | LCCN 2023052565 (ebook) |
   ISBN 9781264803125 (paperback; alk. paper) | ISBN 9781264804986 (ebook)
Subjects: MESH: Headache Disorders | Facial Pain | Pain Management—methods
Classification: LCC RC392 (print) | LCC RC392 (ebook) | NLM WL 342 |
   DDC 616.8/491—dc23/eng/20240202
LC record available at https://lccn.loc.gov/2023052564
LC ebook record available at https://lccn.loc.gov/2023052565

McGraw Hill books are available at special quantity discounts to use as premiums and sales promotions or for use in corporate training programs. To contact a representative, please visit the Contact Us pages at www.mhprofessional.com.

To my beloved daughter, Adelia, and my cherished wife, Nazrin, whose love lights my journey.

To my mother, for her relentless support and guidance in my educational and professional paths.

—Sait Ashina

Contents

Contributors

Zubair A. Ahmed, MD
Assistant Professor of Neurology
Headache Section, Department of
  Neurology
Center for Neurologic Restoration
Neurologic Institute, Cleveland Clinic
Cleveland Clinic Lerner College of
  Medicine
Case Western Reserve University
Cleveland, Ohio

Jessica Ailani, MD, FAHS,
  FAAN, FANA
Professor of Clinical Neurology
Director of MedStar Georgetown
  Headache Center
Department of Neurology
Medstar Georgetown University
  Hospital
Washington, DC

Ashley Alex, MD
Clerkship Director, Department of
  Neurology
Assistant Professor of Neurology
Jacobs School of Medicine and
  Biomedical Sciences
University at Buffalo, The State
  University of New York
Buffalo, New York

Hossein Ansari, MD,
  FAAN, FAHS
Director of Headache and Facial
  Pain Clinic
Kaizen Brain Center
La Jolla, California

Department of Neuroscience
University of California
San Diego, California

Karissa Arca, MD
Assistant Professor of Neurology
Department of Neurology
Mayo Clinic Arizona
Scottsdale, Arizona

Hakan Ashina, MD
Research Fellow
Danish Headache Center,
  Rigshospitalet—Glostrup
University of Copenhagen
Copenhagen, Denmark

Sait Ashina, MD
Assistant Professor of Neurology and
  Anesthesia
BIDMC Comprehensive Headache
  Center
Department of Neurology and
  Department of Anesthesia
Critical Care and Pain Medicine
Harvard Medical School
Beth Israel Deaconess Medical
  Center
Boston, Massachusetts

Lars Bendtsen, MD, PhD
Associate Professor of Neurology
Danish Headache Center
Copenhagen University
  Hospital—Rigshospitalet
University of Copenhagen
Copenhagen, Denmark

Thomas Berk, MD
Medical Director
Neura Health
New York, New York

Eric Bhaimia, DO
Assistant Professor of Medicine
Division of Infectious Diseases
Department of Internal Medicine
Rush University Medical Center
Chicago, Illinois

Federico Bighiani, MD
Physician Scientist
Department of Brain and Behavioral
   Sciences
University of Pavia
Headache Science and
   Neurorehabilitation Center
IRCCS Mondino Foundation
Pavia, Italy

Andrew Blumenfeld, MD
Headache Specialist
The Los Angeles Headache Center
Los Angeles, California

Hayrunnisa Bolay, MD, PhD
Professor of Neurology
Department of Neurology and Algology
NÖROM Centre
Gazi University
Ankara, Turkey

Brooklyn A. Bradley, BS
Postgraduate Research Associate
Department of Psychiatry
Yale School of Medicine
New Haven, Connecticut

Rami Burstein, PhD
John Hedley-Whyte Professor of
   Anesthesia

Department of Anesthesia, Critical
   Care and Pain Medicine
Harvard Medical School
Beth Israel Deaconess Medical Center
Boston, Massachusetts

**Larry Charleston, IV, MD,
   MSc, FAHS**
Professor of Neurology
Director, Headache Medicine and
   Facial Pain
Director, Department Faculty
   Development
Department of Neurology and
   Ophthalmology
Michigan State University College of
   Human Medicine
East Lansing, Michigan

Abigail L. Chua, DO
Director of Neurology
Geisinger Wyoming Valley Medical
   Center
Department of Neurology
Geisinger Health Systems
Wilkes-Barre, Pennsylvania

Alison V. Crum, MD
Professor of Ophthalmology and
   Neurology
Department of Ophthalmology and
   Neurology
University of Utah School of Medicine
John A. Moran Eye Center
Salt Lake City, Utah

Roberto De Icco, MD
Research Scientific
Department of Brain and Behavioral
   Sciences
University of Pavia
Headache Science and
   Neurorehabilitation Center

IRCCS Mondino Foundation
Pavia, Italy

Hans-Christoph Diener, MD, PhD
Professor of Neurology
Department of Neuroepidemiology
Institute for Medical Informatics,
    Biometry and Epidemiology
University Duisburg-Essen
Essen, Germany

Kathleen B. Digre, MD
Distinguished Professor of Neurology
    and Ophthalmology
Department of Neurology and
    Ophthalmology
University of Utah School of Medicine
John A. Moran Eye Center
Salt Lake City, Utah

Thien Phu Do, MD, PhD
Resident Physician
Department of Neurology,
Copenhagen University
    Hospital—Herlev and Gentofte
Herlev, Denmark

David W. Dodick, MD
Professor Emeritus
Department of Neurology
Mayo Clinic
Phoenix, Arizona

Patrick Ebbert, MD
Neurology Resident
Department of Neurology
Icahn School of Medicine at
    Mount Sinai
New York, New York

Deborah I. Friedman, MD, MPH
Key-Whitman Eye Center
Dallas, Texas

Adjunct Faculty
Thomas Jefferson University
Philadelphia, Pennsylvania

**Peter J. Goadsby, MD, PhD,
    DSc, FRS**
Professor of Neurology
NIHR-King's Clinical Research Facility
    and Wolfson SPRRC
Institute of Psychiatry, Psychology and
    Neuroscience
King's College London, United
    Kingdom
Professor Emeritus of Neurology
Department of Neurology
University of California
Los Angeles, California

Frederick A. Godley, III, MD, FACS
University Otolaryngology,
    Providence, Rhode Island
Clinical Assistant Professor
    of Surgery
Warren Alpert Medical School, Brown
    University
Providence, Rhode Island

Robert Charles Goodrich, MD
Neurology Resident
Wake Forest University School of
    Medicine
Winston-Salem, North Carolina

Brian M. Grosberg, MD, FAHS
Professor of Neurology
Director, Hartford Healthcare
    Headache Center
Program Director, Headache and
    Facial Pain Fellowship
Ayer Neuroscience Institute
University of Connecticut School of
    Medicine
West Hartford, Connecticut

Audrey L. Halpern, MD
Director of the Manhattan Center for
    Headache & Neurology
Clinical Assistant Professor of Neurology
Department of Neurology
NYU Grossman School of Medicine
New York, New York

James Hawkins, Med-HPE, DDS, MS
Orofacial Pain Department Chair
Naval Postgraduate Dental School
Naval Medical Leader and Professional
    Development Command
Associate Professor of the
    Postgraduate Dental College
Uniformed Services University of the
    Health Sciences
Bethesda, Maryland

Nada Hindiyeh, MD
Director of Headache Neurology
Metrodora Institute
West Valley City, Utah

Niki Holtzman-Hayes, MD
Headache Medicine Fellow
Montefiore Headache Center
Albert Einstein College of Medicine
Bronx, New York

Caitlin Hussey, NP
Headache Specialist Nurse Practitioner
BIDMC Comprehensive Headache
    Center
Department of Anesthesia, Critical
    Care and Pain Medicine
Harvard Medical School
Beth Israel Deaconess Medical Center
Boston, Massachusetts

Susan Hutchinson, MD
Advisor and Director of Medicine

Haven Headache & Migraine Center
Irvine, California

Dana Ionel, DO
Assistant Professor of Neurology
Department of Neurology
University of Kentucky College of
    Medicine
Lexington, Kentucky

Adelene Jann, MD
Headache Medicine Specialist
Integrative Headache Medicine
    of New York
New York, New York

Madisen Janssen, DO, MBA
Neurology Resident Physician
Department of Neurology
University of Minnesota
Minneapolis, Minnesota

Rigmor Jensen, MD, PhD
Professor of Neurology
Danish Headache Center
Department of Neurology
Rigshospitalet Glostrup
Faculty of Health and Medical
    Sciences
University of Copenhagen
Copenhagen, Denmark

Eric A. Kaiser, MD, PhD
Assistant Professor of Neurology
Department of Neurology
University of Pennsylvania
Philadelphia, Pennsylvania

Robert Kaniecki, MD
Associate Professor of Neurology
UPMC Headache Center
Department of Neurology

University of Pittsburgh School of
Medicine
Pittsburgh, Pennsylvania

**Siddharth Kapoor, MD, MBA, FAHS,
FAES**
Associate Professor of Neurology
Director, Headache Medicine
Program Director, Headache Medicine
Fellowship
Department of Neurology
University of Kentucky College of
Medicine
Lexington, Kentucky

Yury Khelemsky, MD
Associate Professor of Anesthesiology
Department of Anesthesiology, Peri-
operative and Pain Medicine
Department of Neurology
Icahn School of Medicine at Mount
Sinai
New York, New York

Sebastian Koch, MD
Chief of Stroke Program
Professor of Clinical Neurology
Department of Neurology
Miller School of Medicine
University of Miami
Miami, Florida

Athena Kostidis, MD
Clinical Associate Professor of
Neurology
Director, Headache Medicine
Fellowship
Department of Neurology
Loyola University Medical Center
Loyola University of Chicago Stritch
School of Medicine
Maywood, Illinois

Deena E. Kuruvilla, MD, FAHS
Medical Director
Westport Headache Institute
Westport, Connecticut

Jane Lee, MD
Neurology Resident
Department of Neurology
Donald and Barbara Zucker School of
Medicine at Hofstra/Northwell
Great Neck, New York

Morris Levin, MD
Professor and Director
UCSF Headache Center
Department of Neurology
University of California
San Francisco, California

Richard B. Lipton, MD
Professor of Neurology, Professor
of Epidemiology and Population
Health, and Professor of Psychiatry
and Behavioral Science
Montefiore Headache Center
Department of Neurology
Department of Epidemiology and
Population Health
Albert Einstein College of Medicine
Bronx, New York

Amanda Macone, MD
Instructor of Neurology and
Anesthesia
BIDMC Comprehensive Headache
Center
Departments of Neurology and
Anesthesia, Critical Care and Pain
Medicine
Harvard Medical School
Beth Israel Deaconess Medical Center
Boston, Massachusetts

Maksym S. Marek, MD, MS
Clinical Instructor of Neurology
Department of Neurology
Keck School of Medicine
University of Southern
   California
Los Angeles, California

Michael Marmura, MD
Associate Professor of Neurology
Jefferson Headache Center
Department of Neurology
Sidney Kimmel Medical College at
   Thomas Jefferson University
Philadelphia, Pennsylvania

Jaclyn M. Martindale, DO
Assistant Professor of Pediatrics and
   Neurology
Wake Forest University School of
   Medicine
Winston-Salem, North Carolina

**Paul G. Mathew, MD, DNBPAS,
   FAAN, FAHS**
Assistant Professor of
   Neurology
Department of Neurology
Harvard Medical School
Mass General Brigham Health
Atrius Health
Cambridge Health Alliance
Boston, Massachusetts

Alexander Mauskop, MD
Director, New York Headache
   Center
Professor of Clinical Neurology
SUNY Downstate Health Sciences
   University
Brooklyn, New York

**Laszlo L. Mechtler, MD, FAAN,
   FEAN, FASN, FAHS**
Professor of Neurology and
   Neuro-Oncology
Department of Neurology and
   Neuro-Oncology
State University of New York at Buffalo
Buffalo, New York

Ioana Medrea, MD, MSc
Assistant Professor of Neurology
Department of Neurology
SUNY Upstate Medical University
Syracuse, New York

Agustin Melo-Carrillo, MD, PhD
Instructor in Anesthesia
Department of Anesthesia, Critical
   Care and Pain Medicine
Harvard Medical School
Beth Israel Deaconess Medical Center
Boston, Massachusetts

Abby Metzler, MD
Assistant Professor of Neurology
Department of Neurology
M Health Fairview Clinics and
   Surgery Center-Minneapolis
University of Minnesota
Minneapolis, Minnesota

Amara Mian, DO
Headache Specialist
Diamond Headache Clinic
Chicago, Illinois

Teshamae S. Monteith, MD
Chief of Headache Division
Associate Professor of Clinical
   Neurology
Department of Neurology

Miller School of Medicine
University of Miami
Miami, Florida

Cynthia Morris, MD
Assistant Professor of Neurology
Department of Neurology
Saint Louis University School of
  Medicine
SSM Health Cardinal Glennon
  Children's Hospital
Saint Louis, Missouri

Natalia Murinova, MD, MHA
Clinical Professor of Neurology
Director, Headache Center
Department of Neurology
University of Washington School
  of Medicine
Seattle, Washington

Stephanie Nahas, MD
Associate Professor
Director, Headache Fellowship Program
Jefferson Headache Center
Department of Neurology
Sidney Kimmel Medical College at
  Thomas Jefferson University
Philadelphia, Pennsylvania

Umer Najib, MD, FAAN, FAHS
Associate Professor of Neurology and
  Vice Chair for Clinical Operations
Director, WVU Headache Center and
  Headache Medicine Fellowship
  Program
Director, RNI Transcranial Magnetic
  Stimulation Program
Department of Neurology
Rockefeller Neuroscience Institute
West Virginia University
Morgantown, West Virginia

Lauren R. Natbony, MD, FAHS
Medical Director, Integrative Head-
  ache Medicine of New York
Assistant Clinical Professor of
  Neurology, Headache and
  Facial Pain
Department of Neurology
Icahn School of Medicine at Mount
  Sinai
New York, New York

Seniha Nur Ozudogru, MD
Assistant Professor of Clinical
  Neurology
Department of Neurology
Perelman School of Medicine
University of Pennsylvania
Philadelphia, Pennsylvania

Anna Pace, MD
Assistant Professor of Neurology
Department of Neurology
Division of Headache and
  Facial Pain
Icahn School of Medicine at
  Mount Sinai
New York, New York

Simy Parikh, MD
Assistant Professor of Neurology
Jefferson Headache Center
Department of Neurology
Sidney Kimmel Medical College at
  Thomas Jefferson University
Philadelphia, Pennsylvania

Sara Pavitt, MD
Assistant Professor of Neurology and
  Pediatrics
Chief of the Headache Program
Department of Neurology
University of Texas at Austin

Dell Children's Medical Center
   of Central Texas
Austin, Texas

Jelena M. Pavlovic, MD, PhD
Associate Professor of Neurology
Montefiore Headache Center
Department of Neurology
Albert Einstein College of Medicine
Bronx, New York

Juliette Preston, MD, MS
Associate Professor
Director, OHSU Headache Center
Oregon Health & Science University
Portland, Oregon

Melissa Rayhill, MD, FAHS, FAAN
Associate Professor of Neurology
Jacobs School of Medicine and
   Biomedical Sciences
University at Buffalo, The State
   University of New York
Buffalo, New York

Nina Riggins, MD, PhD
President of Brain Performance Center
   and Research Institute
San Diego, California

Jennifer Robblee, MD, MSc, FRCPC
Assistant Professor of Neurology
Department of Neurology
Lewis Headache Center
Barrow Neurological Institute
St. Joseph's Hospital and Medical
   Center
Phoenix, Arizona

**Carrie E. Robertson, MD,
   FAHS, FAAN**
Associate Professor of Neurology

Department of Neurology
Mayo Clinic
Rochester, Minnesota

Christopher L. Robinson, MD, PhD
Resident Physician Scientist
Department of Anesthesia, Critical
   Care and Pain Medicine
Harvard Medical School
Beth Israel Deaconess Medical Center
Boston, Massachusetts

**Pedro Augusto Sampaio
   Rocha-Filho, MD, PhD**
Professor of Neurology
Division of Neuropsychiatry
Centro de Ciências Médicas
Universidade Federal de Pernambuco
   (UFPE)
Hospital Universitario Oswaldo Cruz
Universidade de Pernambuco
Recife, Brazil

Marcela Romero-Reyes, DDS, PhD
Clinical Professor, Director, Brotman
   Facial Pain Clinic
Department of Neural and Pain
   Sciences
University of Maryland, Baltimore
School of Dentistry
Baltimore, Maryland

Noah Rosen, MD
Associate Professor of Neurology
Department of Neurology
Donald and Barbara Zucker School
   of Medicine at Hofstra/Northwell
Great Neck, New York

**Soma Sahai-Srivastava, MD,
   FANA, FAHS**
Professor of Clinical Neurology

Director, Headache and Neuralgia
   Program
Departtment of Neurology
Keck School of Medicine
University of Southern California
Los Angeles, California

Shayna Y. Sanguinetti, MD
Assistant Professor of Neurology
Department of Neurology
Donald and Barbara Zucker
   School of Medicine at Hofstra/
   Northwell
Great Neck, New York

Aaron Schain, PhD
Instructor of Anesthesia
Department of Anesthesia, Critical
   Care, and Pain Medicine
Harvard Medical School
Beth Israel Deaconess Medical Center
Boston, Massachusetts

Fallon Schloemer, DO
Associate Professor
Director, Headache Medicine
   Program
Medical Director, Froedtert & The
   Medical College of Wisconsin
   Neurosciences Clinic
Associate Program Director,
   Neurology Residency Program
Department of Neurology
HUB for Collaborative Medicine
Medical College of Wisconsin
Milwaukee, Wisconsin

Todd J. Schwedt, MD
Professor of Neurology
Department of Neurology
Mayo Clinic
Phoenix, Arizona

Henrik Schytz, MD, PhD
Department of Neurology, Danish
   Headache Center
Copenhagen University
   Hospital—Rigshospitalet
Copenhagen, Denmark

Meagan D. Seay, DO
Assistant Professor of Neurology and
   Ophthalmology
Department of Neurology and
   Ophthalmology
University of Utah School of Medicine
John A. Moran Eye Center
Salt Lake City, Utah

Robert E. Shapiro, MD, PhD
Professor Emeritus
Department of Neurological Sciences
University of Vermont
Burlington, Vermont

Roni Sharon, MD
Director of Department of Headache
   and Facial Pain
Sheba Medical Center
Sackler School of Medicine at
   Tel-Aviv University
Ramat Gan, Israel

Huma U. Sheikh, MD
NY Neurology Medicine, PC
Assistant Professor of Neurology
Department of Neurology
Mount Sinai Beth Israel
Icahn School of Medicine at Mount
   Sinai
New York, New York

Stephen D. Silberstein, MD
Professor of Neurology
Director of Jefferson Headache Center

Department of Neurology
Sidney Kimmel Medical College at
    Thomas Jefferson University
Philadelphia, Pennsylvania

**Rashmi B. Halker Singh, MD,
    FAHS, FAAN**
Associate Professor of Neurology
Department of Neurology
Mayo Clinic
Scottsdale, Arizona

Peter B. Soh, MD, MPH
Medical Director
Soh Headache Center, LLC
Omaha, Nebraska

Andrew M. Strassman, PhD
Associate Professor of Anesthesia
Department of Anesthesia, Critical
    Care, and Pain Medicine
Harvard Medical School
Beth Israel Deaconess Medical Center
Boston, Massachusetts

Lauren Doyle Strauss, DO
Associate Professor of Pediatrics
    and Neurology
Wake Forest University School of
    Medicine
Winston-Salem, North Carolina

Stewart J. Tepper, MD, FAHS
Professor of Neurology
Dartmouth Headache Center
Lebanon, New Hampshire
Department of Neurology
Geisel School of Medicine at
    Dartmouth
Hanover, New Hampshire
Vice President

The New England Institute for
    Neurology and Headache
Stamford, Connecticut

Gretchen E. Tietjen, MD
Professor Emerita of Neurology
Department of Neurology
University of Toledo College
    of Medicine and Life Sciences
Toledo, Ohio

Istvan Tomaschek, MD
Staff Neurologist
Dent Neurologic Institute
Buffalo, New York

Nicholas Tzikas, MD, MPH
Assistant Professor of Clinical
    Neurology
Department of Neurology, Yale-New
    Haven Hospital
Yale School of Medicine
New Haven, Connecticut

Julio R. Vieira, MD, MS
Assistant Professor of Neurology
Department of Neurology
Albert Einstein College
    of Medicine
Bronx, New York
Nuvance Health Neuroscience
    Institute
Kingston, New York

Brinder Vij, MD
Associate Professor of Clinical
Department of Neurology and
    Rehabilitation Medicine
University of Cincinnati College of
    Medicine
Cincinnati, Ohio

Raissa Villanueva, MD, MPH
Associate Professor of Neurology and
   Dentistry
Chief, URMC Headache Center
Department of Neurology
University of Rochester Medical
   Center
Rochester, New York

Maria Dolores Villar-Martinez, MD
Fellow
NIHR-King's Clinical Research
   Facility and Institute of Psychiatry,
   Psychology and Neuroscience
King's College
London, United Kingdom

Marianna Vinokur, DO
Assistant Professor of Neurology

Mount Sinai Headache and
   Facial Pain Center
Department of Neurology
Icahn School of Medicine at
   Mount Sinai
New York, New York

Ailing Eileen Yang, MD
Resident Physician
Department of Neurology
Beth Israel Deaconess Medical Center
Harvard Medical School
Boston, Massachusetts

Eileen Yu, BS
Medical Student
Case Western Reserve University
   School of Medicine
Cleveland, Ohio

Preface

Headache is the most prevalent neurological condition in the general population and one of the most common pain conditions in the world. Headache can also be a symptom of various neurological and medical diseases.[1] Migraine, a primary headache disorder, affects over 1 billion people in the world, and approximately 39 million Americans suffer from migraine.[2,3] Tension-type headache (TTH) is the most prevalent neurological disorder worldwide.[4] Headache disorders including migraine and TTH can be debilitating and associated with impaired quality of life. Healthcare providers often encounter patients with various headache conditions in clinics, on wards, and in urgent care centers or emergency rooms. Headache disorders are commonly diagnosed and managed by neurologists in the United States, but internists, family physicians, and specialists from other medical specialties may also be involved in the care of patients with headache. Advanced practice practitioners including nurse practitioners and physician assistants have been extensively involved in the evaluation and management of patients with headache disorders in the United States. The chief complaint of headache accounts for up to 19% of outpatient neurology office visits and is among the top three chief complaints presenting in the emergency rooms and leading to neurological consultation.[5] Headache diseases or syndromes have been recognized as an Accreditation Council for Graduate Medical Education (ACGME) neurological core milestone. The neurology residents are expected to gain and document proficiency in headache disorders during their residency training.

The book covers epidemiology, pathophysiology, diagnosis, and treatment of primary and secondary headache disorders and facial pain disorders described in the third and latest edition of the *International Classification of Headache Disorders* (ICHD-3) (Table 1).[6] The ICHD-3 is synchronized with the 10th edition of the *International Classification of Diseases* (ICD-10). The headache classification provides operational diagnostic criteria, with explicit rules regarding the combinations of features or symptoms required to establish a correct diagnosis. Other topics covered are anatomy and physiology of headache pain, special treatments, and procedures. Finally, headache in special populations and special topics are also presented in the book. Each chapter finishes with a chapter summary (bullet points), relevant references and web links if applicable.

References

1. Headache Classification Committee of the International Headache Society (IHS). The International Classification of Headache Disorders, 3rd edition. *Cephalalgia.* 2018;38(1):1-211.

2. GBD 2021 Nervous System Disorders Collaborators. Global, regional, and national burden of disorders affecting the nervous system, 1990-2021: a systematic analysis for the Global Burden of Disease Study 2021. *Lancet Neurol.* 2024;23(4):344-381.

3. GBD 2017 US Neurological Disorders Collaborators; Burden of Neurological Disorders Across the US From 1990-2017: A Global Burden of Disease Study. *JAMA Neurol.* 2021;78(2):165-176.

4. Ashina S, Mitsikostas DD, Lee MJ, et al. Tension-type headache. *Nat Rev Dis Primers.* 2021;7(1):24.

5. Hansen CK, Fisher J, Joyce N, Edlow JA. Emergency department consultations for patients with neurological emergencies. *Eur J Neurol.* 2011;18:1317-1322.

6. Robbins MS. Diagnosis and management of headache: a review. *JAMA.* 2021;325: 1874-1885.

Web Links

1. https://ichd-3.org/
2. https://ichd-3.org/wp-content/uploads/2016/08/ICHD-3-Code-vs-ICD-10-NA-Code.pdf

Table 1. Basic organization of the third edition of the *International Classification of Headache Disorders* (ICHD-3).

Part One: The Primary Headaches
1. Migraine
2. Tension-type headache
3. Trigeminal autonomic cephalalgias (including cluster headache)
4. Other primary headache disorders
Part Two: The Secondary Headaches
5. Headache attributed to trauma or injury to the head and/or neck
6. Headache attributed to cranial and/or cervical vascular disorder
7. Headache attributed to nonvascular intracranial disorder
8. Headache attributed to a substance or its withdrawal
9. Headache attributed to infection
10. Headache attributed to disorder of homoeostasis
11. Headache or facial pain attributed to disorder of the cranium, neck, eyes, ears, nose, sinuses, teeth, mouth, or other facial or cervical structure
12. Headache attributed to psychiatric disorder
Part Three: Painful Cranial Neuropathies, Other Facial Pain, and Other Headaches
13. Painful lesions of the cranial nerves and other facial pain
14. Other headache disorders

Headache Classification Committee of the International Headache Society (IHS). *The International Classification of Headache Disorders,* 3rd edition, 1–211. Copyright © 2018 by (International Headache Society). Reprinted by Permission of SAGE Publications.

PART I

Introduction

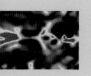

CHAPTER

1

History and Physical Examination

Ailing Eileen Yang, Thien Phu Do, and David W. Dodick

Headache is the most common neurologic symptom. In the United States, it is one of the top five reasons for emergency department visits.[1] Diagnosis of headache primarily relies on medical history because there are no validated biomarkers for most headache disorders. A confirmatory physical examination is often required. Investigations such as neuroimaging are seldom necessary to rule out secondary causes. The clinical presentation of many serious secondary causes of headaches can be similar to that of the most common primary headache disorders, which may complicate the diagnostic process. Therefore, a detailed history and focused physical examination are essential. *The International Classification of Headache Disorders*, 3rd edition (ICHD-3), provides diagnostic criteria for both primary and secondary headache disorders.[2] A comprehensive medical history and physical examination facilitate the application of these criteria, allowing for differentiation between primary and secondary headaches and guiding further workup and medical management.

History

When evaluating a patient with a headache, it is advisable to begin with an open-ended question such as "Can you describe what your headaches feel like?" and then implement a structured approach to assess the pain. The PQRST mnemonic (Box 1-1) is a widely used method for systematically evaluating pain. An appropriate medical history for headaches should include information about the number and types of headaches, age of onset, timing and characteristics of onset, duration and frequency of episodes, location and characteristics of pain, factors that worsen or alleviate the pain, accompanying symptoms, and history of medication use.

Clinicians need to be aware of potential pitfalls when taking a patient's medical history since patients may have varying levels of insight into their symptoms. Therefore, it is recommended to ask questions methodically and directly. For example, to illustrate the sudden onset of a thunderclap headache, clinicians can use snapping or other cues to emphasize the

Box 1-1. PQRST Pain Assessment		
P	Palliating or Provoking factors (triggers)	Positional, Valsalva maneuver (e.g., cough, sneeze, strain), exertional (e.g., walking, climbing stairs), menstruation, substances (e.g., caffeine, marijuana)
Q	Quality	Sharp, dull, achy, stabbing, throbbing
R	Region	Holocephalic, unilateral, regional
	Radiation	To orbits, sinuses, jaw, neck, trapezius
S	Severity (pain scale)	0 (no pain) to 10 (worst pain you have ever felt)
	Symptoms, associated	Photophobia, phonophobia, nausea/vomiting, vision changes, pulsatile tinnitus, autonomic features (e.g., lacrimation, rhinorrhea, conjunctival injection)
T	Timing	Age of onset, time to maximal intensity (e.g., thunderclap), duration, frequency

temporal relationship between the absence of the headache and its peak intensity. Determining the circumstances surrounding the headache occurrence may also provide useful information. Patients with a known primary headache disorder should be cautiously asked about changes in the frequency and phenotype of their headaches, which can often be identified by asking what prompted them to seek medical attention. Headache diaries are useful for recording and organizing the pattern of headaches in patients with a longstanding history.

Several screening tools are available to aid in the diagnostic process. The SNNOOP10 mnemonic covers 15 red flags in the medical history and physical examination that are indicators for further investigation.[3] These features must be actively inquired about when taking a medical history (Box 1-2). Secondary headaches, such as those caused by giant cell arteritis, neoplasms, subarachnoid hemorrhage, idiopathic intracranial hypertension, and intracranial hypotension, are examples of relevant conditions.

The remainder of the medical history for headache should include prior evaluation, prior treatments (acute, preventive, and non-pharmacologic), current medications, allergies, past medical history (such as hypercoagulability, sleep disorders, and mood disorders), family history (of headache disorders and hypercoagulability), and social history (tobacco/vaping, alcohol, recreational drugs, caffeine, diet, exercise, sleep habits, work conditions, and life stressors). Unlike other fields of medicine where investigative techniques may sometimes replace the need for a comprehensive history, in headache medicine, history plays a crucial role in arriving at the correct diagnosis. Taking a headache history is an art that requires practice, and it can be improved with repetition and experience.

Physical Examination

To accurately diagnose headache disorders, physical examination is a critical component (Box 1-3).[4] Confirmatory physical examination findings are usually sufficient, and neuroimaging is generally not required to rule out a secondary etiology. However, specific physical exam findings may provide important clues for certain headache disorders. The physical examination for a patient presenting with a headache should include a general neurologic examination with a focus on the head, eyes, ears, nose, and throat region. For instance, pericranial muscle tenderness may indicate tension-type headache, while scalp tenderness, particularly at the temples, and reduced temporal artery pulsations may suggest giant cell arteritis. Papilledema may be indicative of idiopathic intracranial hypertension, and focal neurologic deficits may suggest an intracranial lesion.

Box 1-2. SNNOOP10 Headache Red Flags

S	Systemic signs/symptoms
N	Neurologic signs/symptoms, focal
N	Neoplasm history
O	Older age of onset >50 years
O	Onset, sudden
P10	Precipitation with Valsalva maneuver (e.g., cough, sneeze, strain)
	Positional
	Pregnancy
	Pattern change
	Painful eye with autonomic features
	Post-traumatic onset of headache
	Pathology of the immune system such as HIV
	Pain medication overuse or new drug use
	Papilledema
	Progressive headache

Box 1-3. Focused Physical Examination in a Patient with Headache

Vital Signs

Head, Eyes, Ears, Nose, and Throat (HEENT) Exam

- Examine the scalp, neck, dentition, and bite
- Palpate the scalp, sinuses, temporomandibular joint, jaw, neck, and shoulder
- Test range of motion of neck and shoulder

Neurologic Exam

- Mental status including mood
- Cranial nerves: pupils, funduscopic exam, extraocular movements, visual fields, facial symmetry and sensation, and palate/tongue
- Motor strength including upper motor exam (arm extensors and leg flexors)
- Reflexes and plantar response
- Coordination: finger-to-nose, heel-to-shin
- Gait

If red flags are detected in the medical history and focal signs are observed during the examination, further diagnostic testing is necessary.[4] In cases where a secondary headache is suspected, magnetic resonance imaging (MRI) of the brain is typically preferred to rule out intracranial pathology. Magnetic resonance angiography (MRA) and magnetic resonance venography (MRV) of the head and neck may be preferred to rule out dissection, vasculitis, aneurysm, cerebral venous sinus thrombosis, and other vascular-related disorders.

Diagnostic Considerations

To effectively manage headache disorders, accurate diagnosis is crucial, and it is important to address any unmet needs of the patient. Given the high prevalence of headache in the general population, it is essential to take a systematic approach when interviewing patient who presents with headache. Since headache is a symptom and not a diagnosis, it is vital to obtain a detailed clinical history of the patient's headache experience to accurately correlate with an ICHD-3 diagnosis. This approach can help patients with a primary headache disorder engage in meaningful discussions with their healthcare providers about the pathophysiology of their disorder and available treatment options. Similarly, patients with a suspected secondary headache disorder can receive further neurologic evaluation to address the underlying cause.

Summary

- *The International Classification of Headache Disorders*, third edition (ICHD-3), categorizes headaches as primary or secondary headache disorders.
- Medical history is essential in diagnosing headaches due to limited biomarkers.
- Physical examination usually confirms diagnosis, and neuroimaging is rarely needed to identify secondary headache disorders.
- Serious secondary headaches can have similar clinical presentations as primary headaches.

REFERENCES

1. Liberman AL, Prabhakaran S, Zhang C, Kamel H. Prevalence of neurological complaints in US emergency departments, 2016-2019. *JAMA Neurol.* 2023;80(2):213-215.
2. Headache Classification Committee of the International Headache Society (IHS). *The International Classification of Headache Disorders*, 3rd edition. *Cephalalgia.* 2018;38(1):1-211.
3. Do TP, Remmers A, Schytz HW, et al. Red and orange flags for secondary headaches in clinical practice: SNNOOP10 list. *Neurology.* 2019;92(3):134-144.
4. Dodick DW. Diagnosing secondary and primary headache disorders. *Continuum (Minneap Minn).* 2021;27(3):572-585.

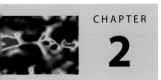

Diagnostic Imaging Studies

Istvan Tomaschek and Laszlo L. Mechtler

Although imaging studies are not always necessary for the diagnosis of primary headache disorders, they become essential when a secondary cause for headache is suspected.[1,2] This is important particularly due to the fact that secondary headaches can mimic primary headache disorders as they may present with a similar phenotype. Imaging becomes imperative if any "red flags" are present in the history or during a physical exam (see Chapter 1). Additional reasons clinicians may order imaging studies include, but are not limited to, patient expectations, medico-legal concerns, and even limitations on physical examination through telemedicine or a language barrier. This in turn may result in increased incidental findings, often leading to further workup, cost, and patient stress that may be unnecessary.

Types of Imaging Tests for Headache

Multiple imaging studies are available and commonly utilized by physicians when evaluating headaches (Table 2-1).[1] The main modalities include computed tomography (CT), magnetic resonance imaging (MRI), myelography, ultrasound (US), and X-ray. Depending on the setting and clinical suspicion, certain diagnostic tools are more suitable than others. For example, a head CT scan may be a more appropriate study over a brain MRI when assessing for an acute subarachnoid hemorrhage (SAH), or recent head trauma, in the emergency department; however, MRI is preferential to CT when evaluating for a suspected secondary cause of a trigeminal autonomic cephalalgia (TAC) involving the pituitary or cerebellopontine angle. American Academy of Neurology does not recommend performing electroencephalography (EEG) for headaches. EEG has no advantage over clinical evaluation and examination in diagnosing headaches, and it does not improve outcomes but increases costs.

Computed Tomography

CT uses X-ray as the basis of imaging. The amount of attenuation through the body's different tissues is measured and represented in a two-dimensional gray-scale image. Multiple consecutive slices are placed together, allowing for a three-dimensional view. When comparing CT to MRI, CT is faster, cheaper, and more available than MRI. Head CT is the standard of care in acute settings. The majority of abnormalities causing headaches can be identified on CT, particularly acute hemorrhage (including SAH), acute trauma, or osseous irregularities.[1,3] The sensitivity for acute SAH is higher in head CT than brain MRI (Figure 2-1). CT can also be utilized to assess vasculature specifically. Both the arterial system and the venous system can be visualized by CT angiography (CTA) and CT venography (CTV), respectively (Figures 2-2 and 2-3a and b). This is of particular importance when working up headaches secondary to vasculature pathologies such as cerebral aneurysm, carotid/vertebral dissection, reversible cerebral vasoconstriction syndrome (RCVS), vasculitis, and dural venous sinus thrombosis or stenosis.

Table 2-1. Imaging Studies Used in the Evaluation of Headaches

	Head CT	CTA Head/ Neck	Myelogram	MRI/MRA/MRV	MRI Cervical Spine
Use	Assess acute SAH or head trauma	Assess arterial dissections and aneurysms	Assess spinal stenosis and cerebrospinal fluid (CSF leaks)	Assess pathology of brain and vessels	Assess the integrity of the spinal column
Advantages	Fast	Fast	Fast	Detailed image	Detailed image
	Low cost	Low cost	Low cost	No radiation exposure	No radiation exposure
Risks/ disadvantages	Radiation exposure	Radiation exposure	Radiation exposure	Contraindications to ferromagnetic material	Contraindications to ferromagnetic material
	Reduced image quality		Requires lumbar puncture (CT myelogram)	Uncooperative patient	Uncooperative patient

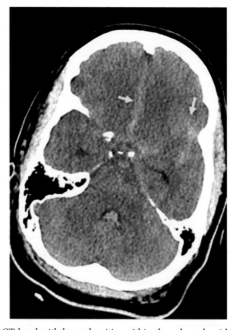

Figure 2-1. Axial noncontrast CT head with hyperdensities within the subarachnoid space (basal cisterns, left sylvian fissures, anterior interhemispheric fissure) in a 35-year-old male with an apoplectic "worst headache of my life." An aneurysm was found on the head CTA that caused the subarachnoid hemorrhage.

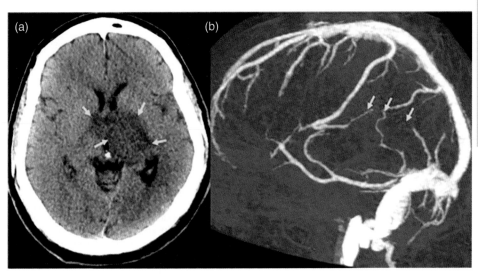

Figure 2-2. Postpartum vein of Galen thrombosis. A 25-year-old female with severe sudden onset of headaches. (a) Axial noncontrast CT showing evidence of bithalamic hypodensities consistent with venous infarct and (b) 3-D maximum intensity projection images from CT venography demonstrating lack of enhancement in the vein of Galen and straight sinus due to the thrombosis.

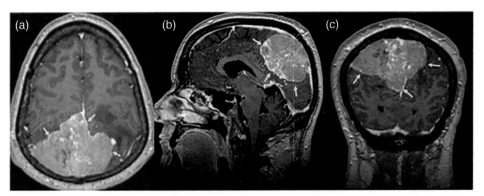

Figure 2-3. Large convexity meningioma (WHO grade 1) in the right parietooccipital region extending through the midline to the left parietal convexity. T1-weighted images with contrast show the lesion in the (a) axial, (b) sagittal, and (c) coronal planes. A 40-year-old male with progressive disabling headaches worse upon awakening and with coughing/sneezing. Postoperatively headaches resolved.

The disadvantages of CT include radiation exposure and decreased sensitivity and specificity with non-SAH intracranial lesions. Two millisieverts, equal to 100 chest radiographs, is the average radiation produced by one head CT. Ionized radiation exposure leads to an increased risk of developing malignancies such as leukemia and cancers of the breast, lung, thyroid, and stomach. Moreover, as compared to MRI, CT has a decreased sensitivity and specificity of non-SAH intracranial lesions, and, therefore, certain pathologies such as neoplasms, ischemia, and meningeal abnormalities can be missed with CT.

Magnetic Resonance Imaging

MRI uses magnetic fields to detect the change in rotation of protons within tissues. This change of rotation throughout various tissues is then translated into a detailed image. Given that MRI does not use radiation, it is considered to be a safer alternative to CT. It has an increased sensitivity and specificity compared to CT for non-SAH intracranial lesions, and, therefore, is favored over CT, when working up headaches.[2,3] For the assessment of posterior fossa lesions, vascular pathology, neoplasm, inflammation, infection, or meningeal abnormalities, MRI is the preferred means of imaging (Figures 2-3 and 2-4).[3]

Detailed images of the arterial and venous systems can also be obtained through MRI. This includes magnetic resonance angiography (MRA) and magnetic resonance venography (MRV). This can be particularly useful in the evaluation for secondary headaches with an underlying vascular etiology. Arterial pathology such as aneurysm, dissection, RCVS, and vasculitis can be assessed with MRA (Figure 2-4). Venous pathology including cortical vein thrombosis and dural venous sinus thrombosis or stenosis can be appreciated with MRV. In patients suffering from neck and head trauma, an MRI of the cervical spine is useful to rule out atlantoaxial instability and post-traumatic cervical disk disease. In addition, paraspinal spasm can be seen by straightening the normal lordotic curvature of the cervical spine.

MRI is indicated in those with an abnormal physical examination and nonacute headache or a history that is atypical of migraine. Contrast can be administered for initial imaging of suspected TAC, chronic headache with increased frequency and/or new features, trigeminal neuralgia, new daily persistent headache, headaches with a positional component, and exertional headaches and in patients with a history of cancer, immunosuppression, or underlying infectious disease. MRI with contrast is not entirely without risk. Potential risks include allergic-like reactions, anaphylactic reactions, and nephrogenic systemic fibrosis in those with underlying kidney dysfunction.

Although MRI is often the preferred means of imaging, it is not always an option. This could be secondary to cost, availability, claustrophobia, inability of patients to remain still, or other contraindications. MRI is contraindicated in patients with certain foreign objects within their body, including noncompatible pacemakers or defibrillators, ferromagnetic aneurysm clips, certain neurostimulation devices, and metallic objects such as shrapnel or ear implants.

Myelogram

Myelography utilizes X-ray or CT with contrast in the dural sac to assess the integrity of the spinal canal and the thecal sac. This imaging test is beneficial in the workup of patients with headaches

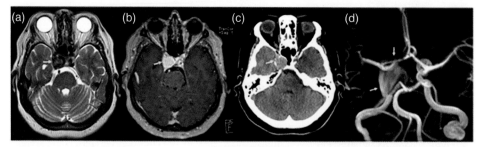

Figure 2-4. Giant cavernous ICA aneurysm. A 55-year-old with an 18-month history of throbbing right-sided headaches not associated with nausea or photophobia. (a) T2-weighted axial images show a mass with a heterogeneous signal within the cavernous sinus on the right. (b) T1-weighted contrast-enhanced study shows ovoid homogenous enhancement of an aneurysm. (c) Nonenhanced CT of the head shows peripheral calcification and ovoid mild hyperdensity. (d) MRA confirms the diagnosis of a cavernous segment internal carotid giant aneurysm on the right.

thought to be secondary to a cerebral spinal fluid (CSF) leak somewhere in the thecal sac or nerve root sleeves (Figure 2-5).[4,5] CSF leaks can be spontaneous or secondary to trauma, surgery, connective tissue disorders, or tears in the dura from lumbar punctures or other procedures where the dura may be compromised. Myelograms are typically ordered for those patients who have a contraindication to MRI, who need further imaging to locate the site of the leak(s) for potential surgery, or in those cases where the suspicion for low-pressure headache is high but MRI was inconclusive. MR myelography is a relatively new imaging sequence technique that can produce myelogram-like images of the thecal sac by MR imaging. MR myelography is a less invasive means of evaluating dural tears.

Ultrasound

US imaging has a pivotal role in medicine; however, its use in headache treatment is less frequent than MRI or CT. The US waves are generated by piezoelectric crystals and detected by the head of the US transducer. These waves bounce back to the head of the US transducer from the different tissues in the body, and the receiver will record the waves. Depending on the type of tissue and its density, these waves return to the receiver with varying acoustic impedance. This difference in acoustic impedance is what is measured and depicted on a gray-scale image.

US imaging is usually utilized when evaluating patients with giant cell arteritis (GCA) (see Chapter 22). It is particularly helpful in those cases when there is a high suspicion for GCA, but erythrocyte sedimentation rate and C-reactive protein are within normal limits and there is a negative superficial temporal artery biopsy. Superficial temporal artery US looks for a "halo sign," which is a hyperechoic, noncompressible ring around the arterial lumen representing inflammation (Figure 2-6). As the "halo sign" is rarely seen in other forms of vasculitis, it has a sensitivity of up to 87% and specificity of up to 96% in GCA.[6] The test is fast and inexpensive, but the outcome is dependent on the skills of the technician. US can also be used for the evaluation of carotid and vertebral artery dissections.

Conventional X-ray

Conventional X-ray is not commonly used in routine headache workup. However, it can be utilized in assessing fractures of the skull or other osseous structures of the head or neck, which may be an underlying cause for a secondary headache. Further workup with CT, MRI, myelography, or US can aid in the diagnosis.

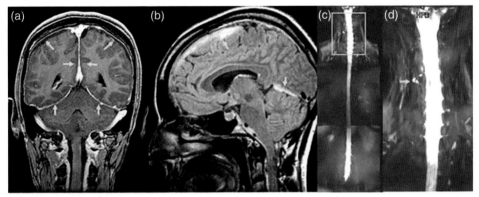

Figure 2-5. Intracranial hypotension after trauma. A 37-year-old involved in a motor vehicle accident suffered a whiplash injury followed by positional headaches. (a) T1-weighted contrast study shows diffuse pachymeningeal enhancement. (b) Sagittal T2-weighted FLAIR shows evidence of subdural effusions. (c) MR myelography shows evidence of a right-sided C3-C4 meningeal diverticula (perineural cyst) and CSF leak. (d) Enhanced view of Figure 2-5(c). Headaches resolved with the cervical blood patch.

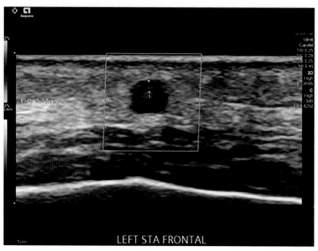

Figure 2-6. Ultrasound color duplex cross section images of the left superficial temporal artery (STA) showing increased intima-media thickening (hypoechoic ring = halo sign).

Summary

- Imaging tests are imperative when evaluating for the secondary causes of headaches.
- Head CT is useful for acute hemorrhage (including SAH), trauma, or osseous irregularities.
- MRI is more specific for posterior fossa lesions, vascular pathology, neoplasm, inflammation, infection, or meningeal abnormalities over CT.
- Myelography is particularly advantageous in visualizing CSF leaks within the thecal sac or nerve root sleeves.
- US of the superficial temporal artery can be used in those patients where the suspicion for giant cell arteritis is high.
- X-ray, although not commonly used in the workup for headaches, can be beneficial for assessing the integrity of the osseous structures of the head or neck.
- EEG is not recommended for the evaluation of headache.

REFERENCES

1. Evans RW, Burch RC, Frishberg BM, et al. Neuroimaging for migraine: the American Headache Society systematic review and evidence-based guideline. *Headache*. 2020;60:318-336.
2. Mitsikostas DD, Ashina M, Craven A, et al. European Headache Federation consensus on technical investigation for primary headache disorders. *J Headache Pain*. 2015;17:5.
3. Whitehead MT, Cardenas AM, Corey AS, et al. ACR Appropriateness Criteria® headache. *J Am Coll Radiol*. 2019;16:S364-S377.
4. Kim DK, Carr CM, Benson JC, et al. Diagnostic yield of lateral decubitus digital subtraction myelogram stratified by brain MRI findings. *Neurology*. 2021;96:e1312-e1318.
5. Schievink WI. Spontaneous intracranial hypotension. *N Engl J Med*. 2021;385:2173-2178.
6. Karassa FB, Matsagas MI, Schmidt WA, Ioannidis JP. Meta-analysis: test performance of ultrasonography for giant-cell arteritis. *Ann Intern Med*. 2005;142:359-369.

WEBSITES

1. The American Society of Neuroimaging: https://www.asnweb.org
2. The International Classification of Headache Disorders: https:ichd-3.org
3. Radiopaedia: https://radiopaedia.org

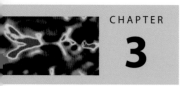

Headaches: Diagnostic Laboratory Studies

Seniha Nur Ozudogru and Juliette Preston

Diagnostic laboratory studies, such as blood tests, urine tests, and CSF studies, are not routinely needed for the evaluation of headaches.[1] However, laboratory studies can be helpful in differentiating headache subtypes and are necessary when secondary causes of headache are suspected (see Chapter 1).[2] The need for laboratory tests is determined based on a detailed medical history and physical examination, including a neurological exam. Careful consideration should be given to the selection of laboratory studies based on the specific headache presentation, as different atypical features may require different sets of tests (Table 3-1).

Blood Tests

Routine blood work, such as complete blood count (CBC) and complete metabolic panel (CMP), can be obtained in new patients with no recent blood tests to establish a baseline and in patients on long-term medications that necessitate monitoring.

CBC: Anemia, infection, inflammation, or certain types of cancer, such as lymphoma or leukemia, can cause abnormalities in the CBC, which may be associated with secondary headaches. CBC monitoring, including white cell count and platelet levels, is recommended for patients on antiepileptic medications, such as carbamazepine and valproic acid.

CMP: Secondary headaches may be associated with dysfunction of the liver or kidneys. Several medications used to manage headaches may potentially be hepatotoxic and cause liver enzyme abnormalities, such as acute hepatocellular injury resulting from acetaminophen, nonsteroidal anti-inflammatory drugs (NSAIDs), and valproic acid, or acute cholestasis reported with NSAIDs and tricyclic antidepressants. Renal function tests (BUN and creatinine) may be necessary to monitor renal function in patients taking potentially nephrotoxic medications such as NSAIDs, angiotensin-converting enzyme inhibitors, angiotensin receptor blockers, and lithium. In addition, sodium levels should be monitored in patients taking carbamazepine or oxcarbazepine.

Thyroid function tests: Thyroid function tests are not typically included in routine headache evaluations. However, hypothyroidism and, in rare cases, hyperthyroidism have been associated with headaches. If thyroid dysfunction is suspected, thyroid function tests can be ordered.

Inflammatory markers: Routine assessment does not include these tests. However, in patients over 50 with suspected giant cell arteritis/temporal arteritis, C-reactive protein (CRP) or erythrocyte sedimentation rate (ESR) may be ordered. When a primary headache disorder (such as migraine, tension-type, or cluster headache) changes in characteristics, becomes refractory to treatment, or presents with atypical features such as joint pain and rash, systemic diseases should be investigated. Patients with migraine may have a higher frequency of systemic inflammatory diseases. A small joint inflammatory arthritis with morning stiffness and swelling of hands, wrists, metatarsalgia, family history of rheumatoid arthritis, and Raynaud's phenomenon may indicate a need for checking inflammatory

Table 3-1. Diagnostic Laboratory Studies for Evaluation of Headache

Clinical Manifestations	Studies to Consider	Possible Conditions
New acute or thunderclap headache, "worse headache of my life"	CSF: RBC, test for xanthochromia	Subarachnoid hemorrhage
New headache in a patient older than 50 years, with new visual symptoms (transient/permanent monocular visual loss), jaw claudication, unexplained fever, weight loss	Blood tests: ESR, CRP, CBC, CMP	Temporal arteritis
New headache with visual disturbances such as bitemporal hemianopia, diplopia, or decreased visual acuity	Blood tests: serum prolactin, serum IGF-1, plasma corticotropin (ACTH) Urine test: 24-hour urinary free cortisol	Sellar masses (such as pituitary adenoma, craniopharyngioma)
New headache in an immunosuppressed patient	Blood tests: CBC, CMP, HIV test Lumbar puncture: opening pressure CSF: cell count, glucose, protein, Gram stain, bacterial culture	Toxoplasmosis, brain abscess, meningitis, CNS malignancy
New headache in pregnancy or post-partum, with hypertension and visual disturbances	Blood tests: CBC, CMP Urine test: protein	Preeclampsia, eclampsia, HELLP syndrome Posterior reversible encephalopathy syndrome
New headache associated with fever, altered mental status, +/− nuchal rigidity	Blood tests: CBC, CMP Blood culture Lumbar puncture: opening pressure CSF: cell count, glucose, protein, Gram stain, bacterial culture	Meningitis or encephalitis
New headache associated with visual disturbances (transient visual loss, double vision), pulsatile tinnitus, worsened with lying supine	Lumbar puncture: opening pressure (>250 mm H_2O) Imaging: brain MRI with MRV without contrast Eye exam: fundoscopic exam and visual field testing	Idiopathic intracranial hypertension
New headache, triggered by exertion, in patients with vascular risk factor	EKG Blood tests: troponin, CBC, CMP Stress test	Cardiac cephalalgia
Worsening headache during or at the end of the menstrual cycle	Blood test: ferritin	End-menstrual migraine

ACTH: adrenocorticotropic hormone; CBC: complete blood count; CMP: comprehensive metabolic panel; CRP: C-reactive protein; CSF: cerebrospinal fluid; EKG: electrocardiogram; ESR: erythrocyte sedimentation rate; HELLP: Hemolysis, elevated liver enzymes, low platelet; HIV: human immunodeficiency virus; IGF-1: insulin-like growth factor-1; MRI: magnetic resonance imaging; MRV: magnetic resonance venography; RBC: red blood cell markers, including antinuclear antibody test. Vascular workup including antiphospholipid antibodies such as anticardiolipin, antibeta2 glycoprotein 1, lupus anticoagulant, and antineutrophil cytoplasmic antibodies should be considered in patients with a history of miscarriages, transient ischemic attack, family history of early-age stroke (<50 years old), or migraine with prolonged aura (>60 min). In patients with gastrointestinal complaints and headaches, irritable bowel syndrome and inflammatory bowel diseases, including celiac disease, can be suspected as they can be associated with migraine headaches. Diagnostic blood tests should include tissue transglutaminase IgA and total IgA. If IgA deficiency is present, deamidated gliadin peptide–IgG testing may be necessary to diagnose celiac disease.

Diagnostic Lumbar Puncture and CSF Studies

Lumbar puncture (LP) is an essential diagnostic tool when headaches due to central nervous system (CNS) infections or subarachnoid hemorrhage are suspected, especially in the setting of negative computed tomography (CT) scans (Table 3-1).[3] Thunderclap headache or the worst headache of a patient's life should raise suspicion for subarachnoid hemorrhage. Even if a patient has a known history of a chronic primary headache disorder, an acute severe headache or an unusually severe headache should prompt consideration of subarachnoid hemorrhage. The sensitivity of the CT scan for subarachnoid hemorrhage decreases, especially when the CT scan is performed more than 6 hours after the onset of the headache and if the patient has anemia. Headaches associated with fever, altered mental status, meningeal signs, or seizures are common symptoms of meningitis, and LP is recommended.

LP is also useful for diagnosing headaches due to CNS malignancies and demyelinating diseases. It provides important information for diagnosing many nonurgent headache-associated conditions, such as idiopathic intracranial hypertension (IIH), intracranial hypotension, CNS lymphoma, autoimmune encephalitis, neurosarcoidosis, and paraneoplastic syndromes. When IIH is suspected based on clinical presentation, LP should be performed even if papilledema is absent on the physical examination to show high opening pressure with normal cerebrospinal fluid (CSF) studies.[4]

Although there are no absolute contraindications to LP, caution should be exercised if the patient has thrombocytopenia; is suspected of having increased intracranial pressure, spinal epidural abscess, or bleeding disorders; or is on anticoagulant therapy.[3] It is generally advised not to perform an LP in patients with coagulation defects with active bleeding, severe thrombocytopenia (platelet counts <50,000 to 80,000/μL), or an international normalized ratio (INR) >1.4, without correcting the underlying coagulation abnormalities. The most serious complication of LP is cerebral herniation. Head CT is indicated prior to performing an LP if there are signs of elevated intracranial pressure such as altered mental status, papilledema, focal neurological deficits, patients presenting with seizures or in the setting of trauma, and elderly patients aged 50 years or older to prevent cerebral herniation. It is important not to delay the treatment of bacterial meningitis while waiting to perform head CT and LP. Other common complications of LP include postdural puncture/LP headache, infection, bleeding, radicular pain, epidural hematoma, paraparesis, and back pain.

The classical approach to order CSF studies includes four tubes. Samples in tubes 1 and 4 are used for cell count and differential count, tube 2 is for glucose and protein levels, and tube 3 is for Gram stain, culture, and sensitivity. At some institutions, only three tubes are sent for analysis, and tube 4 is reserved for special studies when indicated. In this approach, studies are sent from tubes as follows: tube 1 for protein and glucose levels; tube 2 for Gram stain, culture, and sensitivity; and tube 3 for cell count and differential. The difference in RBC count between tubes 1 and 4 can be used to differentiate between a traumatic tap and a subarachnoid hemorrhage. Normal CSF is clear and colorless. Changes in the white blood cell (WBC) count and red blood cell (RBC) count can alter the color of the CSF. The breakdown of hemoglobin causes pink (oxyhemoglobin) color.

Genetic Testing

Genetic testing can be ordered in patients with migraine who present with motor symptoms and are suspected to have hemiplegic migraine. Different subtypes of hemiplegic migraine can be associated with specific gene mutations. For example, mutations in the CACNA1A gene (coding for a calcium channel) on chromosome 19 are associated with familial hemiplegic migraine type 1 (FHM1), while mutations in the ATP1A2 gene (coding for a K/Na-ATPase) on chromosome 1 are associated with FHM2. FHM3 is associated with mutations in the SCN1A gene (coding for a sodium channel) on chromosome 2. Mutations of CaCNA1A can also be seen with episodic ataxia type 2 (EA2) and spinocerebellar ataxia 6 (SC6). FHM1, EA2, and SC6 are all associated with cerebellar atrophy. Additionally, mutations in the PRRT2 gene and SLC4A4 gene have been associated with FHM, while PRRT2 gene mutation has been linked to benign familial infantile epilepsy and paroxysmal kinesigenic dyskinesia 1, and SLC4A4 gene mutation has been associated with proximal renal tubular acidosis with ocular abnormalities.

Genetic testing may help establish a diagnosis of hemiplegic migraine in sporadic cases without a family history or when the attack severity or symptoms differ from those of affected relatives. However, the yield of genetic testing in patients with adult-onset hemiplegic migraine is generally low.

Urine Tests

A urine test may be useful in the evaluation of a patient with a headache when a diagnosis of pheochromocytoma is suspected. Catecholamine levels (epinephrine, norepinephrine, and dopamine) need to be measured as this type of tumor can produce one or more catecholamines. Metanephrine levels also need to be assessed, as metanephrine and normetanephrine are metabolites of catecholamines. In cases with a low index of suspicion, consider 24-hour urinary fractionated catecholamines and metanephrines. In cases with a high index of suspicion, consider checking fractionated metanephrines in the plasma (which are optimally drawn over 30 minutes with patients in a supine position).

The 24-hour urinary free cortisol is one of the first-line diagnostic tests for patients with headaches and suspected Cushing's syndrome. Creatinine clearance should be obtained along with the 24-hour urinary free cortisol, as its validity is based on normal renal function. Note that patients with lower creatinine clearance will have lower cortisol excretion.

In pregnant patients reporting persistent or severe headaches, urine should be assessed for proteinuria (Table 3-1). Proteinuria, a new onset of hypertension with or without signs of end-organ dysfunction, is considered the classic sign of preeclampsia.

Summary

- Patients presenting with a new onset of headache with no recent blood tests should have a set of baseline laboratory data including CBC and comprehensive metabolic panel.
- The need for additional blood tests, including inflammatory markers such as CRP and/or ESR, may be determined based on the patient's clinical presentation, including suspicion of temporal arteritis.
- The diagnostic LP is indicated for the evaluation of secondary headaches, such as those due to suspected subarachnoid hemorrhage, CNS infection, and IIH.
- Genetic testing can be considered for patients with suspected hemiplegic migraine without family history or when the attack severity or symptoms differ from those of affected relatives.
- Urinary testing can be important to exclude headaches due to pheochromocytoma and preeclampsia.

REFERENCES

1. Loder E, Cardona L. Evaluation for secondary causes of headache: the role of blood and urine testing. *Headache.* 2011;51(2):338-345.
2. Cocores AN, Monteith TS. Headache as a neurologic manifestation of systemic disease. *Curr Treat Options Neurol.* 2022;24(1):17-40.
3. Johnson KSS, D. J. Lumbar puncture: technique, indications, contraindications, and complications in adults. In Aminoff MJ, UpToDate Retrieved January 22, 2023, from https://wwwuptodatecom/contents/lumbar-puncture-technique-indications-contraindications-and-complications-in-adults2022.
4. Friedman DI. Headaches due to low and high intracranial pressure. *Continuum (Minneap Minn).* 2018; 24(4, Headache):1066-1091.

WEBSITES

1. Lumbar puncture video (by NEJM): https://www.nejm.org/doi/full/10.1056/nejmvcm054952
2. https://www.merckmanuals.com/medical-calculators/CSF_WBC.htm

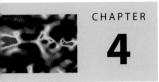
CHAPTER

4

Anatomy and Physiology of Head Pain

Andrew M. Strassman and Aaron Schain

Headache is a subjective symptom, and many different types of headache disorders exist. However, all headaches may share common anatomical pathways and physiology. Understanding anatomy and physiology of head pain is important for clinicians evaluating and treating patient with headache disorders.[1]

Neuroanatomy and Physiology of Pain

The body possesses a sensory system that is specialized for the detection of intense, potentially tissue-damaging stimuli, a process that has been termed nociception.[1] This nociceptive system is capable of evoking the perception of pain, as well as the somatic, autonomic, and endocrine responses that can accompany pain. The pain system may be divided into (a) the peripheral sensory apparatus for detecting noxious stimuli and transmitting this information to the central nervous system (CNS); (b) the multisynaptic central ascending pathways that subserve the reflexive, behavioral, emotional, and perceptual responses evoked by such stimuli; and (c) the central neural pathways responsible for pain modulation, both excitatory and inhibitory. The nociceptive system can also be strongly modulated by the sensory systems that detect nonnoxious thermal and mechanical stimuli. As a result of the multiple modulatory influences exerted on the system, as well as the sustained alterations in intrinsic neuronal properties that can be induced by injurious stimuli, the relationship between stimulus intensity and pain is highly variable.

Nociceptive Pathways

The first-order neurons in the somatosensory system are primary afferent neurons that have their cell body in the dorsal root ganglia or trigeminal (Gasserian) ganglion, a peripheral axonal process in the peripheral nerve, and a central axonal process in the dorsal root or the trigeminal nerve root. The central axonal process enters the CNS and synapses on second-order neurons in the spinal or medullary dorsal horn (trigeminal nucleus caudalis or TNC). The second-order neurons in turn have ascending axonal projections to third-order neurons in the thalamus and other brain regions involved in pain transmission and modulation. It has been suggested that the higher-order projection system may be subdivided into separate components subserving the affective versus sensory-discriminative components of pain, where the affective component is subserved in part by projections from the medial thalamus to the cingulate cortex, while the sensory-discriminative component is subserved by projections from the lateral thalamus/ventrobasal complex to the primary somatosensory cortex.

Nociceptors and Afferent Innervation

The skin is innervated by separate populations of sensory fibers that are specialized for the detection of either noxious or nonnoxious intensities of stimulation. Nociceptors, which selectively respond to noxious stimulus intensities, have axons that are slowly conducting, thinly myelinated A-delta or unmyelinated C-fibers. Mechanoreceptors respond maximally to innocuous intensities of mechanical stimulation and are predominantly rapidly conducting A-beta fibers. Thermoreceptors, which are A-delta and C-fibers, respond maximally to innocuous thermal stimuli and are subdivided into separate populations of warm and cold receptors. Visceral tissues generally lack the full spectrum of sensory modalities represented in the skin and in some cases appear to have a selectively nociceptive sensory function in that the innervation is activated only under potentially injurious conditions, and the only sensation that is evoked by such activation is pain. A distinctive feature of visceral pain is the referral to a characteristic region of the body surface (e.g., the left chest and shoulder, in cardiac pain). As discussed next, the pain evoked from the intracranial meninges may be considered an example of pain in the trigeminal system that is in some ways analogous to visceral pain.

Central Nociceptive Pathways

Primary afferent mechanoreceptors, thermoreceptors, and nociceptors each have axonal projections that terminate centrally in the dorsal horn. The dorsal horn in turn contains three classes of neurons that each receive their main peripheral sensory input from one of these three classes of primary afferent neurons and are called low-threshold mechanoreceptors, thermoreceptors, and nociceptive-specific neurons, respectively. However, the dorsal horn also contains another type of neuron, the wide-dynamic-range neuron, which receives a convergent input from both primary afferent nociceptors and mechanoreceptors. As a result of this convergent multimodal input, wide-dynamic-range neurons respond to both innocuous and noxious stimulus intensities, with higher discharge rates for noxious than nonnoxious stimulation, and have a nociceptive function.

Trigeminal System and Central Neural Pathways for Head Pain

The sensory innervation of the head and face originates from the trigeminal ganglion, as well as the upper cervical (C1-C2) dorsal root ganglia (for the posterior head regions) (Figure 4-1). The trigeminal ganglion differs anatomically from the dorsal root ganglia in that it has three divisions: ophthalmic (first), maxillary (second), and mandibular (third). The first two divisions are sensory, while the third division is mixed, both motor and sensory. The first-order primary afferent neurons of the trigeminal ganglion project centrally through the trigeminal root to terminate on second-order neurons in the brainstem trigeminal nuclear complex. Nociceptive primary afferents terminate primarily in the most caudal subdivision of this nuclear complex, TNC. TNC has been termed the medullary dorsal horn because it is anatomically an extension of the spinal dorsal horn and is similar to the spinal dorsal horn in its anatomical and physiological organization.

Peripheral Nociceptors and Sources of Head Pain

The trigeminal nerve supplies the major somatosensory innervation to the tissues of the anterior head and face, including skin, intraoral mucosa, tooth pulp, sinuses, temporomandibular joint, pericranial muscle (e.g., masseter, temporalis, and lateral and medial pterygoid muscles), periosteum, and cornea.[2]

In addition to this extracranial innervation, the trigeminal nerve has a much smaller intracranial component that provides a sensory innervation to the cranial meninges. This meningeal sensory innervation supplies both the major cerebral arteries, which carry the blood supply to the brain, and the dural venous sinuses, which carry the venous drainage from the brain. The dural (meningeal) arteries are also heavily innervated, as well as the entire expanse of cranial dura, including areas away from the major dural blood vessels. Thus it should be emphasized that the meningeal innervation not only is strictly vascular but also includes extravascular tissue. The sensory innervation of the cerebral arteries is primarily restricted to the proximal branches of the Circle of Willis

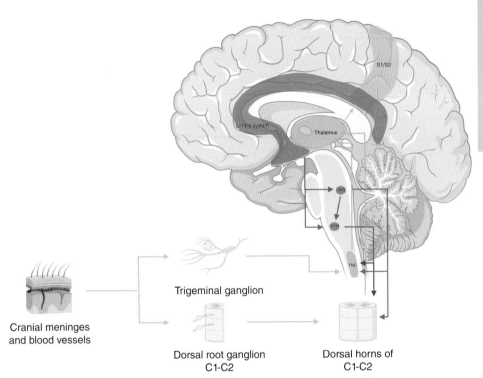

Figure 4-1. Neuroanatomy of head pain. PAG: periaqueductal gray; RVM: rostral ventromedial medulla; S1: primary somatosensory area; S2: secondary somatosensory area; TNC: trigeminal nucleus caudalis.

(e.g., the middle cerebral artery) and the intracranial portion of the carotid and vertebral arteries. The cerebral arteries are invested with sensory fibers only in their course through the pia (the innermost layer of the meninges) that covers the outer surface of the brain and lose this innervation when they exit the pial layer to penetrate the brain parenchyma. Direct mechanical or electrical stimulation of meninges evokes painful, headache-like sensations that are referred to regions of the face and head, analogous to the referral exhibited by pain originating from visceral tissues of the body. For stimulation sites on the supratentorial meninges, the area of pain referral is commonly in the periorbital and temporal region, whereas sensations evoked from more posterior intracranial sites, such as the intracranial portion of the vertebral artery, are referred to the occipital region. Both the sensory innervation and pain sensitivity within the cranium are restricted to the meningeal covering around the outside of the brain and do not extend to the brain itself or its intrinsic blood vessels.

Because the meninges are the only intracranial sites from which pain can be evoked, headaches that accompany intracranial pathologies (e.g., meningitis, subarachnoid hemorrhage, tumor) are thought to result from meningeal stimulation and consequent activation of meningeal sensory fibers. Migraine headache, although not accompanied by any detectable pathology, shares certain clinical features with headaches of intracranial origin, and a large body of evidence now supports a critical role for the meningeal sensory innervation in the headache of migraine.[3] The trigeminal primary afferent neurons that innervate the meninges are predominantly slowly conducting A-delta and C-fibers, and have nociceptive properties, in that they are activated by noxious mechanical, thermal, or chemical stimulation of the cranial dura, including the application of inflammatory mediators. In addition to becoming activated, the neurons become sensitized by inflammatory mediators, expressed as an increased sensitivity to mechanical stimuli.

Peripheral Sensitization and Head Pain

The property of mechanical sensitization is of great relevance for understanding the clinical symptoms of migraine, in particular, those symptoms that indicate the presence of an exaggerated intracranial mechanosensitivity.[3] In migraine, as well as in certain headaches that accompany intracranial pathologies such as meningitis, the headache is worsened by coughing, straining, or sudden head movement. Such activities would be expected to increase intracranial pressure or otherwise change the distribution of mechanical forces within the intracranial space. Such symptoms are evidence of an intracranial mechanosensitive sensory system that, during clinically occurring headaches, can develop abnormally elevated sensitivity that results in activation and generation of pain by normally innocuous intracranial mechanical forces.

Central Pain Processing and Sensitization in Head Pain

Sensory inputs from the head, face, and upper neck are transmitted centrally to neurons in the medullary and upper cervical dorsal horn. Sensory inputs from the dura converge centrally on a subpopulation of dorsal horn neurons that also receive inputs from a facial receptive field, which is commonly in the periorbital region, and is usually nociceptive, either wide-dynamic-range or nociceptive-specific. Such convergence of peripheral sensory inputs from separate deep and superficial tissues onto individual dorsal horn neurons is also found in neurons of the spinal dorsal horn and is regarded as the neural basis for the phenomenon of referred pain originating from deep or visceral tissues. The facial receptive fields of dorsal horn neurons that respond to dural stimulation are consistent with a role for these neurons in mediating the pain evoked by dural stimulation in that their distribution strongly overlaps with the area of dural-evoked pain referral in humans, and the receptive fields are primarily nociceptive. In addition, sensitization of such central neurons, which can be induced by sustained nociceptive input such as from the dural application of inflammatory mediators, results in a state of prolonged neuronal hypersensitivity, with marked enhancement of the responses to stimulation of both the facial and dural receptive fields. This phenomenon of central sensitization of dorsal horn neurons with convergent inputs from deep tissues is thought to be the basis for the phenomenon of referred visceral hyperalgesia and, in the meningeal sensory pathway, provides a mechanism to explain the facial cutaneous allodynia that can occur in migraine.[4]

Central Pain Modulatory Pathways

In addition to the nociceptive transmission system described earlier that conveys nociceptive information from peripheral tissues to the spinal cord and higher brain levels, the brain contains a descending modulatory system that exerts powerful influences, both inhibitory and excitatory, on nociceptive transmission and pain perception. The power of these descending influences is shown by the profound analgesia that can be produced by electrical stimulation or microinjection of morphine at specific brainstem sites, most notably the midbrain periaqueductal gray (PAG). PAG neurons do not project directly to the spinal cord but instead excite neurons in other brainstem regions, such as the rostral ventromedial medulla (RVM), that have direct spinal projections. Brainstem neurons that contain the biogenic amine neurotransmitters serotonin and noradrenaline also contribute to this descending modulatory system and exert direct influences on spinal nociceptive transmission.

Summary

- The trigeminal nociceptive pathway plays a significant role in mediating pain in the head and craniofacial regions.
- Sources of head pain include peripheral nociceptors in the skin, bones (periosteum), mucosa (oral cavity and sinuses), muscles, meninges, and cranial, intracranial, and neck blood vessels.

- The trigeminal ganglion contains the cell body's first-order primary afferent neurons that send peripheral axonal branches to supply the sensory innervation of the craniofacial tissues and central axonal branches that synapse on second-order neurons in the upper cervical and medullary dorsal horn/TNC.

- The sensory innervation of the meninges is thought to mediate the pain of headaches of intracranial origin, including migraine: the primary afferent input from the meninges converges on second-order dorsal horn neurons with facial receptive fields that overlap the region of pain referral evoked by meningeal stimulation.

- Sensitization of these second-order neurons by sustained meningeal afferent input is thought to be the basis for the cutaneous facial allodynia that can accompany migraine headaches.

REFERENCES

1. Messlinger K, Dostrovsky JO, Strassman AM. Anatomy and physiology of head pain. In: Olesen J, Goadsby PJ, Ramadan N, Tfelt-Hansen P, Welch KM, eds. *The headaches*. 3rd ed. Philadelphia: Lippincott, Williams & Wilkins; 2005: 95-119.
2. Edvinsson L, Abel M. Anatomy of muscles, tendons, joints, blood vessels, and meninges. In: Olesen J, Goadsby PJ, Ramadan N, Tfelt-Hansen P, Welch KM, eds. *The headaches*. 3rd ed. Philadelphia: Lippincott, Williams & Wilkins; 2005: 71-109.
3. Ferrari MD, Goadsby PJ, Burstein R, et al. Migraine. *Nature Reviews Disease Primers*. 2022;8(1):2.
4. Chichorro JG, Porreca F, Sessle B. Mechanisms of craniofacial pain. *Cephalalgia*. 2017;37(7):613-626.

PART II

Primary Headaches

SECTION A: MIGRAINE

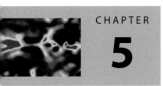

CHAPTER

5

Migraine: Epidemiology, Diagnosis, and Classification

Simy Parikh, Stephanie Nahas, and Richard B. Lipton

Migraine is a neurological disease and ranks as the second-most common primary head-ache. It is characterized by episodic attacks and is generally considered a chronic disorder with a variable natural history. Over time, migraine may evolve into a state in which attacks occur more frequently, with symptoms occurring on more days than not. A migraine is often mistaken for a sinus or tension-type headache (TTH). The head pain associated with migraine, as well as its associated symptoms, can be debilitating and significantly impact the quality of life of those affected. Therefore, it is essential to promptly diagnose and manage migraine to prevent the disability associated with the disorder.

Epidemiology

Incidence and Prevalence

According to population studies, the incidence of migraine ranges from 8.1 to 23.8 per 1000 person-years, with a higher overall incidence among women compared to men.[1] The onset of migraine typically occurs before the age of 35 years, with the highest peak incidence occurring between 20 and 24 years of age for women and 15 and 19 years of age for men. The 1-year global prevalence of migraine is estimated to range from 9 to 35. In the United States, the prevalence of migraine is approximately 12–13% of the population overall, with 18% of those diagnosed being women and 6% being men, resulting in a female-to-male prevalence ratio of 3:1. Chronic migraine affects 1% to 2% of the global population, with 2.5% of individuals with episodic migraine transforming to chronic migraine each year (Figure 5-1).

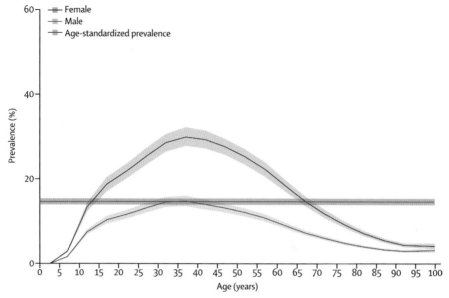

Figure 5-1. Global prevalence of migraine by age and sex in 2016. Prevalence is expressed as the percentage of the population that is affected by the disease. Shaded areas show 95% uncertainty intervals. Values are plotted at the midpoint of 5-year age categories. Global age-standardised prevalence is 14·4% (95% CI 13·8–15·0). (Reproduced with permission from Ashina M, Katsarava Z, Do TP, et al. Migraine: epidemiology and systems of care. *Lancet.* 2021;397(10283):1485-1495.)

Burden

Migraine imposes a considerable burden on individuals and society. According to the 2019 Global Burden of Diseases study,[2] headache disorders are among the top three causes of "disability-adjusted life years" for both men and women, with migraine accounting for 7.3% of all disability. Headache disorders were the primary cause of disability in individuals under 50 years of age, and migraine was the leading cause of disability in women. Poorly controlled migraine can result in missed workdays. Moreover, migraine's detrimental impact extends beyond economic considerations to affect perceived success, relationships, financial stability, quality of life, and even family planning.

Risk Factors

Migraine is a complex and multifactorial disorder.[3,4] Family studies have suggested a genetic influence, as the disorder is more prevalent among family members. First-degree relatives of individuals with migraine without and with aura have an increased risk of 1.9 to 3.8 times for developing migraine, respectively.[4] Twin studies have also supported a genetic component, with significantly higher pairwise concordance rates observed in monozygotic twins (0.28-0.34) compared to dizygotic twins (0.12-0.18), after accounting for environmental factors. Based on these studies, the heritability of migraine is estimated to be around 42%. Other factors, such as demographic and lifestyle factors, have also been linked to migraine. Women between the ages of 30 and 49 years from lower-income households have a higher risk for migraine. Additionally, moderate evidence suggests that obesity, noncephalic pain, frequent nausea, cutaneous allodynia during attacks, snoring, and poor acute medicine efficacy may be potential risk factors for migraine progression to a state where exacerbations occur on more days than not.[3] Strong evidence also supports increased headache frequency, depression, and overuse of acute migraine or headache medication as risk factors for progression.

Comorbidities

Comorbidities may arise due to shared genetic and environmental risk factors associated with the development of both migraine and comorbid conditions. Migraine increases the likelihood of certain comorbidities, such as stroke, epilepsy, and psychiatric disorders.[5] Even individuals with migraine who do not have established cardiovascular disease are at significantly increased risk of peripheral artery disease and stroke. Those with migraine are also at a higher risk of being diagnosed with epilepsy, and individuals with epilepsy are more likely to have migraine than those without either condition (Chapter 21). Psychiatric diseases, such as anxiety and affective disorders, including major depressive disorder or panic disorder, are also associated with migraine. Migraine is the most common comorbidity in those with postural orthostatic tachycardia (Chapter 38).

Diagnostic Criteria and Classification

Migraine diagnosis is based on clinical history and symptoms, with neuroimaging being unnecessary for those with normal neurological exams and lacking atypical features or red flags (Chapter 1). No definitive tests or biological markers exist for migraine diagnosis, but the use of a diagnostic headache diary is recommended. The third edition of the *International Classification of Headache Disorders* (*ICHD-3*) provides diagnostic criteria for migraine and its subtypes, including migraine with or without aura and episodic or chronic migraine based on headache frequency (Boxes 5-1 and 5-2).[6] Migraine with brainstem aura, formerly known as basilar-type migraine, may present with symptoms such as vertigo, dysarthria, diplopia, and confusion and may also include loss of consciousness.[6] Probable migraine can be diagnosed when not all diagnostic criteria are met. A three-item diagnostic tool called ID-Migraine, tested in primary care settings, identifies photophobia, incapacity, and nausea (PIN) as the strongest predictors of migraine diagnosis (Box 5-3).[7] A positive score on any two of the three items has a sensitivity of 0.81, a specificity of 0.75, and a positive predictive value of 0.93. Special types of migraine, including status migrainosus and hemiplegic migraine, are discussed in Chapters 9 to 12.

Symptoms

Migraine is a complex disorder that extends beyond headaches.[8] In the ictal or attack phase, it is characterized by prodromal symptoms, head pain, aura (in those with migraine with aura), and postdromal symptoms. Prodromal symptoms can include irritability, changes in bowel and urinary habits,

---

Box 5-1. ICHD-3 Diagnostic Criteria for Migraine Without Aura

A. At least five attacks fulfilling criteria B through D

B. Headache attacks lasting 4 to 72 hours (untreated or unsuccessfully treated)

C. Headache has at least two of the following four characteristics:
   1. Unilateral location
   2. Pulsating quality
   3. Moderate or severe pain intensity
   4. Aggravation by or causing avoidance of routine physical activity (e.g., walking or climbing stairs)

D. During headache at least one of the following:
   1. Nausea or vomiting
   2. Photophobia and phonophobia

E. Not better accounted for by another ICHD-3 diagnosis

Reproduced with permission from Headache Classification Committee of the International Headache Society (IHS). The International Classification of Headache Disorders, 3rd edition. *Cephalalgia*. 2018; 38(1):1–211.

Primary Headaches

Box 5-2. ICHD-3 Diagnostic Criteria for Migraine with Aura

A. At least two attacks fulfilling criteria B and C

B. One or more of the following fully reversible aura symptoms:
1. Visual
2. Sensory
3. Speech or language
4. Motor
5. Brainstem
6. Retinal

C. At least three of the following six characteristics:
1. At least one aura symptom spreads gradually over 5 or more minutes
2. Two or more aura symptoms occur in succession
3. Each individual aura symptom lasts 5 to 60 minutes
4. At least one aura symptom is unilateral
5. At least one aura symptom is positive
6. The aura is accompanied, or followed within 60 minutes, by headache

D. Not better accounted for by another ICHD-3 diagnosis

Reproduced with permission from Headache Classification Committee of the International Headache Society (IHS). The International Classification of Headache Disorders, 3rd edition. *Cephalalgia*. 2018; 38(1):1–211.

Box 5-3. ID-Migraine

During the last 3 months, have you ever had any of the following symptoms concerning your headache pain?
1. Did you ever feel nauseous when you had headache pain?
2. Did the light trouble you (much more than when there is no headache)?
3. Did your headache ever limit your ability to work, study, or do something you needed to, for at least 1 day?

changes in energy, and excessive yawning. Postdromal symptoms can include severe fatigue and changes in energy. Individuals with severe attacks and central sensitization resulting from activated nociceptive neurons in the trigeminal nucleus caudalis may exhibit cutaneous allodynia. Cutaneous allodynia, which manifests as pain in response to nonnoxious stimuli on the skin, is more prevalent in transformed or chronic migraine (up to 68%) than in episodic migraine (up to 63%).[9] It is a marker of more severe disease and is exhibited in individuals with severe attacks and central sensitization due to activated nociceptive neurons in the trigeminal nucleus caudalis. The interictal phase is the time between migraine attacks, during which migrainous symptoms are absent.

Differential Diagnosis

Box 5-4 shows common differential diagnoses for migraine. Migraine equivalents often occur prior to the initial onset of migraine associated with head pain. Examples of migraine equivalents in childhood include infantile colic, benign paroxysmal torticollis, benign paroxysmal vertigo, abdominal migraine, and cyclical vomiting.[6] The differential diagnosis of migraine includes other primary headache disorders, such as TTH and trigeminal autonomic cephalalgias (TACs) (Chapters 13-15).[6,10]

Box 5-4. Differential Diagnoses of Migraine	
Primary Headache	**Secondary Headache**
Tension-type headache	Infection
Cluster headache	Malignancy
Paroxysmal hemicrania	Stroke
Hemicrania continua	Vascular lesion
Short-lasting unilateral neuralgiform headache	Mass lesion
	Disorders of cerebrospinal fluid (CSF) pressure

Similarly to migraine, TTH can present with moderate head pain and can have chronic episodes. However, unlike migraine, TTH is mainly characterized by bilateral pain and pericranial tenderness. In contrast to migraine, TTH is not aggravated by exertion and does not have nausea or vomiting or more than one of photophobia or phonophobia. An individual can have both migraine and TTH. TACs, such as cluster headache and paroxysmal hemicrania, share the unilateral headache feature with migraine but also display distinct parasympathetic autonomic symptoms (e.g., rhinorrhea, lacrimation, pupillary changes) on the side of the headache. Pharmacological treatment response differs between migraine and TACs. In those with abnormal neurological exams or atypical features, such as those meeting the SNNOOP10 criteria, secondary headache must be considered, and further diagnostic testing may be required to exclude other conditions such as infections, malignancies, strokes, Cerebrospinal fluid (CSF) pressure disorders, or vascular or mass lesions (Chapters 1-3).

Summary

- Migraine is a prevalent primary headache, affecting approximately 12 to 14% of the general population.
- Women are at higher risk for migraine (female-to-male ratio of 3:1).
- Migraine has a substantial impact on individuals and society worldwide and is one of the most common causes of disability for both men and women.
- Risk factors for migraine progression or chronification include increased frequency of headache days, depression, and overuse of acute migraine/headache medication.
- The ICHD-3 classification criteria is a useful tool for diagnosing migraine with or without aura.
- Neuroimaging is unnecessary for diagnosing migraine in individuals with a normal neurological examination and without atypical features or red flags.
- Common comorbidities associated with migraine include stroke, epilepsy, and psychiatric disorders including depression and anxiety.

REFERENCES

1. Ashina M, Katsarava Z, Do TP, et al. Migraine: epidemiology and systems of care. *Lancet.* 2021; 397(10283):1485-1495.
2. Steiner TJ, Stovner LJ, Jensen R, et al. Migraine remains second among the world's causes of disability, and first among young women: findings from GBD2019. *J Headache Pain.* 2020;21(1):137.
3. Buse DC, Greisman JD, Baigi K, Lipton RB. Migraine progression: a systematic review. *Headache.* 2019;59(3):306-338.
4. Ashina M, Terwindt GM, Al-Karagholi MA, et al. Migraine: disease characterisation, biomarkers, and precision medicine. *Lancet.* 2021; 397(10283):1496-1504.

Primary Headaches

5. Wang SJ, Chen PK, Fuh JL. Comorbidities of migraine. *Front Neurol.* 2010;1:16.

6. Headache Classification Committee of the International Headache Society (IHS): *the International Classification of Headache Disorders,* 3rd edition. *Cephalalgia.* 2018 jan;38(1):1-211.

7. Lipton RB, Dodick D, Sadovsky R, et al. A self-administered screener for migraine in primary care: the ID Migraine validation study. *Neurology.* 2003;61(3):375-382.

8. Ferrari MD, Goadsby PJ, Burstein R, et al. Migraine. *Nature Reviews Disease Primers.* 2022;8(1):2.

9. Bigal ME, Ashina S, Burstein R, et al. Prevalence and characteristics of allodynia in headache sufferers: a population study. *Neurology.* 2008;70(17):1525-1533.

10. Onan D, Younis S, Wellsgatnik WD, et al. Debate: differences and similarities between tension-type headache and migraine. *J Headache Pain.* 2023;24:92. https://doi.org/10.1186/s10194-023-01614-0

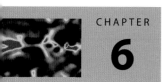

Migraine: Pathophysiology

Agustin Melo-Carrillo and Rami Burstein

Basic and clinical research conducted over the past several years has improved our understanding of the pathophysiological mechanisms of migraine.[1] Migraine is not just headache and may involve different phases: prodrome, aura, headache phase, postdrome, and interictal phase. It affects multiple cortical, subcortical, and brainstem areas that regulate autonomic, affective, cognitive, and sensory functions. In some cases, the headache begins with no warning signs, but, in other cases, the headache may be preceded by a prodromal phase that includes fatigue, euphoria, depression, irritability, food cravings, constipation, neck stiffness, increased yawning, and/or abnormal sensitivity to light, sound, and smell, and an aura phase that includes a variety of focal cortically mediated neurological symptoms that appear just before and/or during the headache phase. Symptoms of migraine aura develop gradually, feature excitatory and inhibitory phases, and resolve completely. Positive and negative symptoms may present as scintillating lights and scotomas when affecting the visual cortex, paresthesia and numbness of the face and hands when affecting the somatosensory cortex, tremor and unilateral muscle weakness when affecting the motor cortex or basal ganglia, and aphasia when affecting the speech area.[2] The pursuing headache can last a few hours to a few days. As the headache progresses, it may be accompanied by a variety of autonomic (nausea, vomiting, nasal/sinus congestion, rhinorrhea, lacrimation, ptosis, yawning, frequent urination, and diarrhea), affective (depression and irritability), cognitive (attention deficit, difficulty finding words, transient amnesia, and reduced ability to navigate in familiar environments), and sensory (photophobia, phonophobia, osmophobia, muscle tenderness, and cutaneous allodynia) symptoms.

In many cases, migraine attacks are likely to begin centrally, in brain areas capable of generating the classical neurological symptoms of prodromes and aura, whereas the headache phase begins with consequential activation of meningeal nociceptors at the origin of the trigeminovascular system (Figure 6-1).

Genetics

Family history points to a genetic predisposition to migraine.[1,3] A genetic association with migraine was first observed and defined in patients with familial hemiplegic migraine (FHM) (Chapter 10). The three genes identified with FHM encode proteins that regulate glutamate availability in the synapse. FHM1 (CACNA1A) encodes the pore-forming $\alpha 1$ subunit of the P/Q-type calcium channel, FHM2 (ATP1A2) encodes the $\alpha 2$ subunit of the Na+/K+-ATPase pump, and the FHM3 (SCN1A) encodes the $\alpha 1$ subunit of neuronal voltage-gated Nav1.1 channel. Collectively, these genes regulate transmitter release, glial ability to clear (reuptake) glutamate from the synapse, and the generation of action potentials. Since these early findings, large genome-wide association studies have identified 13 susceptibility gene variants for migraine with and without aura, of which 3 regulate glutaminergic neurotransmission (MTDH/AEG-1 gene downregulates glutamate transporter, LPR1 modulates synaptic transmission through the *N*-methyl D-aspartate (NMDA) receptor,

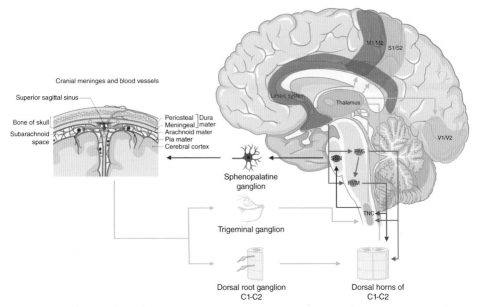

Figure 6-1. Pathophysiology of migraine. M1: primary motor cortex; M2: secondary motor cortex; PAG: peri-aqueductal gray; RVM: rostral ventromedial medulla; S1: primary somatosensory area; S2: secondary somatosensory area; SSN: superior salivatory nucleus; TNC: trigeminal nucleus caudalis; V1: primary visual cortex (striate cortex); V2: secondary visual cortex.

and MEF-2D gene regulates the glutamatergic excitatory synapse), and 2 regulate synaptic development and plasticity (ASTN2 gene involves in structural development of cortical layers, and FHL5 gene regulates cAMP-sensitive cAMP response element binding (CREB) proteins involved in synaptic plasticity). These findings provide the most plausible explanation for the "generalized" neuronal hyperexcitability of the migraine brain. In the context of migraine, increased activity in glutamatergic systems can lead to excessive occupation of NMDA receptors, which in turn may amplify and reinforce pain transmission and the development of allodynia and central sensitization. Network-wise, widespread neuronal hyperexcitability may also be driven by thalamocortical dysrhythmia; defective modulatory brainstem circuits that regulate excitability at multiple levels along the neuraxis; and inherently improper regulation/habituation of cortical, thalamic, and brainstem functions by limbic structures such as the hypothalamus, amygdala, nucleus accumbens, caudate, putamen, and globus pallidus. Given that 2 of the 13 susceptibility genes regulate synaptic development and plasticity, it is reasonable to speculate that some of the networks mentioned earlier may not be properly wired to set a normal level of habituation throughout the brain, thus explaining the multifactorial nature of migraine. Along this line, it is also tempting to propose that at least some of the structural alterations seen in the migraine brain may be inherited and, as such, may be the "cause" of migraine rather than being secondary to (i.e., being caused by) the repeated headache attacks. But this concept awaits evidence.

Prodromes

In the context of migraine, prodromes are symptoms that precede the headache by several hours and sometimes days.[1] Examination of symptoms that are most commonly described by patients points to the potential involvement of the hypothalamus (fatigue, depression, irritability, food cravings, and yawning), brainstem (muscle tenderness and neck stiffness), cortex (abnormal sensitivity to light, sound, and smell), and limbic system (depression and anhedonia) in the prodromal phase of a migraine attack.[1,4] Recently, much attention has been given to the hypothalamus because it plays a key role in many aspects of human circadian rhythms and in the continuous effort to maintain homeostasis. Because the migraine brain is extremely sensitive to deviations from homeostasis, it seems reasonable that hypothalamic neurons that regulate homeostasis and circadian cycles are at the origin of some of the migraine prodromes. These include orexinergic, melanin-concentration hormone, dopaminergic, and histaminergic neurons in the perifornical, dorsomedial, lateral, and tuberomammillary hypothalamic nuclei—all known for playing an important role in responses to sleep deprivation, fasting, and stress.

Cortical Spreading Depression

Both clinical and preclinical studies suggest that migraine aura is caused by cortical spreading depression (CSD), a slowly propagating wave of depolarization/excitation (2-5 mm/min), followed by hyperpolarization/inhibition in cortical neurons and glia.[5] In the cortex, the initial membrane depolarization is associated with a large efflux of potassium; influx of sodium and calcium; release of glutamate, adenosine triphosphate (ATP) and hydrogen ions; neuronal swelling; upregulation of genes involved in inflammatory processing; and a host of changes in cortical perfusion and enzymatic. Outside the brain, activation of pial and dural macrophages and dendritic cells and caspase-1—a potential initiator of inflammation involving high-mobility group protein B1 (HMGB1) and interleukin 1 beta (IL-1β), nuclear factor κB (NF-κB), and cyclooxygenase-2 (COX2) could all contribute to the activation of meningeal nociceptors and the release of calcitonin gene–related peptide. Collectively, such alterations in functions of meningeal immune cells and expression of inflammatory molecules around meningeal nociceptors may provide the link between CSD and activation of the trigeminovascular pathway or aura and headache. Studies in animals show that CSD initiates delayed and immediate activation of peripheral and central trigeminovascular neurons in a fashion that resembles the classical delay and occasional immediate onset of headache after aura.

Trigeminovascular Pathway: From Activation to Sensitization

Neuroanatomy

The trigeminovascular pathway conveys nociceptive information from the meninges to the brain (Chapter 4).[6] The pathway originates in trigeminal ganglion neurons whose peripheral axons reach the pia, dura, and large cerebral arteries and whose central axons reach the nociceptive dorsal horn laminae of the spinal trigeminal nucleus (SpV) or trigeminal nucleus caudalis. In the SpV, the nociceptors converge on neurons that receive additional input from the periorbital skin and pericranial muscles. The ascending axonal projections of trigeminovascular SpV neurons transmit monosynaptic nociceptive signals to (a) brainstem nuclei such as the ventrolateral periaqueductal gray, reticular formation, superior salivatory, parabrachial, cuneiform, and the nucleus of the solitary tract; (b) hypothalamic nuclei such as the anterior, lateral, perifornical, dorsomedial, suprachiasmatic, and supraoptic; and (c) basal ganglia nuclei such as the caudate-putamen, globus pallidus, and substantia innominata. These projections may be critical for the initiation of nausea, vomiting, yawning, lacrimation, urination, loss of appetite, fatigue, anxiety, irritability, and depression by the headache itself. Additional projections of trigeminovascular SpV neurons are found in the thalamic ventral posteromedial (VPM), posterior (PO), and parafascicular nuclei. Relay trigeminovascular thalamic neurons that project to the somatosensory, insular, motor, parietal association, retrosplenial, auditory, visual, and olfactory cortices are in a position to construct the specific nature of migraine pain (i.e., location, intensity, and quality) and many of the cortically mediated symptoms that distinguish between migraine headache and other pains. These include transient symptoms of motor clumsiness, difficulty focusing, amnesia, allodynia, phonophobia, photophobia, and osmophobia.

Origin of Pain and Peripheral Sensitization

In migraine with aura, the onset of the headache phase of a migraine with aura coincides with the activation of meningeal nociceptors at the peripheral origin of the trigeminovascular pathway.[7] Whereas the vascular, cellular, and molecular events involved in the activation of meningeal nociceptors by CSD are not well understood, a growing body of data suggests that transient constriction and dilatation of pial arteries and the development of dural plasma protein extravasation, neurogenic inflammation, platelet aggregation, mast cell degranulation, macrophage activation, and migration of dendritic cells can introduce to the meninges pro-inflammatory molecules that alter the molecular environment in which meningeal nociceptors exist and render them hyperexcitable, hyperactive, and hyperresponsive. While it is not clear how other migraine triggers end up activating the meningeal nociceptors, current evidence for the efficacy of migraine prophylactic drugs that do not cross the blood–brain barrier supports the notion that activation of meningeal nociceptors is essential for the initiation of the headache by events such as mild head trauma, stress, lack of sleep, or any one of the many well-recognized migraine triggers.

Central Sensitization

When activated in the altered molecular environment described earlier, peripheral trigeminovascular neurons become sensitized (their response threshold decreases and their response magnitude increases) and begin to respond to dura stimuli to which they showed minimal or no response at baseline. When central trigeminovascular neurons in laminae I and V of SpV and the thalamic PO/VPM nuclei become sensitized, their spontaneous activity increases, their receptive fields expand, and they begin to respond to innocuous mechanical and thermal stimulation of cephalic and extracephalic skin areas as if it were noxious. The human correlates of the electrophysiological measures of neuronal sensitization in animal studies are evident in contrast analysis of blood-oxygen-level-dependent (BOLD) signals registered in fMRI scans of the human trigeminal ganglion, spinal trigeminal nucleus, and the thalamus, all measured during migraine attacks.[8] The clinical manifestation of peripheral sensitization during migraine, which takes about 10 minutes to develop, includes the perception of throbbing headache and the transient intensification of headache while bending over or coughing, activities which momentarily increase intracranial pressure. The clinical manifestation of sensitization of central trigeminovascular neurons in the SpV, which takes 30 to 60 minutes to develop and 120 minutes to reach full extent, includes the development of cephalic cutaneous allodynia signs such as scalp and muscle tenderness and hypersensitivity to touch. The clinical manifestation of thalamic sensitization during migraine, which takes 2 to 4 hours to develop, also includes extracephalic allodynia signs that cause patients to remove tight cloth and jewelry and avoid being touched, massaged, or hugged.

Central sensitization might also play a role in the transformation of episodic migraine to chronic migraine.[9] With repeated migraine attacks, the central nervous system becomes more sensitized, increasing the frequency and severity of migraine episodes, progressing to a chronic state.

Postdrome and Interictal Phase

The migraine postdrome and interictal phases of migraine are the least studied and least understood phases of the condition. After the storm of a migraine attack subsides, its impact continues to be felt during the postdrome and interictal phases. The postdrome phase, often referred to as the "migraine hangover," is characterized by a range of symptoms that persist even after the headache has waned. Fatigue, difficulty concentrating, mood changes, and a general sense of malaise are common companions during this phase. As if unraveling the intricate threads of the migraine's aftermath, individuals may find themselves navigating through a mental fog that casts a shadow on their cognitive and emotional well-being. This phase, often overlooked, underscores the lingering toll that migraines can take. In contrast, the interictal phase denotes the time between migraine attacks. Far from a neutral hiatus, this phase represents a period of susceptibility and heightened reactivity to potential triggers. Neurological and sensory systems remain in a state of flux, potentially contributing to the unpredictability of when the next migraine episode might strike. Understanding and addressing these phases is crucial for comprehensive migraine management, ensuring that the full spectrum of the migraine experience is acknowledged and managed effectively.

Summary

- Migraine is not just a headache and may involve different phases: prodrome, aura, headache phase, postdrome, and interictal phase.

- Family history indicates a genetic link to migraines, with genes tied to FHM and other variants affecting neurotransmission and synaptic development, suggesting reasons for the migraine brain's hyperexcitability.

- Migraine affects multiple cortical, subcortical, and brainstem areas that regulate autonomic, affective, cognitive, and sensory functions.

- In many cases, migraine attacks are likely to begin centrally, in brain areas capable of generating the classical neurological symptoms of prodromes and aura, whereas the headache phase begins with consequential activation of meningeal nociceptors.

- Migraine aura is caused by CSD, a slowly propagating wave of depolarization/excitation (2-5 mm/minute) followed by hyperpolarization/inhibition in cortical neurons and glia.

- Central sensitization develops during migraine attacks, manifesting with cutaneous allodynia, and is a risk factor for the transformation of migraine from episodic to chronic forms.

REFERENCES

1. Ferrari MD, Goadsby PJ, Burstein R, et al. Migraine. *Nature Reviews Disease Primers.* 2022;8:2.

2. Cutrer FM, Olesen J. Migraine with aura and their suforms. In: Olesen J, Goadsby PJ, Ramadan N, Tfelt-Hansen J, Welch KM, eds. *The headaches.* USA: Lippincott, Williams and Wilkins; 2006; 407-421.

3. Harder AVE, Terwindt GM, Nyholt DR, van den Maagdenberg A. Migraine genetics: status and road forward. *Cephalalgia.* 2023;43:3331024221145962.

4. May A, Burstein R. Hypothalamic regulation of headache and migraine. *Cephalalgia.* 2019;39: 1710-1719.

5. Noseda R, Burstein R. Migraine pathophysiology: anatomy of the trigeminovascular pathway and associated neurological symptoms, CSD, sensitization and modulation of pain. *Pain.* 2013;154(suppl 1): 10.1016/j.pain.2013.1007.1021.

6. Ashina M, Hansen JM, Do TP, et al. Migraine and the trigeminovascular system—40 years and counting. *Lancet Neurol.* 2019;18:795-804.

7. Olesen J, Burstein R, Ashina M, Tfelt-Hansen P. Origin of pain in migraine: evidence for peripheral sensitisation. *Lancet Neurol.* 2009;8:679-690.

8. Ashina S, Bentivegna E, Martelletti P, Eikermann-Haerter K. Structural and functional brain changes in migraine. *Pain Ther.* 2021;10:211-223.

9. Louter MA, Bosker JE, van Oosterhout WPJ, et al. Cutaneous allodynia as a predictor of migraine chronification. *Brain.* 2013;136:3489-3496.

Primary Headaches

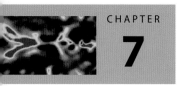

CHAPTER

7

Migraine: Acute Treatment

Ioana Medrea and Stewart J. Tepper

A migraine attack is frequently disabling, and a day lived with migraine is as disabling as a day lived with dementia, quadriplegia, or acute psychosis. A treatment that resolves the attack can prevent that disability. Additionally, there is a toll of ongoing uncontrolled attacks, and those with ineffective acute therapy tend to develop more headaches over time and risk migraine chronification, that is, transformation of episodic to chronic form.

General Treatment Principles

Patient Education

Education is an integral part of migraine treatment. If patients understand their condition, they are more likely to adhere to treatment. Providers need to emphasize that migraine is a disorder of the brain involving dysregulation in sensory processing with a hereditary predisposition to decreasing the threshold for generating headaches. This propensity to generate headaches is generally life long, but the frequency of attacks is variable throughout life based on the interaction between genetics and the environment. It is important to set realistic expectations because there is no absolute cure for migraine. As highlighted in Box 7-1, an optimal treatment should get the patient pain free by 2 hours, with no recurrence in the next 22 hours and no need for more treatment, either rescue or the initial treatment taken again. If this is not possible, then the duration of the episode should be shortened, and pain and disability lessened. Finally, both safety and tolerability are crucial.

Treatment Monitoring

Providers must tailor the treatment to the goals and expectations of the patient in every assessment. They should advise patients to regularly use a headache diary. A completed diary simplifies the assessment of response to therapy, the frequency of acute medication use is easily verified, and this improves communication. At each visit, the response to medications and the tolerability of these medications should be discussed. The risk of acute medication overuse needs to be clearly communicated with patients when most acute medication is being prescribed. There is a risk of migraine chronification if acute medications containing opioids and barbiturates are used 4 to 8 days per month, but due to the high risk of chronification with even fewer days of use, most headache clinicians avoid these medications for acute treatment altogether.[1-3] Use of combination analgesic

---

Box 7-1. Goals of Acute Treatment of Migraine

1. Render patient headache free at 2 hours and free of most bothersome symptoms
2. Otherwise, should decrease the duration of the headache, decrease pain, and decrease disability
3. Ideally should have no headache recurrence and no need for additional treatment

---

formulations and triptans should be less than 10 days per month and less than 2 to 3 days per week, to avoid development of medication overuse headache (MOH) (Chapter 28).[4] Nonsteroidal anti-inflammatory drugs (NSAIDs) taken in monotherapy may be linked to transformation to MOH at 15 or more days per month.[2,4] Gepants do not appear to be associated with MOH or transformation to chronic migraine (CM), and, in fact, frequent use leads to reduced number of migraine attacks and even prevention.[4]

Nonpharmacological Treatment

Nonpharmacological approaches can be very important adjuvants to acute medications. Some recommended interventions are rest in a quiet dark place, hydration, ice, deep breathing/relaxation, behavioral methods, biofeedback, and use of noninvasive neuromodulation devices (Chapters 46 and 47).

Pharmacological Treatment

Matching patients' need to therapy is critical, and this stratified care is superior to nonspecific step care when directly compared. In step care, nonspecific treatments is used as the first line in all comers, and care is escalated after failure of first-line medications. In stratified care, treatment is varied based on the severity of pain or other bothersome features of attack, using triptans, for example, for severe attacks and NSAIDs only for moderate attacks. These strategies for migraine have not been rigorously evaluated. Disability can be a surrogate marker for disease severity, and significant migraine impact dictates the use of migraine-specific acute treatment. Nonspecific migraine treatments can be used synergistically with specific migraine treatments for enhanced benefit. Patients with significant nausea or vomiting can be prescribed nonoral parenteral therapy.

Disease Nonspecific Treatments

Acute medications can be nonspecific, in which case they can work on other pain and primary headache disorders or migraine-specific and targeted to the specific primary headache disorder. Disease nonspecific acute treatments include analgesics, NSAIDs, antiemetics, steroids, barbiturates, and opioids. The use of barbiturates and opioids for the acute treatment of migraine is not recommended for patients with primary headache disorders because these medications commonly lead to difficult-to-control MOH and can lead to dependence and addiction. These are detailed in Table 7-1.

Analgesics

Over-the-counter analgesics and prescription formulations are commonly used for acute migraine treatment. Some are indicated in mild to moderate attacks, and there can be significant benefits from these nonspecific analgesics. NSAIDs are commonly used for many indications, including analgesia, antipyretic, antithrombotic, and anti-inflammatory indications. Their activity depends on the degree of selective inhibition of the cyclo-oxygenase enzyme (COX), also known as prostaglandin synthase. NSAIDs work by interfering with the transformation of arachidonic acid to prostaglandins, prostacyclin, and thromboxane. COX-1 enzyme inhibition leads to the loss of normal platelet aggregation and gastric protection, whereas COX-2 enzyme inhibition leads to decreased inflammation. NSAIDs mediate their mechanisms of action at multiple sites, reducing meningeal neurogenic inflammation, trigeminal neuron and trigeminal nucleus caudalis (TNC) activation, and hypothalamic activation (Figure 7-1). NSAIDs should not be used in patients with a history of gastric ulcer, bleeding, or severe gastritis; a history of gastric bypass; uncontrolled hypertension; or renal failure. Side effects include nausea, gastrointestinal upset, ulcers, and the risk of upper gastrointestinal bleeding, abdominal discomfort, diarrhea, constipation, and tinnitus.

Some commonly used NSAIDs and their dosages are listed in Table 7-1. Use of shorter-acting NSAIDs such as ibuprofen is recommended only in patients with infrequent headaches, in doses

Table 7-1. Disease Nonspecific Acute Treatments of Migraine

Drug	MDD	American Guidelines	Canadian Guidelines	AE	Contraindications	When to Consider
ASA 500-1000 mg PO every 4-6 hours	4 g	A	Strong, high-quality evidence	+	History of renal failure, gastric bypass, or ulcer/severe gastritis	Healthy adults, mild-moderate headache
Acetaminophen/paracetamol 1000 mg PO/IV every 6 hours	4 g	A	Strong, high-quality evidence	+	Significant liver disease	Healthy adults, mild-moderate headache
Acetaminophen/aspirin/ caffeine 500/500/130 mg PO every 4-6 hours		A	Strong, high-quality evidence	+	History of renal failure, gastric bypass, or ulcer/severe gastritis	Healthy adults, mild-moderate headache
Ibuprofen 400-600 mg PO every 4-6 hours	2.4 g	A	Strong, high-quality evidence	+	History of renal failure, gastric bypass, or ulcer/severe gastritis	Healthy adults, mild-moderate headache
Naproxen 500 mg PO every 12 hours	1 g	A	Strong, high-quality evidence	+	History of renal failure, gastric bypass, or ulcer/severe gastritis	Healthy adults, mild-moderate headache
Diclofenac 50 mg, 100 mg PO every 6 hours	200 mg	A	Strong, high-quality evidence	+	History of renal failure, gastric bypass, or ulcer/severe gastritis	Healthy adults, mild-moderate headache
Ketoprofen 100 mg PO every 6-8 hours	300 mg	B		+	History of renal failure, gastric bypass, or ulcer/severe gastritis	Healthy adults, mild-moderate headache
Flurbiprofen 100 mg PO every 6-8 hours	300 mg	B		+	History of renal failure, gastric bypass, or ulcer/severe gastritis	Healthy adults, mild-moderate headache
Ketorolac 30 mg, 60 mg IV/IM every 6 hours	120 mg	B		+	History of renal failure, gastric bypass, or ulcer/severe gastritis	Status migrainosus
Indomethacin 25 mg, 50 mg PO/PR every 4-6 hours	200 mg			+	History of renal failure, gastric bypass, or ulcer/severe gastritis	Status migrainous
Celecoxib 120 mg liquid daily	120 mg			+	History of renal failure, gastric bypass, or ulcer/severe gastritis	Healthy adults, mild-moderate headache

Drug	MDD	American Guidelines	Canadian Guidelines	AE	Contraindications	When to Consider
MgSO$_4$ 1-2 g IV daily	2 g	B		+	Renal failure	Migraine with aura
Valproate 400-1000 mg IV every 6-12 hours	2000 mg	C		++	Liver disease	When migraine persistent >72 hours and DHE contraindicated
Dexamethasone 4-16 mg IV every 4-6 hours	16 mg	C		++		Status migrainosus in conjunction with another therapy
Metoclopramide 10 mg PO/ IV every 4-6 hours	40 mg	B	Strong, moderate-quality evidence	++	Akathesia with antidopaminergic medications	When significant nausea or failure of another therapy can add on
Chlorpromazine 12.5 mg IV	25 mg	B		++	Akathesia with antidopaminergic medications	When significant nausea or failure of another therapy can add on
Prochlorperazine 10 mg IV/IM or 25 mg PR every 4-6 hours	40 mg PO or 100 mg PR	B		+	Akathesia with antidopaminergic medications	When significant nausea or failure of another therapy can add on
Butalbital-containing medications		C	Strong to not use, low-quality evidence	+	Should not be used	Not recommended
Opiates including tramadol		B	Weak, low- to moderate-quality evidence	+	Should not be used	Not recommended

AE: Adverse Effects, ASA: Acetylsalicylic Acid (Aspirin), DHE: Dihydroergotamine, IM: Intramuscular, IV: Intravenous, MDD: maximum daily dose, MgSO4: Magnesium Sulfate, PO: Per Os (Orally), PR: Per Rectum

Primary Headaches

Acute Migraine Treatment and Migraine Pathophysiology

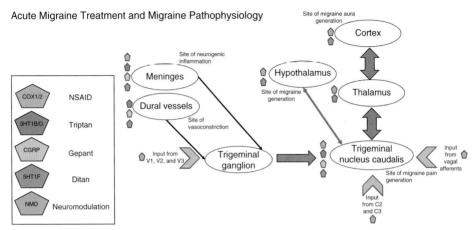

Figure 7-1. Proposed sites of action of acute migraine treatments. V1—ophthalmic branch of the trigeminal nerve, V2—maxillary branch of the trigeminal nerve, V3—mandibular branch of the trigeminal nerve, C2 and C3—cervical afferent sensory fibers, CGRP—calcitonin gene–related peptide, ditan—class of medications used for migraine acute therapy selectively binding the 5HT1F receptor, gepant—calcitonin gene–related peptide receptor small-molecule antagonists used for acute treatment of migraine, NSAID—nonsteroidal anti-inflammatory drug.

of 400 to 600 mg. Quicker-onset formulations such as diclofenac sodium dissolvable powder (U.S. brand name CAMBIA), liquid celecoxib (U.S. brand name ELYXYB), both FDA approved for acute treatment of migraine, or ketorolac nasal spray (U.S. brand name SPRIX), FDA approved for pain, are available and effective, but access can be a problem. In patients with more frequent headaches (>10 days per month as a higher risk of chronification) or longer-lasting migraine, a longer-acting NSAID such as naproxen can be selected. Another formulation to consider if patients have severe nausea or vomiting and require an NSAID is an indomethacin suppository.

Anti-emetics

Anti-emetics are commonly used when there is significant nausea or vomiting. There is associated gastric stasis with migraine, and neuroleptics can help with nausea and gastric stasis. There are oral, suppository, and injectable formulations. These can also be added to other acute therapies for the treatment-resistant headaches. Possible side effects of neuroleptics include sedation, akathisia, and, rarely, dystonia. Pretreatment with diphenhydramine or anticholinergic agents can minimize the more serious of these side effects. Metoclopramide can be a first-line treatment for nausea. Additionally, prochlorperazine or promethazine suppositories can be used in patients with vomiting for at-home rescue. Finally, serotonin (5HT)$_3$ antagonists such as ondansetron and granisetron can be better tolerated than traditional neuroleptics and are commonly used for the treatment of nausea without vomiting.

Disease-Specific Treatments

Migraine-specific treatments are outlined in Table 7-2.

Nonselective Serotonin 5HT Agonists

Nonselective serotonin 5HT agonists were the first migraine-specific therapies introduced. Ergotamine and dihydroergotamine (DHE) are in this class. Both can inhibit the reuptake of noradrenaline at sympathetic nerve endings, but DHE is better tolerated. They are agonists at 5HT$_{1A}$, 5HT$_{1B}$,

Table 7-2. Disease-Specific Acute Treatments of Migraine

Drug	MDD	American Guideline	Canadian Guideline	AE	Contraindications	When to Consider
Ergots						
Ergotamine/caffeine 1/100 mg every 4-6 hours	6 mg/day and 10 mg/week	B	Weak (not recommended), moderate-quality evidence	+++	Cardiac, peripheral vascular, or cerebral disease	
DHE 0.5-1 mg IV/IM every 4-6 hours	3 mg/day, 6 mg per week	B	Weak, moderate-quality evidence	++	Cardiac, peripheral vascular, or cerebral disease	Resistant status migrainous
DHE 2 mg NS daily	2 mg/day at most twice per week	A	Weak, moderate-quality evidence	++	Cardiac, peripheral vascular, or cerebral disease	Migraine resistant to triptans or frequent recurrence
DHE 1.45 mg NS (Truedhesa), can repeat at 1 hour	2.9 mg/day at most twice per week	NA	NA		Cardiac, peripheral vascular, or cerebral disease	Migraine resistant to triptans or frequent recurrence
Triptans						
Sumatriptan 50 mg, **100 mg PO repeat at 2 hours,** 5 mg, 10 mg, **20 mg NS repeat at 1 hour,** 22 mg nasal powder, 3 mg, 4 mg, **6 mg SC** repeat at 1 hour	200 mg PO, 40 mg NS, 12 mg SC	A	Strong, high-quality evidence	++	Cardiac or cerebral disease risk	Healthy adults moderate–severe headache
Zolmitriptan **2.5 mg, 5 mg PO,** 2.5 mg, **5 mg NS, can repeat at 2 hours**	10 mg PO or NS	A	Strong, high-quality evidence	++	Cardiac or cerebral disease risk	Healthy adults moderate–severe headache
Rizatriptan 5 mg, **10 mg PO, can repeat at 2 hours**	20 mg PO recommend, as per manufacturer 30 mg	A	Strong, high-quality evidence	++	Cardiac or cerebral disease risk	Healthy adults moderate–severe headache

(Continued)

Table 7-2. Disease-Specific Acute Treatments of Migraine (*Continued*)

Drug	MDD	American Guideline	Canadian Guideline	AE	Contraindications	When to Consider
Naratriptan **2.5 mg PO, can repeat at 2 hours**	5 mg PO	A	Strong, high-quality evidence	+	Cardiac or cerebral disease risk	Healthy adults moderate–severe headache
Almotriptan 6.25 mg, **12.5 mg PO, can repeat at 2 hours**	25 mg PO	A	Strong, high-quality evidence	+	Cardiac or cerebral disease risk	Healthy adults moderate–severe headache
Frovatriptan **2.5 mg PO, can repeat at 2 hours**	5 mg PO	A	Strong, high-quality evidence	++	Cardiac or cerebral disease risk	Healthy adults moderate–severe headache
Eletriptan 20 mg, **40 mg PO, can repeat at 2 hours**	80 mg PO	A	Strong, high-quality evidence	++	Cardiac or cerebral disease risk	Healthy adults moderate–severe headache
Gepants						
Rimagepant 75 mg PO, can repeat at 48 hours	75 mg per 48 hours	NA	NA	+	Concomitant use of strong CYP3A4 inhibitors, severe hepatic impairment and renal failure	Cardiac or cerebral disease risk
Ubrogepant 50 mg, **100 mg** PO, can repeat at 2 hours	200 mg PO	NA	NA	+	Concomitant use of strong CYP3A4 inhibitors, severe hepatic impairment and renal failure	Cardiac or cerebral disease risk
Zavegepant 10 mg NS, can repeat at 24 hours		NA	NA	+	Concomitant use of strong CYP3A4 inhibitors, severe hepatic impairment and renal failure	Cardiac or cerebral disease risk

Drug	MDD	American Guideline	Canadian Guideline	AE	Contraindications	When to Consider
Ditans						
Lasmiditan 50 mg, **100 mg** and can consider 200 mg	One dose daily	NA	NA	++	Renal failure	Cardiac or cerebral disease risk, do not need to drive, or Gepant failure
Neuromodulation						
tSNS 60 minutes		NA	NA	+	Implanted electrical devices such as pacemaker or ICD	Intolerance to medications, pregnancy, MO/MOH
sTMS 2-4 pulses, repeat every 15 minutes for 2 hours until the attack terminates		NA	NA	+	Implanted electrical devices such as pacemaker or ICD	Frequent aura, intolerance to medications, pregnancy, MO/MOH
nVNS 3x2 minutes, can repeat once at 2 minutes		NA	NA	+	Implanted electrical devices such as pacemaker or ICD	Intolerance to medications, pregnancy, MO/MOH
REN 45 minutes		NA	NA	+	Implanted electrical devices such as pacemaker or ICD	Intolerance to medications, pregnancy, MO/MOH
CO-TNS 60 minutes		NA	NA	+	Implanted electrical devices such as pacemaker or ICD	Intolerance to medications, pregnancy, MO/MOH

The optimal dose is bolded in this table. MDD—maximum daily dose, AE—adverse effects, PO—per OS, IV—intravenous, SC—subcutaneous, MO—medication overuse, MOH—medication overuse headache, NA—not applicable, NS—nasal spray, PR—per rectum, ditan—class of medications used for migraine acute therapy selectively binding the 5HT1F receptor, gepant—small-molecule CGRP receptor antagonists used for acute treatment of migraine, +—adverse effects as appreciated by authors, eTNS—external trigeminal neurostimulation, sTMS—single singlepulse transcranial magnetic stimulation, nVNS—noninvasive vagal nerve stimulation, REN—remote electrical neuromodulation, CO-TNS—combined occipital and supraorbital transcutaneous nerve stimulation.

Primary Headaches

$5HT_{1D}$, $5HT_{1E}$, and $5HT_{1F}$ receptors. DHE is associated with less nausea compared to ergotamine. DHE is commonly used in the treatment of refractory migraine in patients with no cardiovascular risk factors. It can be administered as a spray, intramuscularly or subcutaneously, or intravenously. It has a low headache recurrence rate (<20%), and for this reason the intravenous formulation is the treatment of choice for resistant status migrainous, often given in multiple repetitive doses with an anti-emetic such as metoclopramide (Chapter 9). DHE nasal spray can be the first line in select patients with migraine, especially in morning migraine, in patients who need a nonoral treatment and in long-duration attacks such as menstrual migraine. DHE nasal spray can also be very helpful when triptans are not effective or are associated with headache recurrence. Adverse events include rhinorrhea which is a side effect of DHE nasal spray, and when given intramuscularly or intravenously, nausea and vomiting are the most common side effects, along with abdominal pain, diarrhea, and leg cramps. Rarely ergots can precipitate cardiac or cerebral vascular events, and there are reports of venous clots with central line administration. Contraindications for ergots include cardiac, peripheral vascular, and cerebrovascular disease.

Triptans

Triptans are selective agonists at $5HT_{1B/D}$ receptors. Their mechanisms of action are multiple as outlined in Figure 7-1 and include inhibition of neurotransmitter and calcitonin gene–related peptide (CGRP) release, reduction of pain signaling from trigeminal nerves to the TNC, reduced neurogenic inflammation by reducing trigeminal sensory nerve activation, and vasoconstriction of CGRP-dilated vessels.[3] The triptans and their dosages are listed in Table 7-2. There are seven triptans approved for the acute treatment of migraine in the United States: sumatriptan, zolmitriptan, rizatriptan, naratriptan, almotriptan, frovatriptan, and eletriptan.[5,6]

If tolerated, triptans are the first-choice treatment in adults with severe migraine headaches with no increased risk of vascular disease. There are two types of triptans, those that with quicker onset of benefit, shorter duration of effect, and generally higher efficacy rates (sumatriptan, zolmitriptan, rizatriptan almotriptan, and eletriptan) and those that have slower onset with less recurrence but generally lower efficacy rates (naratriptan and frovatriptan). In patients with less frequent headaches and rapid onset of severe headaches, the faster-onset, higher-efficacy triptans such as sumatriptan 100 mg or rizatriptan 10 mg are generally selected. In patients where there is a longer time to peak intensity, and/or longer-duration migraine, a triptan with a slower onset, lower recurrence rate, and better tolerability such as naratriptan 2.5 mg can be used. Additionally, although not FDA approved for this indication, naratriptan and frovatriptan are often used twice a day for 5 to 7 days for mini prevention of menstrual migraine. If other triptans are not effective, or if there is significant nausea or vomiting, nasal spray or injectable formulations can also be considered. Common triptan side effects include tingling in fingertips or on lips, flushing, chest, throat, neck pain or tightness, dizziness or drowsiness, nausea, or drowsiness in some cases. Additionally, injection-site pain is seen with subcutaneous sumatriptan injection, and taste disturbance is common with nasal spray formulations. Rizatriptan is the only FDA-approved triptan for children aged 6 to 17. Smaller children weighing 20 to 39 kg are approved for lower-dose rizatriptan at 5 mg (see also Chapter 49). Almotriptan is FDA approved for children aged 12 to 17. Contraindications to triptans include cardiovascular or stroke history and history of arrhythmia and should be avoided in patients with a high cardiovascular risk.

Ditans

Lasmiditan is currently the only available ditan and works as an agonist at $5HT_{1F}$ receptors, which have no known vascular effects. These receptors are located at multiple locations peripherally at the trigeminal nerve preventing CGRP release and centrally at the TNC, upper brainstem, hypothalamus, thalamus, and cortex, decreasing pain signaling (Figure 7-1). Lasmiditan can be considered for acute use in those with a history of cardiovascular disease. The central effects of lasmiditan require a driving restriction for 8 hours after dosing, and other central side effects can include dizziness, some nausea, and drowsiness. Lasmiditan is contraindicated in patients with renal failure.

Gepants

Gepants are small-molecule antagonists of CGRP receptors that block peripheral CGRP-mediated meningeal neurogenic inflammation and CGRP-induced vasodilation (Figure 7-1). There are two oral medications in this class currently available for acute therapy: rimegepant and ubrogepant. Zavegepant is a gepant nasal spray for the acute treatment of migraine. As noted, gepants do not appear to carry the risk for transformation to CM and MOH, and rimegepant is also FDA approved for preventive use (Chapter 8). Gepants do not carry a warning prohibiting use in those with vascular disease, as they prevent vasodilation but do not cause vasoconstriction. They are better tolerated than most triptans and can be used when triptans are not tolerated, ineffective, or contraindicated. Rare gepant side effects include nausea, constipation, and drowsiness. Gepants are contraindicated in renal failure and hepatic disease and should not be used with potent CYP3A4 inhibitors. The use of a risk score such as Framingham is generally adequate to assess the risk of cardiovascular disease. Gepants or lasmiditan become first-line acute migraine-specific treatments when risk is elevated.

Device Treatment

Multiple noninvasive neuromodulation devices are currently FDA cleared for the acute treatment of migraine (see also Chapter 46). These include external trigeminal neurostimulation (eTNS, brand name CEFALY), single-pulse transcranial magnetic stimulation (sTMS, brand name sTMS MINI), noninvasive vagal nerve stimulation (nVNS, brand name GAMMACORE), remote electrical neuromodulation (REN, brand name NERIVIO), and combined occipital and supraorbital transcutaneous nerve stimulation (CO-TNS, brand name RELIVION). Nonpharmacological therapies may be preferred in some patients. There are those who prefer these modalities of treatment or have poor tolerance or contraindications to pharmacological treatments. In women who are planning to get pregnant or are pregnant, or lactating noninvasive neuromodulation may be useful, with no apparent or known risk of harm to a developing fetus or baby. Additionally, in patients with acute medication overuse, this class of interventions may be useful in addition to behavioral approaches. Neuromodulation modifies neuronal activity by electrical or magnetic activity of these devices through inhibitory mechanisms. These devices reduce pain levels by manipulating central or peripheral pain processing pathways as shown in Figure 7-1.

Treatment Considerations

There are no direct comparisons of triptans, gepants, and ditans. Indirect comparisons suggest that most triptans have higher rates of 2-hour pain freedom than lasmiditan, rimegepant, and ubrogepant. Lasmiditan, especially at higher doses, has more side effects, as do certain triptans (sumatriptan, zolmitriptan, rizatriptan, and eletriptan). Thus, it is reasonable to use triptans as first-line acute therapy for moderate to severe migraine and to recommend gepants in those with cardiovascular disease and intolerance to or failure of triptans. Lasmiditan can also be considered in those with cardiovascular disease and failure with gepants or triptans if the patient does not need to drive within 8 hours of taking medication. In addition to being a reasonable first line for headache, when triptan therapy is inadequate or contraindicated, NSAIDs and other analgesics or anti-emetics can be added to a triptan for enhanced effect. In individuals with frequent headaches ($\geq$10 headache days per month), one approach is for the patient to select days when they need to be functional to use the acute medications that can cause MOH such as triptans or NSAIDs and on other days use treatments less likely to cause MOH such as gepants and noninvasive neuromodulation devices.

Headache recurrence can occur with triptans in 15 to 40% of patients, and taking the same triptan for the recurrence is a reasonable first step. In case of triptan failure or no response to triptan, there are multiple different recommended rescue plans. NSAID and triptan combination is commonly used in triptan failure and using a long half-life NSAID such as naproxen is recommended. Treatment with NSAID and dopamine antagonist (anti-emetic) especially if IV or IM, such as a ketorolac and meto-clopramide "migraine cocktail," is often used in an emergency department setting (see Chapter 9). Home treatments with self-injection or nasal spray of ketorolac or DHE and promethazine supposi-tory can be effective. Suppository indomethacin can also be considered for triptan failure when com-bined with a dopamine antagonist (anti-emetic) in patients hesitant to self-inject. DHE, given its lower recurrence rate, is often used in triptan failure or headache recurrence, provided 24 hours have elapsed since triptan use, and can be administered in monotherapy at home by nasal spray, injected at home or parenterally in an infusion center or as an inpatient (see Chapter 9). DHE can be combined with an anti-emetic if nausea is a limiting side effect. Corticosteroid courses starting with prednisone 60 mg or dexamethasone 12 mg and quickly tapering over 3 to 5 days might be considered in cases of refractory migraine or status migrainosus (see Chapter 9). For the treatment of refractory migraine and headache using infusion treatments, refer to Chapter 45.

Summary

- Patient education about disease, goals, and expectations of acute treatment is of paramount importance.
- Counselling on acute medication overuse and how to use stratified care and rescue strategies are essential to success; limit use of acute medications (except gepants) to 9 days per month or less to avoid MOH.
- Use of migraine-specific treatment for attacks with headache-related disability is recommended.
- Triptan is the first-line acute treatment for attacks with disability in the absence of vascular disease.
- Treatment with gepants, lasmiditan, and neuromodulation is recommended in cases of intol-erance and contraindication to, and failure with triptans; the use of butalbital-containing com-bination medications or opioids in acute migraine treatment is discouraged.
- Consider NSAIDs with injection or suppository anti-emetic dopamine antagonists or DHE nasal spray or injection in those with triptan failure.

REFERENCES

1. Ailani J. Acute migraine treatment. *Continuum (Minneap Minn).* 2021;27(3):597-612.
2. Ailani J, Burch RC, Robbins MS; Board of Directors of the American Headache Society. The American Headache Society Consensus Statement: update on integrating new migraine treatments into clinical practice. *Headache.* 2021;61(7):1021-1039.
3. Worthington I, Pringsheim T, Gawel M, et al. Canadian Headache Society Guideline: acute drug therapy for migraine headache. *Can J Neurol Sci.* 2013;40(S3):S1-S3. doi:10.1017/S0317167100118943.
4. Ashina S, Terwindt GM, Steiner TJ, et al. Medica-tion overuse headache. *Nat Rev Dis Primers.* 2023 Feb 2;9(1):5. doi:10.1038/s41572-022-00415-0.
5. Marmura MJ, Silberstein SD, Schwedt TJ. The acute treatment of migraine in adults: the American Headache Society evidence assessment of migraine pharmacotherapies. *Headache J Head Face Pain.* 2015;55(1):3-20.
6. Yang CP, Liang CS, Chang CM, et al. Comparison of new pharmacologic agents with triptans for treatment of migraine: a systematic review and meta-analysis. *JAMA Netw Open.* 2021;4(10):e2128544-e2128544.

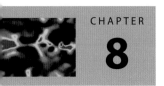

CHAPTER

8

Migraine: Preventive Treatment

Jessica Ailani, Marianna Vinokur, and Stephen D. Silberstein

Migraine is a disabling headache condition that individuals often try to manage on their own until the burden of the disease surpasses the effectiveness of home remedies. Up to 20% of people with frequent migraine attacks do not seek treatment with a healthcare provider, and, when they do, less than 10% receive appropriate care.[1] Although 40% of individuals with migraine are eligible for treatments to reduce disability, only 16% are on preventive therapies.[2] When migraine leads to disability, it is important to start a conversation with patients about available options, including preventive treatment, to improve their functioning and reduce the burden of disease. The burden of migraine extends beyond missed work days and encompasses presentism, missed social and family events, neglected household chores, anxiety about future attacks, and increased reliance on acute treatments to prevent further impact. Consensus statements and guidelines by various national societies discuss when preventive treatment should be started for migraine. They all agree that disability should be the primary factor when making the decision to discuss prevention.[3] It has been shown that preventive treatment reduces the need for office and outpatient visits, emergency department visits, use of diagnostic imaging such as CT scans and MRI, and overall utilization of migraine medications.

General Treatment Principles

The preventive treatment of migraine is indicated in people with frequent, disabling attacks.[3] This treatment is taken even in the absence of a headache, to reduce the frequency, duration, or severity of attacks in the longer term. Additional benefits include improving responsiveness to acute attack treatment and reducing overall disability. Timely initiation of preventive treatment may avert the transformation of episodic to chronic migraine and result in reductions in healthcare and resource consumption. Migraine varies widely in its frequency, severity, and impact on patients' quality of life. A migraine treatment plan should consider not only the patient's diagnosis, symptoms, and any coexistent or comorbid conditions but also the patient's expectations, needs, and goals. Setting realistic expectations for the patient is essential for success. A headache diary can help track progress while adjusting medications and eliminate recall bias. A patient's attitudes toward taking a daily medication, as well as their trust in the healthcare system as a whole, are important considerations in building a patient-physician relationship and affect adherence to a treatment plan. The duration a person with migraine remains on prevention is unclear. In the past, oral prevention may have been recommended for only 6 to 9 months. However, currently, it is recommended that patients should be treated for 6 months, at least with traditional oral agents, with the option to continue for 12 months. If headaches are well controlled, medication may be tapered and discontinued. Dose reduction may provide a better risk-to-benefit ratio.

Although monotherapy is preferred, polypharmacy is sometimes necessary to achieve adequate migraine control. Antidepressants are often used with beta-blockers or calcium channel blockers, and topiramate or divalproex sodium may be used in combination with any of these medications. However, controlled trials are still needed to determine the true advantage of the combination treatments in episodic and chronic migraine. Antidepressants are frequently prescribed alongside beta-blockers or calcium channel blockers, and topiramate or divalproex sodium may be combined with any of these medications. However, further controlled trials are necessary to ascertain the actual benefits of combination treatments for both episodic and chronic migraine.

The U.S. Headache Consortium Guidelines outlines indications for preventive treatment for migraine.[4] When selecting a preventive therapy, considerations such as efficacy, adverse events, and coexisting or comorbid conditions guide the choice.[3] Usually, the medication is initiated at a low dose and gradually escalated until therapeutic effects are observed or the maximum effective dose is reached, unless the medication has only one available dose. A complete therapeutic trial may span from 3 to 6 months. Women who can become pregnant should have a conversation with their healthcare provider regarding contraception options.[3]

Patient Education

The initial phase of any preventive treatment involves lifestyle optimization, which includes prioritizing factors such as adequate sleep, hydration, exercise, and stress management, all of which are vital in reducing migraine disability.

Nonpharmacological Treatment

In addition to lifestyle modification, behavioral treatments have good evidence in improving migraine disability and frequency (Chapter 47). There are many behavioral treatments that can be explored, but those with the best evidence in migraine prevention include progressive muscle relaxation, guided meditation, biofeedback, and cognitive-behavioral therapy. Progressive muscle relaxation and guided meditation can be easily prescribed to patients as they are simple and relatively inexpensive, with some resources even available for free. Biofeedback phone apps are starting to become more widely available if patients are unable to meet with a biofeedback therapist in person for sessions. Cognitive-behavioral therapy can be particularly beneficial for patients with comorbid anxiety or those struggling with medication overuse.

Emerging behavioral therapies like mindfulness-based stress reduction and acceptance and commitment therapy are currently being investigated for their impact on migraines. Preliminary studies have shown a reduction in migraine-related disability without a significant change in migraine days, making them valuable tools to enhance functional outcomes for patients with more resistant forms of the disease.

Acupuncture has gained a greater evidence base in migraine prevention over time and is a therapeutic option that can be offered to patients to help reduce migraine frequency.[5] The optimal number of acupuncture sessions required before noticeable improvement in migraines varies and lacks a consensus.

Pharmacological Treatment

Pharmacological preventive treatments for migraine encompass nutraceuticals (Chapter 47), traditional preventive treatments (Table 8-1), and the more recent calcitonin gene-related peptide (CGRP)-targeting treatments (Table 8-2).

Nutraceuticals

Magnesium deficiency has been suggested to increase susceptibility to migraine. Additionally, data suggest that magnesium intake is inadequate in a large percentage of the population. There is Grade C

Table 8-1. Traditional Preventive Pharmacological Treatments for Migraine

Class	Drug	Dose	Class Evidence	Adverse Effects	Contraindications	When to Consider
ACE-inhibitors	Lisinopril	10-20 mg/day	C	Cough, dizziness	Hypotension, orthostasis, angioedema, pregnancy	Comorbid hypertension, CKD, DMII
ARBs	Candesartan	16-32 mg/day	C	Dizziness, fatigue, hyperkalemia	Hypotension, orthostasis, angioedema, pregnancy	Comorbid hypertension
Beta-blockers	Propranolol	60-120 mg/day	A	Exercise intolerance, hypotension, bradycardia	Depression, hypotension, bradycardia	Comorbid essential tremor, generalized and social anxiety, HTN
	Timolol	20-30 mg/day	A	Exercise intolerance, hypotension, bradycardia	Hypotension, orthostasis, bradycardia	Rarely used in clinical practice
	Nadolol	40-80 mg per day; maximum 240 mg/day	B	Bradycardia	Hypotension, orthostasis, bradycardia	Rarely used in clinical practice
	Metoprolol	25-100 mg/day	A	Bradycardia		Unlikely to affect asthma because highly cardioselective
Calcium channel blockers	Verapamil	120-240 mg/day	U	Constipation, peripheral edema	Hypotension, orthostasis	May be useful in hemiplegic and basilar migraine Consider comorbid cluster headache
	Nimodipine	40 mg TID	U/not better than placebo	Hypotension, bradycardia, vertigo, flushing, abdominal discomfort	Hypotension Avoid hepatic impairment CYP3A4 inducers	

(Continued)

Primary Headaches

Table 8-1. Traditional Preventive Pharmacological Treatments for Migraine *(Continued)*

Class	Drug	Dose	Class Evidence	Adverse Effects	Contraindications	When to Consider
	Nifedipine	5-30 mg TID; maximum 120 mg/day	U/not better than placebo	Peripheral edema, dizziness, flushing, weight gain, paresthesia	Strong CYP450 inducers. Hypotension, aortic stenosis. Avoid in the elderly and those with hepatic impairment	Consider in migraine patients with comorbid Raynaud's disease
	Nicardipine	20 mg daily × 7 days and then 20 mg BID	Significantly better than placebo	Dizziness, peripheral edema, N/V, GI upset	Aortic stenosis, heart failure, hypertrophic cardiomyopathy	
Anticonvulsants	Valproate	250-1000 mg BID or 500-1000 mg DR/day	A	Weight gain, hair loss, somnolence, hepatotoxicity, pancreatitis, tremor, thrombocytopenia		Use should be limited by side-effect profile despite efficacy. Monitor CBC and CMP. Avoid in people of childbearing potential
	Topiramate	50-200 mg BID	A	Paresthesia, somnolence, weight loss, cognitive dulling, word-finding difficulties	Nephrolithiasis, glaucoma	May aid in weight loss. Good option for comorbid IIH. May result in fetal cleft lip and palate, recommended to use for concurrent birth control
	Gabapentin	100-900 mg TID	U	Somnolence		Not very effective for headaches despite common use. Benign option for geriatric or medically complex patients. Can be used as a preventive and PRN for rebound headaches. Consider in comorbid anxiety or insomnia

Class	Drug	Dose	Class Evidence	Adverse Effects	Contraindications	When to Consider
	Levetiracetam	500-1000 mg BID	None	Agitation		Questionable efficacy. May be more beneficial as an acute treatment than as a preventive
	Lamotrigine	Start at 25 mg daily and then slowly titrate to 50-100 mg; maximum 300 mg/day	Probably ineffective	Rash, including the risk of Steven Johnson syndrome, giddiness, somnolence, GI intolerance		Effective for patients with migraine aura, comorbid SUNCT/SUNA
TCA	Amitriptyline	10-75 mg nightly	B	Somnolence, dry mouth, constipation, weight gain if taken long term	Narrow-angle glaucoma. May worsen suicidal ideation	Consider in comorbid insomnia, comorbid depression
	Nortriptyline	30-50 mg daily	None		May worsen suicidal ideation	Lower anticholinergic profile than amitriptyline. Can be tried if excessive sleepiness with amitriptyline
SNRI	Venlafaxine	75-150 mg/day	B	GI intolerance at the start, withdrawal syndromes with skipped doses	Hypertension. May worsen suicidal ideation	Consider in comorbid depression or anxiety
	Duloxetine	30-120 mg/day	None	GI intolerance at the start, withdrawal syndrome with skipped doses	May worsen suicidal ideation	Consider in comorbid fibromyalgia or body pain conditions, depression or anxiety

(Continued)

Primary Headaches

Table 8-1. Traditional Preventive Pharmacological Treatments for Migraine *(Continued)*

Class	Drug	Dose	Class Evidence	Adverse Effects	Contraindications	When to Consider
NMDA receptor antagonists	Memantine	10 mg BID	None	Mood change	Insomnia	Well tolerated but inconclusive efficacy
Alpha adrenergic agonist	Tizanidine	2 mg/day to maximum dose; 8 mg TID	Significant reduction vs placebo in headache frequency, severity, and duration	Hypotension, somnolence, dry mouth	Strong CYP1A2 inhibitors Caution with use in the elderly, hepatic or renal insufficiency, hypotension, concurrent CNS depressants, psychiatric comorbidity	Comorbid spasticity, myofascial tightness
Neurotoxin	Onabotulinum-toxin A	155 units injected every 12 weeks	A	Muscle paralysis may result in facial asymmetries, neck pain	Needle-phobia	Requires adherence to 12-week schedule Consider in medication averse, medically complex, and geriatric patients

Level of evidence per 2012 AAN/AHS guidelines if available. Otherwise, evidence based on metanalysis and expert opinion.

ACE: Angiotensin-Converting Enzyme, ARBs: Angiotensin Receptor Blockers, BID: Bis in Die (Twice Daily), CBC: Complete Blood Count, CKD: Chronic Kidney Disease, CMP: Comprehensive Metabolic Panel, CNS: Central Nervous System, CYP1A2: Cytochrome P450 1A2, CYP450: Cytochrome P450, DMII: Diabetes Mellitus Type II, DR: Delayed Release, GI: Gastrointestinal, HTN: Hypertension, IIH: Idiopathic Intracranial Hypertension, N/V: Nausea/Vomiting, NMDA: N-Methyl-D-Aspartate, PRN: Pro Re Nata (As Needed), SNRI: Serotonin-Norepinephrine Reuptake Inhibitor, SUNA: Short-lasting Unilateral Neuralgiform headache attacks with cranial Autonomic symptoms, SUNCT: Short-lasting Unilateral Neuralgiform headache attacks with Conjunctival Injection and Tearing, TCA: Tricyclic Antidepressant, TID: Ter in Die (Three Times Daily).

Table 8-2. CGRP-Targeting Therapies for Migraine Prevention

Class	Medication	Dose	Half-Life	Indication	Side Effect
CGRP mAb	Erenumab	Subcutaneous dosing via single-dose prefilled autoinjector: 70 or 140 mg once monthly	**28 days**	Preventive treatment of migraine in adults	Injection-site reaction
CGRP mAb	Galcanezumab	Subcutaneous dosing via single-dose prefilled autoinjector: Loading dose of 240 mg, followed by 120 mg monthly	**27 days**	Preventive treatment of episodic and chronic migraine in adults. Treatment of episodic cluster headache	Injection-site reaction
CGRP mAb	Fremanezumab	Subcutaneous dosing via single-dose prefilled autoinjector or single-dose prefilled syringe: 225 mg monthly or 675 mg every 3 months	**30 days**	Preventive treatment of migraine in adults	Injection-site reaction
CGRP mAb	Eptinezumab	100 or 300 mg infusion every 12 weeks	**27 days**	Preventive treatment of migraine in adults	Nasopharyngitis, hypersensitivity
Gepant	Rimegepant	75 mg every other day	**11 hours**	Acute treatment of migraine attacks with or without aura. Preventive treatment of episodic migraine	Nausea (2.7%). Stomach pain/indigestion (2.4%)
Gepant	Atogepant	10, 30, or 60 mg once daily	**11 hours**	Preventive treatment of episodic migraine in adult	Nausea, constipation, and fatigue

mAb: monoclonal antibody.

(possibly effective) evidence for dietary magnesium supplementation of 400 to 600 mg for the prevention of migraine. Melatonin 3 mg was found to be more effective for migraine prevention, and as effective as amitriptyline 25 mg, suggesting a potential preventive benefit.

Petasites or butterbur (100-150 mg daily) can reduce migraine attack frequency by 36 to 60%. However, nonpetasite formulations of butterbur have been rarely associated with hepatic toxicity.[6] Riboflavin 400 mg, coenzyme Q10 100 or 300 mg, and feverfew have also been effective in preventing migraine. Increasing dietary n-3 EPA+DHA to 1.5 g/day while maintaining linoleic acid consumption at 7% or decreasing to <1.8% produced biochemical changes that can reduce headache days in those with migraine.[3]

Antihypertensives

Beta-blockers

Propranolol (40-120 mg twice daily), timolol (20-30 mg once daily), bisoprolol (5 mg once daily), and metoprolol (25-100 mg twice daily) have been shown to be efficacious treatments for migraine prevention, with atenolol (50-200 mg daily) and nadolol (40-80 mg daily) also showing more modest efficacy.[5] Although the mechanism by which they impart migraine relief is not completely understood, inhibition of $\beta 1$-mediated effects, which prevents norepinephrine release, is considered the main pathway. This class of medication carries common adverse effects of bronchoconstriction, bradycardia, dizziness, fatigue, exercise intolerance, symptomatic orthostasis, and insomnia and may worsen depression. Classically beta-blockers should be avoided in patients with asthma, bradycardia, hypotension, and congestive heart failure. There has been concern that dosing beta-blockers at night may reduce the risk of developing diabetes. Also, of note, patients concurrently taking propranolol and rizatriptan require the rizatriptan be reduced to a dose of 5 mg.

Calcium Channel Antagonists

Although not FDA approved for migraine, the efficacy of several different agents including verapamil (120-240 mg once daily), nimodipine, nifedipine, and nicardipine has been reported. The most common side effects are constipation and peripheral edema. Verapamil has been described as particularly useful for hemiplegic and basilar migraine. Flunarizine is a calcium channel antagonist, not available in the US, frequently used in some countries for the prevention of migraine. The recommended dose for migraine prevention is 5-10 mg once daily.

Angiotensin-Converting Enzyme Inhibitors and Angiotensin-Receptor Blockers

Although not FDA approved for migraine, lisinopril (10 mg once daily) and candesartan (8-16 mg once daily) have been used and have reduced migraine frequency by about 30-35%. Candesartan has been shown to be noninferior to propranolol for the prevention of migraine.[3] Side effects include hyperkalemia, especially in the setting of renal impairment, hypotension, and orthostasis, but can be useful in patients with comorbid hypertension. Candesartan is teratogenic and should not be used while a woman is family planning or pregnant (black-box warning).

Antidepressants

Although not FDA approved, selective serotonin reuptake inhibitors, serotonin norepinephrine reuptake inhibitors (SNRIs), and tricyclic antidepressants (TCAs) have been used for many years for the prevention of migraine, particularly in patients with coexisting depression and anxiety. Amitriptyline (10-75 mg once daily) is the only TCA shown to be effective for migraine prevention in clinical trials, although nortriptyline (between 25 and 50 mg) is also commonly used with its more tolerable side-effect profile.[5] Common adverse effects of this class are sedation, dry mouth, constipation, and weight gain due to its anticholinergic properties. SNRIs such as venlafaxine (75-225 mg once daily) and duloxetine (20-120 mg once daily) have been shown to have moderate efficacy in preventing migraine. They can cause nausea, vomiting, sweating, tachycardia, urinary retention, and increased blood pressure.

Anticonvulsants

Valproate and topiramate are FDA approved for migraine prevention.[7] They are similarly effective in decreasing migraine frequency, and both have been rigorously verified by numerous trials to demonstrate therapeutic benefit. For topiramate 100 and 200 mg outperformed 50 mg, although side effects intensify as dose increases. Topiramate has multiple mechanisms of action, including inhibition of voltage-dependent sodium channels and high-voltage-activated L-type calcium channels, inhibition of glutamate-mediated excitatory neurotransmission, and increasing gamma-aminobutyric acid (GABA)-A-mediated inhibition, as well as carbonic anhydrase inhibition. Unfortunately, it is less clear which of these mechanisms are the main action by which topiramate is effective against migraine. Similar to topiramate, valproate also affects multiple pathways, from enhancing GABAergic inhibition to inhibition of voltage-dependent sodium and calcium channels. For valproate, a dose–effect correlation has not been established, although 250 to 800 mg daily are commonly used doses. About 50% of patients achieve a ≥50% reduction in headache frequency with these drugs. It has been reported that topiramate was at least as effective as propranolol for migraine prevention. There was no unequivocal evidence of efficacy for any of the other anti-epileptics. Several anticonvulsants, including acetazolamide, gabapentin, carbamazepine, clonazepam, oxcarbazepine, and vigabatrin, were not superior to placebo for episodic migraines, based largely on the metric of ability to reduce headaches by 50%. Lamotrigine was found effective at 4 weeks though ineffective at 12 weeks. There is conflicting evidence regarding the efficacy of levetiracetam, but given its tolerability, a trial may be reasonable if there are no contraindications. Unfortunately, the efficacy of these medications is often overshadowed by tolerability profiles. Valproate is strictly contraindicated in pregnancy due to its known risk of neural tube defects and generally should not be prescribed for women of childbearing. Furthermore, chronic use is associated with hepatotoxicity, alopecia, weight gain, drug-induced pancreatitis, tremor, thrombocytopenia, and polycystic ovaries. Topiramate is associated most commonly with cognitive difficulties, namely word-finding difficulties, peripheral paresthesia, somnolence, weight loss, and appetite suppression. Risk of osteopenia and osteoporosis is associated with long-term use of topiramate. Particularly the cognitive difficulties appear to be dose dependent. Topiramate is also contraindicated during pregnancy due to the risk of cleft palate malformations and should be avoided in patients with a history of nephrolithiasis.

OnabotulinumtoxinA

Pericranial intramuscular injections of onabotulinumtoxinA have been FDA approved since September 2010 for the prevention of chronic migraine. Injections of 155-200 units are administered every 12 weeks into areas innervated by major sensory peripheral nerves (see Chapter 43). Treatment is generally well tolerated by the patients. Adverse effects include neck pain, headache and migraine, muscle aches and pains, ptosis, and head drop. If side effects develop, they are temporary as the toxin is only efficacious for a maximum of 12 weeks postinjection.[8] The proposed mechanism by which onabotulinumtoxinA alleviates migraine is by interrupting vesicle release, via soluble N-ethylmaleimide-sensitive factor activating protein receptor (SNARE) proteins, of not only acetylcholine but neurotransmitters associated with primary headache disorders such as CGRP, substance P, serotonin, glutamate, GABA, norepinephrine, and dopamine.

CGRP-Targeting Medications

CGRP monoclonal antibodies (mAbs) were the first class of preventives specifically developed for the primary indication of preventive treatment of migraine. CGRP mAbs include erenumab, fremanezumab, galcanezumab, and eptinezumab (Table 8-2).[7] The benefit of CGRP mAbs is that most are

Primary Headaches

dosed monthly or quarterly, are effective, and generally have fewer side effects than traditional oral therapies. However, as this class of medications has been available only since 2018, long-term safety data are limited. Given the long half-life of approximately 28 days for most of these medications, there is a long washout period. If a patient is planning for pregnancy or has side effects, this can pose a problem. It is recommended that if a female patient is planning pregnancy, she stop the CGRP mAb about 5 to 6 months before trying to become pregnant to allow the medication to come out of the system. A recent review of safety reports of suspected adverse drug reactions to CGRP mAbs during pregnancy found no concrete maternal toxicities, major birth defects, or increased risk of spontaneous abortion, although the number of adverse drug reactions is limited and there continues to be a lack of long-term safety data. The American Headache Society recommends re-assessing the therapeutic efficacy of CGRP mAb therapy 3 months after initiation of treatment for those administered monthly, although based on the drug, higher dosages may be tried.[3] With the increased utilization of CGRP mAbs, some patients began to report a wear-off effect when they were next due for their treatment. This seemed to be independent of the CGRP mAb being used in clinical practice. Posthoc analysis of clinical trials of erenumab, fremanezumab, and galcanezumab did not show any evidence of wear-off in the trial population. It is possible that, in a trial setting, when patients are given treatment on specific dates and reminders are sent to give treatment, this may help reduce the chance of delays in the treatment. In the real-world setting, clinicians may need to remind patients to set alerts to take treatment every 28 days and ensure limited delay in treatment. In a recent study comparing topiramate and erenumab for the prevention of migraine, erenumab demonstrated a comparatively favorable tolerability and efficacy profile.

Gepants are small molecules targeting the CGRP receptor. They are currently available as two oral medications. One is available as acute treatments can also be used as a preventive medicine (rimegepant). One is indicated only for the preventive treatment of migraine (atogepant). Gepants are not thought to cause medication-overuse headaches and are the first pharmacological treatments that bridge acute and preventive treatment–targeted medications.[8] This is considered a revolution in the care of people with migraine (Table 8-2).

Neuromodulation

Device treatment is a burgeoning area of interest because it offers nonpharmacologic options for migraine prevention for patients who are medication averse, already on hefty medication regimens, or are sensitive to systemic side effects (Chapter 46). Devices are generally well tolerated without major adverse effects. The use of devices is largely cost-prohibitive, summing upward of hundreds to thousands of dollars per year, as the majority of devices are not covered by insurance. Some of the most popular devices cleared for migraine prevention are transcutaneous trigeminal nerve stimulation, noninvasive vagal nerve stimulation, remote electrical nerve stimulation, external combined occipital and trigeminal neurostimulator, and single-pulse transcranial magnetic stimulation (sTMS). The transcutaneous trigeminal nerve stimulation device is applied to the forehead for 20-minute treatments daily to target the supratrochlear and supraorbital nerves. Studies have shown a modest benefit of about 2 monthly headache day reduction compared to the control group and was well tolerated. The noninvasive vagal nerve stimulator is meant to be used twice daily, within 1 hour of waking and at night for 2-minute treatments. First, a conductive gel is applied to the anterolateral neck and a handheld conductive device is subsequently applied. There was approximately a one monthly headache day reduction compared to the sham group, although the trial was terminated early due to the COVID-19 pandemic. sTMS has been used for nearly 30 years to treat other conditions including depression and obsessive-compulsive disorder. This is typically a handheld device consisting of an external coil applied to the occipital scalp, which delivers a magnetic field to interrupt abnormal electrical activity related to migraine. sTMS showed the greatest reduction in headache days compared to the other devices of 3 headache days. The remote electrical nerve stimulator is applied to the upper arm for 45 minutes to treat an acute attack and can also be used every other day for 45 minutes to prevent migraine attacks and has been cleared for use in both episodic and chronic migraine. The external combined occipital and trigeminal neurostimulator is applied to the head for acute treatment of migraine. One treatment is for 40 minutes during a migraine attack. Chapter 46 provides a detailed discussion of the neuromodulation treatment of migraine and headaches.

Summary

- Goal of preventive treatment of migraine include a reduction in the number of headache days and overall headache disability burden.
- The choice of preventive therapy is based on efficacy, adverse events, and coexistent and comorbid conditions.
- Preventive medications should be started and titrated to the most efficacious and tolerable dose, although often a polypharmacy approach may be necessary.
- Preventive treatments for migraine include nutraceuticals; neuromodulation devices; oral medications such as propranolol, candesartan, lisinopril, topiramate, valproate, venlafaxine, and amitriptyline; CGRP mAbs; and gepants.
- OnabotulinumtoxinA is indicated for the treatment of chronic migraine.

REFERENCES

1. Steiner TJ, Stovner LJ, Vos T, Jensen R, Katsarava Z. Migraine is first cause of disability in under 50s: will health politicians now take notice? *J Headache Pain*. 2018;19(1):17.
2. Lipton RB, Nicholson RA, Reed ML, et al. Diagnosis, consultation, treatment, and impact of migraine in the US: results of the OVERCOME (US) study. *Headache*. 2022;62(2):122-140.
3. Ailani J, Burch RC, Robbins MS, the Board of Directors of the American Headache Society. The American Headache Society Consensus Statement: update on integrating new migraine treatments into clinical practice. *Headache*. 2021;61(7):1021-1039.
4. Silberstein SD, Holland S, Freitag F, Dodick DW, Argoff C, Ashman E. Evidence-based guideline update: pharmacologic treatment for episodic migraine prevention in adults: report of the Quality Standards Subcommittee of the American Academy of Neurology and the American Headache Society. *Neurology*. 2012;78(17):1337-1345.
5. Ashina M, Buse DC, Ashina H, et al. Migraine: integrated approaches to clinical management and emerging treatments. *Lancet*. 2021;397(10283):1505-1518.
6. Borlak J, Diener HC, Kleeberg-Hartmann J, Messlinger K, Silberstein S. Petasites for migraine prevention: new data on mode of action, pharmacology and safety. A narrative review. *Front Neurol*. 2022;13:864689.
7. Burch R. Preventive migraine treatment. *Continuum (Minneap Minn)*. 2021;27(3):613-632.
8. Robbins MS. Diagnosis and management of headache: a review. *JAMA*. 2021;325(18):1874-1885.

Primary Headaches

Status Migrainosus

Peter B. Soh and Brian M. Grosberg

Status migrainosus (SM) is described in the third edition of the *International Classification of Headache Disorders* (ICHD-3) as a severe and debilitating migraine attack lasting for more than 72 hours. Patients with SM typically present with headaches of similar quality to previous headache attacks but with the exception of increased severity and prolonged duration. The persistence and/or recurrence of headaches is disabling and can result in presenteeism in daily activities or absenteeism from work or school. Further, recurrence of SM among those with episodic migraine is associated with a greater likelihood of developing chronic migraine. Patients may also have intractable nausea or vomiting, which can lead to subtherapeutic absorption of oral medications and inadequate oral hydration. The associated symptoms of migraine can be as debilitating as the headache. Due to the disability associated with SM, a prompt evaluation is helpful in expediting care.[1]

Epidemiology

Studies on the epidemiology of SM are limited.[2] Approximately 97% of surveyed headache clinicians report seeing SM in practice.[3] A 2013 Nationwide Readmissions Database found that 14.4% of 12,448 hospital admissions for migraine were for the primary diagnosis of SM.[4] The prevalence of SM in a tertiary headache center was found to be 3%. A recent population study reported the incidence of SM[5] as 26.6 per 100,000 with a peak incidence occurring between ages 40 and 49. Moreover, 24.3% of those with aura and 20.6% of those without aura experienced SM.[6] The median age of a patient with SM[7] is 35 years (range: 26-47 years). Patients with SM are predominantly white and female (84.4% and 88.6%, respectively). At the time of the incident SM episode, a majority experienced episodic migraine (63.7%) and migraine without aura (64.3%).[8]

Risk factors for SM include stress, poor sleep, depression, anxiety, overuse of acute headache medications, diet, hormonal factors, dehydration, and subtherapeutic preventive therapy. SM is associated with substantial headache-related disability and socioeconomic impact. The emergency department (ED) visits and inpatient treatment services for migraine cost up to over $1 billion annually in the United States.[9] Among patients using the ED for headache treatment, 19% are frequent ED users and account for 51% of the reported ED visits for the treatment of headaches. Increasing disease burden, depression, and lower socioeconomic status are independent risk factors for ED use for migraine.[10] SM is highly disabling and can worsen comorbidities such as anxiety and depression.

Pathophysiology

The specific pathophysiology of SM has not been identified in the literature. A possible mechanism for SM is the continuous activation of trigeminal nociceptive pathways leading to central sensitization, dysregulation of descending pain modulation, downregulation of serotonergic receptors, and endorphin depletion (see Chapter 6).

Diagnosis and Clinical Characteristics

When evaluating a patient for presumed SM, it is necessary to obtain a thorough clinical history and physical exam. If headache "red flags" are present in history or examination, further evaluation to exclude a secondary cause of headache may necessary (see Chapters 1-3). Headache red flags are succinctly guided by the mnemonic, SNNOOP10 (Chapter 1). Gathering information on temporal progression of symptoms, occurrence of a "thunderclap" presentation (i.e., where the pain peaks in maximal intensity within seconds to minutes), severity and disability of the pain, new associated neurological or systemic symptoms (i.e., confusion, impaired alertness, loss of consciousness, or focal signs), change from typical headache pattern, frequency and dosing of acute medication(s) taken, date of acute medication(s) last used, recent changes in medications or generics, and recent medical illness or injuries provides important data for evaluation and management decisions (Chapter 1).

The ICHD-3 criteria for SM is an unremitting headache, similar in phenotype to previous attacks, in a patient with a history of migraine without aura and/or migraine with aura. The attack persists for at least 72 hours, and the pain and/or associated symptoms are debilitating. Remissions up to 12 hours due to medication or sleep are accepted. Headaches due to medication overuse would negate the diagnosis of SM.

The symptoms of migraine are nonspecific and can be present in many other primary and secondary headache disorders. Many conditions can mimic SM including but not limited to hemorrhagic pituitary adenoma, cervical and vertebral artery dissection, brain abscess, sphenoid sinusitis, reversible cerebral vasoconstriction syndrome, subarachnoid hemorrhage, subdural hematoma, idiopathic intracranial hypertension, brain tumor, intermittent hydrocephalus, meningitis, and acute glaucoma. Primary headache disorders can also mimic SM. If the headache is persistent and side-locked with ipsilateral autonomic features, hemicrania continua is a possible diagnosis. If there is a clear date of onset, and the headache persists for more than 3 months with negative testing, then a new daily persistent headache should be considered.

Treatment

SM can be treated in the outpatient setting but may also require a higher level of care utilizing inpatient or outpatient infusion therapy. Obtaining a clinical history of what has helped the patient in the past can expedite a therapeutic treatment plan that is both safe and effective. Knowing what medications the patient has recently taken can help avoid supratherapeutic dosing of ergot derivatives, neuroleptics, or steroids. Setting realistic expectations with patients is important for safety and perceived therapeutic goals. If a patient has a long-standing baseline daily headache and is currently experiencing an exacerbation, then the goal should be to return to their baseline intensity. In contrast, for patients with episodic migraine who experience SM, the goal should be sustained relief from headache. Figure 9-1 outlines suggested treatment approach for status migrainosus.

Outpatient Treatment

A combination of oral hydration, triptans, ergotamine agents, NSAIDs, acetaminophen, antidopaminergic neuroleptics, gepants, ditans, antiemetics, antihistamines, antiseizure medications, magnesium, steroids, muscle relaxants, or anesthetics can be used in a stratified approach (see also Chapters 7 and 8). Combining classes of medications is often more effective than monotherapy when providing headache care for SM. Dexamethasone, ketorolac, naratriptan, metoclopramide, nerve blocks, or a combination of these therapies can be prescribed or administered in the outpatient setting. Table 9-1 and Figure 9-1 outline suggested therapies for the treatment of SM.

Oral medications may be difficult for a patient to tolerate and take a longer time to reach steady-state concentration than intranasal (IN), subcutaneous (SC), or intramuscular (IM)-delivered medications. Choosing the appropriate delivery of therapy is important to a patient

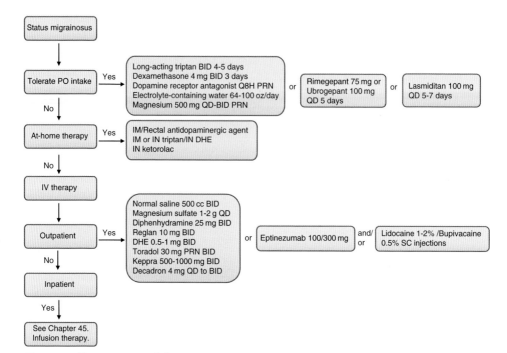

Figure 9-1. Treatment approach for status migrainosus. BID: twice a day; IM: intramuscular; IN: intranasal; IV: intravenous; PO: per os; QD: once a day; SC: subcutaneous.

while concomitantly considering access to the prescribed therapy in terms of availability and affordability. At-home treatment for mild attacks with oral hydration and NSAIDs, acetamino-phen, triptans, gepants, or ditans can avert a severe attack. A stratified approach can use simple analgesics for mild attacks and migraine-specific medications for moderate to severe attacks. Since rimegepant and ubrogepant single-dose data was for the treatment of moderate to severe attacks, this may augment treatment approaches that recommend abortive therapy at the onset of the attack when the attack may start as mild.[11,12] But when attacks are severe upon awakening or severe early on during a headache, SC or IN triptans, or IN or IM dihydroergotamine (DHE), are preferred because of faster therapeutic onset due to the parenteral route of delivery. For intractable nausea and/or vomiting, oral disintegrating, rectal, or IM antidopaminergic medications can be taken or combined with a triptan and/or NSAID at the beginning of an attack. NSAIDs such as ketorolac are often used and available in oral, IM, and IN forms. Liquid celecoxib oral solution (ELYXYB) was FDA approved for the acute treatment of migraine and has a shorter T_{max} (median 0.7 hours) than the capsule form.

If first-line therapy is unsuccessful, second-line at-home treatments can be used before the attack reaches 72-hour duration. There are no robust data for off-label use of medications, but the literature and expert opinions convey higher dosing or frequency such as twice daily for abortive therapies. A trial of naratriptan 2.5 mg twice daily by mouth for 5 days, or lasmiditan 100 mg daily for 5 to 7 days, has been reported to resolve SM. Lidocaine intranasal can also be self-administered at home using viscous lidocaine with a syringe or by spray.[13]

Recurrence of moderate to severe headaches within 24 hours after successful treatment can occur in up to 50% of patients. Positive predictors for recurrence of migraine include female gender, age ≥35 years, and severe baseline headache pain.[14] A course of dexamethasone 4 mg twice daily by

Table 9-1. Outpatient Treatments for Status Migrainosus

Class	Route	Drug Name	Dosing	Caution
Electrolyte	IV, PO	Normal saline	500-1000 ml	Congestive heart failure
		Electrolyte-containing water supplements	64-100 oz/day	
Minerals	IV, PO	Magnesium	500-1000 mg/day in 1 to 2 doses/day	Hypotension, flushing, avoid in hypermagnesemia
Dopamine receptor antagonists	IV, PO, IM	Prochlorperazine	10 mg	Akathisia, extrapyramidal symptoms, prolonged QT interval
		Metoclopramide	10 mg	
	IV, PO	Haloperidol	2.5-5 mg	
		Chlorpromazine	25 mg (oral), 0.1 mg/kg (IV)	
	IM, PR, PO	Promethazine	12.5 or 25 mg	
NSAID	IV, IM IN	Ketorolac	30-60 mg/mL Q8H 3-5 days	Gastritis, kidney disease
			15.75 mg one spray in each nostril Q8H for up to 5 days	
	PO		10 mg with ondansetron 4 mg Q6H for up to 3 days	
		Ibuprofen	600-800 mg	
		Naproxen	500 mg	
		Ketoprofen	75 mg	
		Piroxicam	20 mg	
		Indomethacin	50 mg	
		Diclofenac	50 mg	
Antiepileptics	IV, PO	Valproic acid	500-1000 mg within 15 minutes (IV)	Hyperammonemia and encephalopathy, avoid with hepatic disease, category D with topiramate
			250 mg Q8H (oral)	
	PO	Gabapentin	300-900 mg Q8H	
Ergot alkaloid	IV, IN	DHE	0.5-1 mg	Cardiovascular disease, stroke, peripheral arterial disease
			1.45 mg (precision olfactory delivery)	
			4 mg/mL spray	
Steroids	IV, PO	Dexamethasone methylprednisolone	4-16 mg (IV), 4 mg BID for 3 days (oral) 100-200 mg (IV), medrol dose pack as directed (oral)	Avascular necrosis, abdominal discomfort, emotional lability, insomnia, glucose intolerance
Antihistamine	IV	Diphenhydramine	25 mg	Sedation

Primary Headaches

(Continued)

Table 9-1. Outpatient Treatments for Status Migrainosus (*Continued*)

Class	Route	Drug Name	Dosing	Caution
Triptan	PO	Naratriptan	2.5 mq BID for 5 days	Cardiovascular disease, stroke, peripheral arterial disease
		Almotriptan	12.5 mg	
		Eletriptan	40 mg	
		Frovatriptan	2.5 mg	
		Rizatriptan (tablet or odt)	10 mg	
		Sumatriptan	100 mg	
		Zolmitriptan (tablet or odt)	5 mg	
	IN	Sumatriptan	20 mg	
		Zolmitriptan	5 mg	
	IM	Sumatriptan	6 mg	
Analgesics	PO	Acetaminophen	1000 mg Q8H	
Gepants or ditans	PO	Rimegepant ODT Ubrogepant tablet lasmiditan	75 mg for up to 5 days 50/100 mg for up to 5 days 50/100/200 mg for up to 5-7 days	Separate from use of macrolide antibiotics, antifungals, and grapefruit juice
Muscle relaxants	PO	Cyclobenzaprine	5-10 mg Q8H	Somnolence
		Tizanidine	2-8 mg Q8H	
		Baclofen	5-10 mg Q8H	
Anesthetic	SC	Lidocaine 1.2% Bupivacaine 0.5%	Provider specific	Pregnancy category B category C
Timolol	Ophthalmic	0.25% solution	1 drop/eye for up to 5 days	Asthma, Raynaud's
Calcitonin gene-related peptide monoclonal antibodies (CGRP mAbs)	SC	Erenumab	70/140 mg/month	Limited pregnancy, hypersensitivity reaction
		Fremanezumab	225 mg/month, 675 mg/3 months	Limited pregnancy, hypersensitivity reaction
		Calcanezumab	240 mg loading dose followed by 120 mg/month	Limited pregnancy, hypersensitivity reaction
	IV	Eptinezumab	100/300 mg/3 months	Limited pregnancy, hypersensitivity reaction, constipation, hypertension

Example combination IV therapy: (normal saline 1 L IV, diphenhydramine 25 mg IV, magnesium sulfate 1 g IV, metoclopramide 10 mg IV, DHE 0.5-1 mg IV, levetiracetam 1 g IV, dexamethasone 4 mg, IV) BID.

Prior to treatment, check urine drug screen, pregnancy test (if applicable), CBC, BMP, LFT, magnesium level, and ECG.

BID: twice a day, BMP: basic metabolic panel, CBC: complete blood count, CGRP: calcitonin gene-related peptide, DHE: dihydroergotamine, ECG: electrocardiogram, IM: intramuscular, IN: intranasal, IV: intravenous, LFT: liver function test, NSAID: non-steroidal anti-inflammatory drug, ODT: orally disintegrating tablet, oz: ounce, PO: per os (oral), PR: per rectum (rectal), q6h: every 6 hours, q8h: every 8 hours, SC: subcutaneous.

mouth for 3 days can help prevent the recurrence of headaches. Therefore, combining a triptan with a steroid can be utilized to prevent recurrence and alleviate pain. Antidopaminergic drugs such as metoclopramide, haloperidol, prochlorperazine, promethazine, or chlorpromazine can treat both nausea and pain, but adverse effects can preclude future use. Gepants and ditans are understudied with the treatment of SM, but anecdotal evidence is seen in practice. Table 9-1 lists relative contraindications of treatment suggestions for SM. Increasing or starting new preventive therapy during SM may be necessary if there is preventive medication subtherapy prior to the attack. Additionally, sleep irregularity has been identified as a potentially modifiable risk factor for the recurrence of SM in 1 year. Modifiable risk factors should be addressed when treating the patient.

Interventional Procedural Treatments

Trigeminal branch and occipital nerve blocks can be used for the treatment of SM (Chapter 44). Nerve blocks can be administered alone or in combination with a triptan, intranasal DHE, NSAIDs, an antiemetic, or a steroid. Multiple peripheral cranial nerve blocks with a 1:1 mixture of lidocaine 2% and bupivacaine 0.5% showed an improvement in total headache days, pain-free days, moderate to severe headache days, duration, and severity after 4 weeks.[15] Lidocaine-only multiple cranial nerve blocks seem more likely to achieve pain-free status within 24 hours, and for at least 48 hours, than one-time IM ketorolac or twice daily dosing of naratriptan. Further large-scale studies are needed for the evaluation of multiple cranial nerve blocks. However, because of relatively few potential adverse effects and contraindications, nerve blocks delivered by a trained injector are a safe and effective treatment for SM.

Inpatient Treatment

If at-home treatments are unsuccessful, then procedures or outpatient or inpatient intravenous (IV) therapies may be necessary (Figure 9-1) (Chapter 45). The advantages of IV infusion include avoiding first-pass metabolism, increased bioavailability, and the ability to titrate medications based on clinical side effects. The Raskin protocol provides DHE dosing in an inpatient setting.[16] A modified Raskin protocol of IV DHE 0.5 to 1 mg twice daily for 3 to 5 days with pretreatment of IV metoclopramide can be given in an outpatient infusion site. If dopamine antagonists are intolerable, then pretreatment with IV ondansetron may be considered. There are no studies to support this modified Raskin protocol of IV DHE; however, the authors have seen clinical efficacy and cost–benefit to the patient.

In addition to providing fluid replacement, there is some evidence that IV fluids alone, such as 500 to 1000 mL of 0.9% normal saline solution, can provide headache relief. This therapeutic effect may be possibly due to correcting dehydration, which in itself can trigger migraine.[17] In addition, IV magnesium sulfate can block cortical spreading depression and antagonize N-methyl-D-aspartate receptors. A systematic review of IV 1 gm magnesium sulfate infusion showed potential benefit in pain intensity at 60, 90, and 120 minutes.[18]

Pretreating antidopaminergic or neuroleptic medications with IV lorazepam and/or diphenhydramine may minimize extrapyramidal symptoms (EPS) such as akathisia or a dystonic reaction. NSAIDs such as IV ketorolac can be helpful in treating SM because of their high bioavailability and clinical efficacy. IV steroids, such as dexamethasone or methylprednisolone, can improve head pain and reduce the recurrence of headaches after discharge.[19] Gastrointestinal protection with a histamine blocker or proton pump inhibitor should be considered when administering an NSAID or a steroid.

Currently being studied for acute treatment of SM, IV administration of 100 mg eptinezumab during a migraine attack showed a significant reduction in pain and associated symptoms at 2 hours compared to placebo.[20] The 100% immediate bioavailability postinfusion and rapid response to treatment in some patients are two factors that make eptinezumab particularly attractive for the acute treatment of migraine.

Treatment Considerations

It is important to consider drug-to-drug interactions and potential side effects when deciding what combination of drugs to trial. Unwanted side effects such as akathisia from a neuroleptic may be prevented with careful dosing of the rescue therapy and pretreatment with diphenhydramine or benzodiazepine. Subjecting a patient to adverse side effects may not only bring unwanted symptoms worse than the headache but also deter the patient from using a potentially effective therapy in the future.

Prognosis

Recurrence of headache attacks may also result in repeated hospital ED visits or outpatient encounters, thereby, potentially delaying headache remission, worsening comorbidities, and increasing healthcare costs. A 14.8% recurrence of SM at a median of 58 days following the initial attack has been reported.[8] Up to two-thirds report recurrent headaches within 24 hours after ED discharge, and up to half report functional disability.[21] Before accessing a higher level of care, patients often have taken prescribed or unprescribed therapy and have reached moderate to severe headache intensity. The time to treatment from headache attack onset can be negatively correlated with the pain-free response rate. Treatment within hours of a headache attack has a significantly lower chance of headache-free status than treatment within minutes of the onset of headache.

An average attack duration of 4.8 weeks for patients with SM has been demonstrated. When treated, patients have a median attack duration of 5 days and a mean duration of 8.6 days.[8] Although there are no good data on the average length of SM when untreated, we do know that patients with episodic migraine with SM have a very high propensity to progress to chronic migraine and that recurrence of SM is associated with conversion from episodic to chronic migraine.

Summary

- SM is a complication of migraine and is defined as a severe and debilitating attack lasting for more than 72 hours.
- Obtaining a thorough clinical history and ruling out secondary causes are the most important initial steps before further headache management.
- The goal is to improve the patient's pain and associated symptoms quickly and, if possible, prevent headache recurrence.
- Having a plan in place for treating SM is imperative to avoid unnecessary ED/urgent care visits.
- Treatment of SM includes a combination of therapies that can include NSAIDs, dopamine receptor antagonists, triptans, DHE, gepants, ditans, antiepileptics, minerals, electrolytes, CGRP monoclonal antibodies, and peripheral nerve blocks.

REFERENCES

1. Marcus DA. Treatment of status migrainosus. *Expert Opin Pharmacother.* 2001 Apr;2(4):549-555. doi: 10.1517/14656566.2.4.549. PMID: 11336606.

2. Couch JR, Diamond S. Status migrainosus: causative and therapeutic aspects. *Headache.* 1983; 23(3):94-101.

3. Velickovic Ostojic L, Liang JW, Sheikh HU, Dhamoon MS. Impact of Aura and Status Migrainosus on Readmissions for Vascular Events After Migraine Admission. *Headache.* 2018;58(7):964-972.

4. Beltramone M, Donnet A. Status migrainosus and migraine aura status in a French tertiary-care center: An 11-year retrospective analysis. *Cephalalgia.* 2014;34:633-637.

5. VanderPluym JH, Mangipudi K, Mbonde AA, et al. Incidence of Status Migrainosus in Olmsted County, Minnesota, United States: Characterization and Predictors of Recurrence. *Neurology.* Published online September 29, 2022:10.1212/WNL.0000000000201382.

6. Pryse-Phillips W, Aubé M, Bailey P, et al. A clinical study of migraine evolution. *Headache*. 2006;46:1480-1486.

7. Insinga RP, Ng-Mak DS, Hanson ME. Costs associated with outpatient, emergency room and inpatient care for migraine in the USA. *Cephalalgia*. 2011;31(15):1570-1575.

8. VanderPluym JH, Mangipudi K, Mbonde AA, et al. Incidence of status migrainosus in Olmsted County, minnesota, united states: characterization and predictors of recurrence. *Neurology*. 2023;100(3):e255-e263.

9. Friedman BW, Serrano D, Reed M, Diamond M, Lipton RB. Use of the emergency department for severe headache. A population-based study. *Headache*. 2009;49(1):21-30.

10. Friedman BW, Serrano D, Reed M, Diamond M, Lipton RB. Use of the emergency department for severe headache: a population-based study. *Headache*. 2009;49(1):21-30.

11. Croop R, Goadsby PJ, Stock DA, et al. Efficacy, safety, and tolerability of rimegepant orally disintegrating tablet for the acute treatment of migraine: a randomised, phase 3, double-blind, placebo-controlled trial. *Lancet*. 2019;394(10200):737-745.

12. Lipton RB, Dodick DW, Ailani J, et al. Effect of ubrogepant vs placebo on pain and the most bothersome associated symptom in the acute treatment of migraine: the ACHIEVE II randomized clinical trial. *JAMA*. 2019;322(19):1887-1898.

13. Maizels M. Sphenopalatine ganglion block without a catheter. *Pract Neurol US*. 2021;20(4):39-42.

14. Dodick DW, Lipton RB, Goadsby PJ, et al. Predictors of migraine headache recurrence: a pooled analysis from the eletriptan database. *Headache*. 2008;48(2):184-193.

15. Miller S, Lagrata S, Matharu M. Multiple cranial nerve blocks for the transitional treatment of chronic headaches. *Cephalalgia*. 2019;39(12):1488-1499.

16. Raskin NH. Repetitive intravenous dihydroergotamine as therapy for intractable migraine. *Neurology*. 1986;36(7):995-997.

17. Vécsei L, Szok D, Nyári A, Tajti J. Treating status migrainosus in the emergency setting: what is the best strategy? *Expert Opin Pharmacother*. 2018;19(14):1523-1531.

18. Miller AC, Pfeffer BK, Lawson MR, Sewell KA, King AR, Zehtabchi S. Intravenous magnesium sulfate to treat acute headaches in the emergency department: a systematic review. *Headache*. 2019;59(10):1674-1686.

19. Sumamo Schellenberg E, Dryden DM, Pasichnyk D, et al. Acute migraine treatment in emergency settings. Agency for Healthcare Research and Quality (US); 2012.

20. McAllister P, Winner PK, Ailani J, et al. Eptinezumab treatment initiated during a migraine attack is associated with meaningful improvement in patient-reported outcome measures: secondary results from the randomized controlled RELIEF study. *J Headache Pain*. 2022;23(1):22.

21. Friedman BW, Grosberg BM. Diagnosis and management of the primary headache disorders in the emergency department setting. *Emerg Med Clin North Am*. 2009;27(1):71-viii.

Primary Headaches

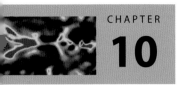

Special Types of Migraine

Teshamae S. Monteith and Sebastian Koch

Migraine is a complicated neurovascular disorder of the brain that can be associated with disturbances in sensory processing and transient neurological symptoms. Special types of migraine exist. These include hemiplegic migraine, retinal migraine, and migrainous infarction (Table 10-1). The last and third edition of *International Classification of Headache Disorders* (ICHD-3) provides formal diagnostic criteria for these entities.[1] The clinical presentations, epidemiology, pathophysiology, and management are explored here for these rare special types of migraine.

Clinical Presentations

Hemiplegic Migraine

Hemiplegic is a subtype of migraine that can be divided into familial and sporadic forms.[1,2] Individuals with familial hemiplegic migraine have first-degree family members who are more likely to have common forms of migraine. Attacks may be associated with typical aura (visual, sensory, speech) and brainstem symptoms, seizures, ataxia, and, rarely, disturbances in consciousness and coma. Acute attacks may also present with fever and CSF pleocytosis. Attacks typically last less than 72 hours but can last up to several weeks in some cases. Even minor head injuries may trigger attacks. Given alternations in consciousness and possible seizures due to cerebral edema, misdiagnosis of epilepsy is common. In addition, shared genetics may exist between the two conditions.

It may be difficult for patients to distinguish between transient neurological deficits characterized by true weakness from that of sensory loss, apraxia, or coordination abnormalities. One way to distinguish between a hemiplegic migraine attack and a transient ischemic attack (TIA) or stroke is to carefully review the onset and evolution of symptoms with the patient and to determine if similar attacks have occurred previously. For example, an attack of gradual onset, particularly with a visual aura and other neurological symptoms, developing subsequently, and followed by a headache would favor a migraine over TIA or stroke. This is particularly true if the patient has experienced these on multiple prior occasions. Imaging characteristics of migraine aura show hypoperfusion is not limited to specific vascular territories but may have perfusion deficits with moderate increases in time-to-peak (TTP). However, hypoperfusion limited to a specific vascular territory and marked increases in TTP or mean transit time are suggestive of acute ischemic stroke.

Other etiologies to consider include the syndrome of transient headache and neurological deficits with cerebrospinal fluid lymphocytosis (HaNDL) (Chapter 26). During the evaluation, it is important to assess the family history of migraine with aura and motor symptoms. Cerebellar signs are the most common findings and occur in up to 20% of families.

Retinal Migraine

Retinal migraine is a subtype of migraine that is characterized by monocular visual disturbances that are fully reversible, typically slowly progressive, and resolve within 60 minutes.[3]

Table 10-1. Diagnostic Criteria of Special Types of Migraine

Diagnosis	ICHD-3 Criteria	Exam Findings and Differential Diagnosis
Hemiplegic migraine	Migraine with aura including motor weakness. A. Attacks fulfilling criteria for *Migraine with aura* and criterion B below B. Aura consisting of both of the following: Attacks fulfilling criteria for 1.2.3 *Hemiplegic migraine* C. At least one first- or second-degree relative has had attacks fulfilling criteria for *Hemiplegic migraine* D. fully reversible motor weakness E. fully reversible visual, sensory and/or speech/language symptoms	Patients with hemiplegic migraine present with unilateral reversible weakness, typical aura, and may have ataxia, brainstem symptoms, confusion, and loss of consciousness. Laboratory studies/genetic testing: • FMH1: CACNA1A gene mutation • FMH2: ATP1A2 gene mutation • FMH3: SCN1A gene mutation • FMH4: possibly PRRT2 Recent PRRT2 variations have been associated with many neurological phenotypes such as epilepsy, sleep disorders, paroxysmal movement disorders, and learning disabilities, in addition to hemiplegic migraine.
– *Sporadic*	No first- or second-degree relative has migraine aura including motor weakness	
– Familial	At least one first- or second-degree relative has had attacks	It is important to exclude such conditions as TIA/stroke, HaNDL, seizures, CADASIL, and migraine with aura.

Retinal migraine	Retinal migraine is described as repeated attacks of monocular visual disturbance, including scintillations, scotomata, or blindness, associated with migraine headache.
	
	A. Attacks fulfilling criteria for 1.2 Migraine with aura and criterion B below
	
	B. Aura is characterized by both of the following:
	  1. fully reversible, monocular, positive, and/or negative visual phenomena (eg, scintillations, scotomata or blindness) confirmed during an attack by either or both of the following:
	    – clinical visual field examination
	    – the patient's drawing of a monocular field defect (made after clear instruction)
	  2. at least two of the following:
	    – spreading gradually over ≥5 minutes
	    – symptoms last 5-60 minutes
	    – accompanied, or followed within 60 minutes, by a headache
	
	C. Not better accounted for by another ICHD-3 diagnosis, and other causes of amaurosis fugax have been excluded
		Headache is likely ipsilateral to the side affected. On the cover–uncover test, the exam will show monocular visual acuity loss and an afferent pupillary defect, with otherwise normal, cranial nerves and neurological examination. Patient may draw the vision loss or field deficit to confirm the loss.
		
		Complications of retinal migraine have been suggested but should be considered with scrutiny: reversible and irreversible central retinal artery occlusion, branch retinal artery occlusion, retinal hemorrhages, and disk edema, ischemic optic neuropathy, choroidal ischemia, dilation of retinal veins, vitreous hemorrhage, stroke, permanent vision loss.
		
		Differential diagnosis transient monocular visual loss includes vascular, ocular, and optic disease. Important secondary causes to rule out are amaurosis fugax, central retinal occlusion, choroidal ischemia, intracranial pressure, orbital apex mass, optic neuritis, giant cell arteritis, dry eye, papilledema, optic nerve compression/anterior ischemic optic neuropathy, and angle closure glaucoma.

Primary Headaches

(Continued)

Table 10-1. Diagnostic Criteria of Special Types of Migraine (*Continued*)

Diagnosis	ICHD-3 Criteria	Exam Findings and Differential Diagnosis
Migrainous infarction	Migrainous infarction occurs when symptoms of an otherwise usual migraine aura persist, and an ischemic lesion is demonstrated by neuroimaging in the appropriate territory. A. A migraine attack fulfilling criteria B and C B. Occurring in a patient with 1.2 *Migraine with aura* and typical of previous attacks except that one or more aura symptoms persist for >60 minutes[1] C. Neuroimaging demonstrates ischemic infarction in a relevant area D. Not better accounted for by another ICHD-3 diagnosis	In the setting of an attack of migraine with aura, patients may present with visual loss, vertigo, ataxia, hemibody sensory changes, hemiparesis as well as other brainstem symptoms. Corresponding clinical findings most frequently include visual field defects, ataxia, hemisensory changes, and hemiparesis. Differential diagnosis to consider are ischemic stroke, hemorrhagic stroke mass lesions such as tumor, subdural and epidural hematoma, seizures with Todd's paralysis, and on occasion metabolic derangements such as hyperglycemia.

CADASIL: Cerebral Autosomal Dominant Arteriopathy Subcortical Infarcts and Leukoencephalopathy, FMH: familial hemiplegic migraine, HaNDL: Headache with neurological deficits and CSF lymphocytosis, ICHD-3: International Classification of Headache Disorders, 3rd Edition, TIA: transient ischemic attack.

Headache Classification Committee of the International Headache Society (IHS). The International Classification of Headache Disorders, 3rd edition, (38(1)) 1–211. Copyright © 2018 by (International Headache Society). Reprinted by Permission of SAGE Publications.

These visual disturbances are followed by headaches, although, historically, headaches may not always be present. According to ICHD-3, retinal migraine is defined as repeated attacks of monocular visual disturbance, including scintillations, scotomata or blindness, and migraine headaches.[1] The ICHD-3 requires attacks meet the criteria for migraine with aura. The deficit can be confirmed by a visual field examination to distinguish monocular visual disturbance from hemianopia. Routine testing includes cover–uncover tests, fundus exams ideally with photography, optical coherence tomography (OCT), OCT angiography, and a visual field exam; findings may be normal or show reversible retinal artery hypoperfusion. In addition, magnetic resonance imaging (MRI) of the brain/orbits, MR angiogram of the brain, carotid duplex, inflammatory markers, and rheumatological panels are warranted. Permanent vision loss as a complication of retinal migraine has been described, but it is not clear if at times these are differing disorders involving the retina, choroid, or optic nerve. Retinal migraine is a diagnosis of exclusion, and secondary causes of transient monocular vision loss should be excluded. These include amaurosis fugax due to carotid artery stenosis, central artery or vein occlusion, and anterior ischemic optic neuropathy.

Migrainous Infarction

Migrainous infarction is a very rare complication of an attack of migraine with aura.[1] Migrainous infarction is associated with the persistence of the usual migraine aura-associated neurological symptoms for more than 60 minutes but with no other cause for the stroke identified. Migrainous infarction, therefore, presents as a complication in the setting of an acute attack of migraine aura, with one or more aura symptoms, and with an ischemic brain lesion demonstrated on neuroimaging with a computed tomography (CT) scan of the head or MRI of the brain with diffusion-weighted imaging. Age and symptoms of nausea and vomiting can be predictors of stroke. These attacks are typically characterized by symptoms stemming from regions of the brain supplied by posterior circulation, predominately the occipital lobes, with involvement of the brainstem on rare occasions. Patients may present with visual loss, vertigo, ataxia, and other brainstem symptoms and the corresponding clinical findings most frequently include visual field defects, ataxia, hemisensory changes, and hemiparesis.

This diagnosis must be distinguished from ischemic stroke co-occurring with migraine, as migraine with aura is associated with double the risk of ischemic stroke. This, at a minimum, requires a careful history to determine the exact nature of the prior aura and current neurological symptoms to ensure that they are indeed the same, as well as extra- and intracranial vascular imaging and a cardiac workup to rule out major cardioembolic sources such as atrial fibrillation and intracardiac thrombi. In younger individuals (less than 50 years of age) with migraine with aura, investigations for the presence of a right to left shunt due to a patent foramen ovale should be performed. A patent foramen ovale is often associated with stroke in younger stroke populations and the prevalence of a patent foramen ovale is higher in patients with migraine with aura. Migrainous infarction is associated with a lower frequency of traditional vascular risk factors with smoking and oral contraceptive use being the most common risk factors present.[4] The issue is further complicated by the fact that headaches are a frequent stroke symptom, seen in up to 27% of strokes, especially in the posterior circulation. Migraine is also associated with other rarer causes of stroke such as cervical dissection, posterior reversible encephalopathy syndrome, and reversible cerebral vasoconstriction syndrome, which at the time of presentation, may not have fully manifested themselves and complicate the diagnostic process. In addition, migraine may be on a continuum with stroke as ischemia may trigger a migraine attack and can make the determination of causality difficult.

Epidemiology

The prevalence of special migraine types has not been extensively evaluated in the population. For hemiplegic migraine, very limited data exist but the sporadic forms of hemiplegic migraine are likely as common as the familial forms. It is estimated that the prevalence is 0.002% for the sporadic and 0.003% for the familial forms of hemiplegic migraine.[5] The exact prevalence of retinal migraine is unknown. It is considered exceedingly rare, although it may be both underdiagnosed and misdiagnosed. Descriptions of the clinical characteristics of migrainous infarction are limited to case reports and small case series in the literature. It has been shown that among 2000 consecutive stroke patients, only 9 met the strict ICHD definition for migrainous infarction.[6] Young women, without traditional vascular risk factors, and strokes in the posterior circulation, represented most patients with migrainous infarction.[7] This aligns well with what is known about subclinical ischemic lesions associated with migraine, which are also more common in young women and also involve the posterior circulation.

Pathophysiology

Knowledge of the pathophysiological mechanisms of special types of migraine is evolving. The monogenic familial and sporadic hemiplegic migraine subtypes due to ion channelopathies are variable in genotypic–phenotypic expression.[2] Investigations with genetic mouse models show increased glutamatergic neurotransmission, cerebral hyperexcitability, and reduced thresholds for cortical spreading depolarization (CSD), the underlying physiological substrate for migraine aura.[8] The first type of familial hemiplegic migraine gene, FHM1, is associated with mutations in the CACNA1A gene (coding for a calcium channel in the presynaptic terminal of excitatory and inhibitory neurons) on chromosome 19. Patients with familial hemiplegic migraine 2 (FHM2) and familial hemiplegic migraine 3 (FHM3) carry mutations in the ATP1A2 gene (coding for an alpha2-subunit, the catalytic site of K/Na-ATPase, expressed on the surface of astrocytic glial cells) on chromosome 1 and SCN1A gene (coding for a sodium channel, expressed on GABAergic neurons and interneurons) on chromosome 2, respectively (Figure 10-1). More recently, PRRT2 has been implicated as the possible fourth familial hemiplegic migraine gene. PRRT2 encodes for a presynaptic protein associated with the exocytosis complex and is a critical component in the calcium-dependent neurotransmitter release.

Mechanisms of retinal migraine are not fully clarified. For migraine with aura, the retinal fiber layer and ganglion cells are significantly thinner than for migraine without aura and controls.[9] Spreading depression (SD) has been identified in vitro in animal (chick) retina and is thought to be a cause of

Primary Headaches

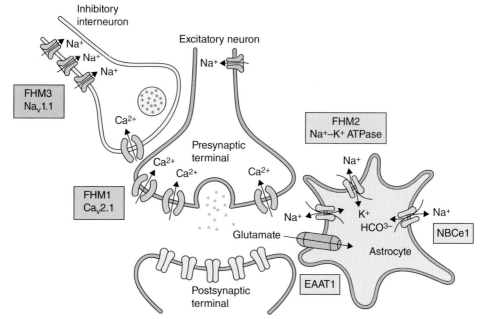

Figure 10-1. Functional roles of proteins encoded by genes involved in familial hemiplegic migraine (FHM) at a central nervous system (CNS) glutamatergic synapse. (Reproduced with permission from Russell MB, Ducros A. Sporadic and familial hemiplegic migraine: pathophysiological mechanisms, clinical characteristics, diagnosis, and management. *Lancet Neurol.* 2011;10(5):457-470.) Na$^+$: sodium; Ca^{2+}: calcium; FHM: familial hemiplegic migraine; K$^+$: potassium; ATPase: adenosine triphosphatase; HCO$_3^-$: bicarbonate; EAAT1: excitatory amino acid transporter; NBCe1: electrogenic sodium bicarbonate cotransporter.

retinal migraine. Retinal SD is mediated by calcitonin gene-related peptide (CGRP) receptors in vitro, but SD has not been identified in the human retina. Historically, vasospasm has also been widely suggested as a potential underlying mechanism of retinal migraine and is evidenced by ictal fundus photography. However, retinal vasospasm is unlikely the underlying mechanism as vasospasm is not consistently present, followed by headache, or symptoms consistent with the migraine diagnosis. Other vascular processes such as endothelial dysfunction, platelet aggregation, blood hypercoagulability, and thrombus formation have been implicated in retinal migraine.

Migrainous infarction typically occurs in the posterior circulation and is also associated with CSD, along with additional vulnerabilities to ischemia. The mechanisms associated with an increased frequency of migraine aura and an increased risk of ischemic stroke are unknown and are likely multifactorial, with neurovascular and hemostatic dysfunction likely being the main contributors. CSD describes waves of cortical depolarization that are initially associated with cortical hyperexcitability followed by inhibition of cortical function. CSD is associated with biochemical and blood flow changes accompanied by oligemia, even though the degree of hypoperfusion does not reach levels usually seen in ischemia.[10] It is theorized that CSD may cause endothelial dysfunction and migraine attacks have been associated with coagulation abnormalities in some individuals. This combination may lead to a prothrombotic state and possibly microemboli. Coupled with oligemia induced by CSD, this may precipitate cerebral infarction in extremely rare instances. The reasons for the predilection of the posterior circulation in migraine and other vascular conditions such as posterior reversible encephalopathy syndrome are uncertain. Anatomic differences have been noted in the posterior circulation, which has less sympathomimetic innervation. How this may translate into an increased ischemic risk with migraine is not known.

Treatment and Prognosis

Hemiplegic migraine requires acute symptomatic treatment and preventive treatment if attacks are frequent or disabling.[2] Due to regional blood flow reductions, triptans and ergotamines are contraindicated in patients with hemiplegic migraine even though there is no scientific evidence to support clinically significant ischemia. Attacks may be treated with nonspecific treatments such as nonsteroidal anti-inflammatory agents, acetaminophen, and neuroleptics/antiemetics. Newer non-vasoconstrictive serotonin 1F receptor agonists, lasmitidan and CGRP receptor antagonists, and gepants are likely safe and effective. Anticonvulsants (topiramate, valproate, lamotrigine), verapamil, and acetazolamide are often used for the prevention of hemiplegic migraine. Evidence-based treatments are lacking. According to the authors' experience and clinic-based studies, lamotrigine may be effective in preventing motor aura. Taken together, hemiplegic attacks are fully reversible and have an excellent prognosis with effective management. The use of aspirin for preventive treatment in the case of prolonged attacks of hemiplegic migraine and retinal migraine has been suggested to prevent ischemic complications but the risk-benefit ratio should be taken into consideration as there is no clinical evidence to support this practice.

Retinal migraine is often treated with anticonvulsants or calcium channel blockers such as verapamil if attacks are frequent (occurring >1 per month).[3] Beta-blockers such as propranolol are typically avoided due to a theoretical concern of precipitating visual loss. Triptans and ergotamines are also avoided due to the potential risk of vasoconstriction.

The treatment of migrainous infarction in the acute setting should not differ from other causes of ischemic stroke, even though a timely diagnosis of ischemia arising out of a migraine attack is challenging. Treatment considerations should include intravenous thrombolysis if there are no contraindications. The effectiveness of intravenous thrombolysis, however, in migrainous infarction is unknown. The risks of thrombolysis may be lower, given the relatively younger age of most patients and lack of comorbidities compared to the usual ischemic stroke population. Similarly, all patients should be emergently screened for a large vessel occlusion and evaluated for mechanical thrombectomy. Secondary prevention includes the use of antiplatelets, reducing any vascular risk factors such as smoking and hypertension, and avoiding estrogen-containing oral preventive medications. In selected patients who have a patent foramen ovale, endovascular closure may be considered for secondary stroke prevention, particularly with large shunting, the presence of an atrial septal aneurysm and the absence of vascular risk factors. For migrainous infarction, the prognosis is generally considered excellent with minor residual symptoms or even total recovery.[7] There are no data to suggest that preventing migraine attacks will prevent migrainous infarction, but it is sensible to consider reducing migraine aura attack frequency and severity to prevent reoccurrence.

Summary

- Hemiplegic migraine may be familial or sporadic and is a consequence of gene mutations that increase susceptibility to CSD and motor aura.

- Retinal migraine is a very rare condition described as recurrent, transient monocular visual loss and may be complicated by permanent visual loss.

- Migrainous infarction is a type of stroke that is associated with the persistence of migraine aura symptoms, which arises out of an otherwise typical migraine attack but with corresponding pathological neuroimaging findings.

- Triptans and ergotamines are avoided in retinal migraine and according to FDA labels, triptans and ergotamines should be avoided in patients with hemiplegic migraine and brainstem aura (formerly known as basilar migraine) due to safety concerns. However, sufficient evidence is lacking for these recommendations.

Primary Headaches

REFERENCES

1. *The International Classification of Headache Disorders.* Headache Classification Committee of the International Headache Society (IHS). *The International Classification of Headache Disorders,* 3rd edition. *Cephalalgia.* 2018;38:1-211.

2. Russell MB, Ducros A. Sporadic and familial hemiplegic migraine: pathophysiological mechanisms, clinical characteristics, diagnosis, and management. *Lancet Neurol.* 2011;10:457-470.

3. Maher ME, Kingston W. Retinal migraine: evaluation and management. *Curr Neurol Neurosci Rep.* 2021;21:35.

4. Serrano F, Arauz A, Uribe R, Becerra LC, Mantilla K, Zermeño F. Long-term follow-up of patients with migrainous infarction. *Clin Neurol Neurosurg.* 2018;165:7-9.

5. Thomsen LL, Eriksen MK, Roemer SF, Andersen I, Olesen J, Russell MB. A population-based study of familial hemiplegic migraine suggests revised diagnostic criteria. *Brain.* 2002;125:1379-1391.

6. Arboix A, Massons J, García-Eroles L, Oliveres M, Balcells M, Targa C. Migrainous cerebral infarction in the Sagrat Cor Hospital of Barcelona stroke registry. *Cephalalgia.* 2003;23:389-394.

7. Laurell K, Artto V, Bendtsen L, et al. Migrainous infarction: a Nordic multicenter study. *Eur J Neurol.* 2011;18:1220-1226.

8. Ferrari MD, Klever RR, Terwindt GM, Ayata C, van den Maagdenberg AM. Migraine pathophysiology: lessons from mouse models and human genetics. *Lancet Neurol.* 2015;14:65-80.

9. Ekinci M, Ceylan E, Cağatay HH, et al. Retinal nerve fibre layer, ganglion cell layer and choroid thinning in migraine with aura. *BMC Ophthalmol.* 2014;14:75.

10. Olesen J, Larsen B, Lauritzen M. Focal hyperemia followed by spreading oligemia and impaired activation of rCBF in classic migraine. *Ann Neurol.* 1981;9:344-352.

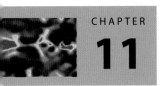

CHAPTER 11

Migraine, Dizziness, and Vestibular Migraine

Carrie E. Robertson and Rashmi B. Halker Singh

The association between dizziness and migraine has been well established and reported.[1] In patients with a history of migraine, it may be tempting to attribute any symptom of dizziness to their migraine without considering alternative explanations. However, both migraine headaches and dizziness are common conditions, suggesting that patients with migraine may at some point present with other causes of dizziness as well. Because the list of possible causes of dizziness is extensive, often with overlapping clinical features, it is only through careful history, examination, and sometimes additional testing, that alternative causes of dizziness can be excluded.

Diagnostic Considerations

The first step in evaluating a patient with dizziness is to have them describe their symptom in greater detail. Some patients use the term "dizzy" to mean that they are unsteady on their feet while walking, which could refer to cerebellar ataxia or sensory ataxia. Others will say they feel "dizzy" when they experience a lightheaded/woozy feeling, or a feeling of presyncope. Finally, some individuals will use this term to describe a true vertigo, meaning they experience a sensation that they are moving or the world around them is moving. Vertigo can be further classified as either a spinning vertigo or a nonspinning vertigo (e.g., rocking, swaying, bobbing, shifting). The description of dizziness can help with the differential diagnoses dramatically. Below are some of the etiologies of dizziness to consider with different descriptions, and some of these are further described in Table 11-1.

Lightheadedness: Anemia, dehydration, medication side effect, hypoglycemia/hyperglycemia, tachycardia (e.g., from postural orthostatic tachycardia, anxiety, medication/drug use, thyroid disease, or arrhythmia), heart failure, hypoxia.

Episodic recurrent spinning vertigo: Benign paroxysmal positional vertigo (BPPV), vestibular migraine, Meniere's disease, superior canal dehiscence.

Persistent/prolonged spinning vertigo: Ischemia (vertebrobasilar infarct/dissection), otitis media, vestibular neuritis, Cogan's syndrome, vestibular schwannoma.

Non-spinning vertigo (e.g., rocking, swaying): Persistent postural perceptual dizziness (PPPD), Mal de Debarquement syndrome.

Unsteadiness/ataxia: Sensory ataxia (e.g., B12 or copper deficiency, demyelinating cord lesion, peripheral neuropathy), cerebellar ataxia (e.g., ischemia to the posterior fossa, epileptic vertigo, demyelinating disease, Episodic Ataxia-2).

If the patient describes episodes that are triggered, this can also be helpful diagnostically. BPPV may be triggered only by changes in position, while superior canal dehiscence may be triggered by loud sounds or Valsalva maneuvers such as coughing or straining. Patients should be questioned about associated cochlear and other neurologic symptoms. This includes any changes in hearing in either or both ears, pulsatile or nonpulsatile tinnitus, aural fullness, oscillopsia (apparent visual movement of stationary objects), autophony (hearing one's own voice or internal sounds, louder than normal), ataxia/dysmetria, diplopia, and systemic symptoms.

Table 11-1. Differential Diagnosis for Vestibular Migraine

Peripheral Vertigo	
Otitis media	Vertigo or dysequilibrium with unilateral hearing loss and possible ear discharge; acute otitis media may have fever, ear pain, and often starts during or just following an upper respiratory infection
Vestibular neuritis	Inflammation of CN 8 presenting with vertigo, imbalance, and nausea; typically peaking within 24-48 hours and lasting several days (may take weeks to months to fully improve)
Meniere's disease	Severe attacks of vertigo lasting 20 minutes to 12 hours, associated with unilateral fluctuating sensorineural hearing loss (low-frequency loss is characteristic), tinnitus, and aural fullness; very severe attacks may cause abrupt loss of balance and falls ("drop attacks")
Cogan's syndrome	Autoimmune syndrome characterized by recurrent inflammation of the eyes and ears, leading to vision loss, bilateral hearing loss, vertigo, with associated systemic symptoms
Perilymphatic fistula	Abnormal communication between inner and middle ear leading to vertigo, with unilateral hearing loss and tinnitus; often follows direct trauma or barotrauma but may also be idiopathic
Vestibular schwannoma	Slowly progressive vertigo or imbalance, often with slowly progressive unilateral hearing loss
Vestibular paroxysmia (vascular compression of CN 8)	Multiple brief (seconds) attacks of vertigo per day, typically responsive to carbamazepine or oxcarbazepine; may have associated tinnitus
Benign paroxysmal positional vertigo (BPPV)	Vertigo comes on without warning, maximal at onset, lasting minutes, without changes in hearing, tinnitus, or aural fullness; and tends to be triggered by changes in position such as turning the head quickly or rolling over in bed; most common type of BPPV is torsional nystagmus on Dix-Hallpike maneuver. May improve with canalith repositioning
Superior canal dehiscence	Abnormal defect in bone covering the semicircular canal; vertigo with possible oscillopsia, autophony, pulsatile tinnitus, or unilateral hyperacusis; often triggered by loud sounds or Valsalva maneuvers (e.g., cough, strain)
Central Vertigo	
Persistent postural-perceptual dizziness (PPPD)	Chronic fluctuating nonvertiginous dizziness and unsteadiness that is often comorbid with migraine and vestibular migraine; symptoms occur without trigger but are often exacerbated by change in position, exposure to moving visual stimuli or complex visual patterns
Vertebrobasilar ischemia or infarct	Abrupt onset symptoms, often with other brainstem symptoms, ataxia, dysarthria, or visual defects; often occurring in older patients or patients with vascular risk factors or cervical trauma
Epileptic vertigo	Isolated ictal vertigo is rare, but brief vertigo (seconds) can be associated with other epileptic symptoms, some of which resemble migraine symptoms (head pressure, visual hallucinations) or other symptoms (nystagmus, tinnitus, dysacusis); may have transient loss of awareness, automatisms, déjà vu, confusion, or epigastric rising

Table 11-1. Differential Diagnosis for Vestibular Migraine (*Continued*)

Demyelinating disease	Vertigo can occur with brainstem lesions; cerebellar ataxia (from lesions in cerebellar pathways) and sensory ataxia (from lesions of proprioceptive pathways) are also sometimes described as dizziness
Episodic ataxia-2	Long-duration attacks (hours to days) of vertigo, ataxia and headache; may respond to acetazolamide
Mal de Debarquement syndrome	Occurs after exposure to passive motion for a prolonged time (boat travel, airplane flight); patients describe persistent perception of self-motion with a sense of swaying or rocking, as if they are walking on uneven ground

CN: cranial nerve.

Dizziness: Symptom of Migraine

As ICHD-3 criteria for vestibular migraine is still being refined, with current proposed criteria listed in the appendix, it is important to note that vestibular migraine is a clinical diagnosis, with no specific laboratory studies or tests that can confirm this diagnosis.[2] Additionally, many more individuals may experience various symptoms of "dizziness" with their migraine attacks without having true vestibular migraine, and it may require careful history taking and possibly a multidisciplinary approach to best help these patients.

Vestibular Migraine

Epidemiology

Individually, migraine and dizziness are both commonly seen conditions, with migraine present in approximately 12% of the population and "dizziness" reported in about 15% to 29% of adults.[3-5] The prevalence of these conditions, the overlapping clinical presentations of various causes of dizziness, and the evolving definition of vestibular migraine, have made the true epidemiology of vestibular migraine difficult to ascertain.

The estimated one-year prevalence of vestibular migraine is 1% to 2.7%,[1] but in clinics that specialize in migraine, the prevalence has ranged from 4% to 10%.[1,6] Vestibular migraine is more common in women, with a female to male ratio of 1.5 to 5:1.[1,7] It is common for migraine headache to present first, sometimes years before the vestibular symptoms start.

Pathophysiology

The exact pathophysiology behind vestibular migraine is still under investigation. Some studies suggest that patients with migraine have a hypersensitivity to vestibular and visual motion stimuli, analogous to their sensitivity to other sensory input, such as light and sound stimuli.[8] Short-lived attacks associated with migraine attacks may be related to migraine aura from a pathophysiology standpoint, as a type of cortical spreading depression involving posterior parietal cortex with subsequent influence on brainstem vestibular nuclei.[9] The same neurotransmitters involved in the pathogenesis of migraine (e.g., calcitonin gene-related peptide [CGRP], serotonin, norepinephrine) may also contribute to altered vestibular excitability through modulation of central and peripheral vestibular neurons leading to prolonged vertigo during the duration of migraine. Altered activity in the vestibular system could lead to transient vestibulo-ocular dysfunction or vestibular hypersensitivity with migrainous features. It has also been suggested that vestibular migraine may be caused by a type of thalamocortical dysregulation, with abnormal sensory modulation or integration within the thalamo-cortical network resulting in dizziness and spatial disorientation.[1,9]

Primary Headaches

Clinical Presentation and Diagnosis

Vestibular migraine is described as episodic spinning or nonspinning vertigo that tends to be unprovoked but is often aggravated by positional changes or visual motion. ICHD-3 appendix criteria for vestibular migraine are described in Box 11-1.[2] Patients have a history of migraine and may experience vertigo episodes just before, during, or between headaches. Vertigo is associated with migrainous symptoms, such as photophobia, phonophobia (2/3 of patients), and visual aura. Mild subjective hearing changes, tinnitus (unilateral or bilateral), and aural fullness may also be present. Episodes of vertigo tend to last minutes to hours, though a subjective unsteadiness and visual motion sensitivity may persist longer.

Diagnosis of vestibular migraine tends to be made through history and examination. ICHD-3 appendix criteria can be used. During an episode of vestibular migraine, patients may have nystagmus, especially if examined using tools that block visual fixation. Patients may also have impaired smooth pursuit and an abnormal vestibular-ocular reflex by head impulse testing. Dysmetria and cerebellar ataxic gait would be atypical and should raise the question of an alternative diagnosis. Between episodes, the examination tends to be normal. If vertigo is very brief and provoked by position, patients should be examined for BPPV with a Dix-Hallpike maneuver. While aural fullness and tinnitus can occur in migraine, prominent fluctuations in hearing, unilateral hearing loss, and changes in pitch or loudness of tinnitus are more suggestive of Meniere's disease. Vestibular testing may show nonspecific abnormalities and is not required for the diagnosis of vestibular migraine. However, it may be helpful in select cases where alternative central or peripheral causes of vertigo are suspected. Audiometry is advised to evaluate for subclinical hearing loss and possible Meniere's disease. If the first episode of dizziness is longer than a few minutes, imaging with an MRI and MRA of the brain with a focus on posterior circulation will help exclude vascular pathology or structural abnormalities of the brainstem or cerebellum. If a peripheral cause of vertigo is suspected, or if there are prominent hearing changes present, a referral to ear, nose, and throat specialist is recommended.

Treatment

Treatment of vestibular migraine resembles treatment for migraine headache, as preventative therapies for migraine may also reduce the frequency and severity of vestibular symptoms.[1] Amitriptyline, propranolol, topiramate, or flunarizine (where available) are often considered first.

Box 11-1. International Classification of Headache Disorders-3 A1.6.6 Vestibular Migraine Criteria

History of Migraine and At Least Five Episodes Fulfilling Criteria A-C:

A. Vestibular symptoms of moderate to severe intensity lasting between 5 minutes and 72 hours
   - Sense of self-motion or motion of visual surroundings
   - Can be triggered by change in head position, complex, or large moving visual stimulus
   - 10% of patients have episodes lasting seconds, 30% last minutes, 30% last hours, and 30% last days

B. At least half of episodes are associated with one of the three migrainous features:
   - Migraine headache (2 of 4 qualities: unilateral, pulsating, moderate-severe, aggravated by exertion)
   - Photophobia/phonophobia
   - Visual aura

C. Not better accounted for by another vestibular disorder

Serotonin-norepinephrine reuptake inhibitors (e.g., venlafaxine) may be considered in patients with prominent vestibular symptoms, especially if they have comorbid persistent postural perceptual dizziness (PPPD) or anxiety/depression. Early evidence suggests onabotulinumtoxinA may be helpful in reducing the vestibular symptoms in addition to headache symptoms. It is not yet clear whether CGRP targeting medications will be helpful for vestibular migraine, but it may be reasonable to consider CGRP monoclonal antibodies (erenumab, galcanezumab, fremanezumab, eptinezumab) or gepants (ubrogepant, rimegepant, atogepant) in selected cases. Acute attacks of vestibular migraine that are prolonged or associated with prominent nausea may respond to dopaminergic antiemetics (promethazine, prochlorperazine, metoclopramide), antihistamines (meclizine, dimenhydrinate, diphenhydramine), or benzodiazepines (diazepam, lorazepam). Triptans are not commonly used for vestibular symptoms associated with migraine but select patients may find triptans to be helpful in reducing the duration of vertigo, especially when associated with headache pain.

Patients with prominent visual motion sensitivity or who have comorbid PPPD may benefit from vestibular rehabilitation, targeting habituation to visual motion stimuli.[10] Comorbid anxiety or depression often also require individualized treatment.

Prognosis

There is limited information in the literature about the prognosis of vestibular migraine. It has been shown that in adults with vestibular migraine, 9 years after initial diagnosis, most (almost 90%) of the patients were still experiencing recurrent vertigo.[11] The frequency was reduced in 56% of patients, increased in 29% of patients, and unchanged in 16%. In patients with migraine, there is some suggestion that patients with associated vestibular symptoms do not do as well as those without vestibular symptoms. However, over the course of an individual's life, vestibular symptoms may fluctuate, sometimes improving with improvement in migraine frequency or severity, or even improving spontaneously.

Summary

- Dizziness is a term that may be used to describe several different sensory experiences, such as lightheadedness, imbalance/unsteadiness, spinning vertigo, and nonspinning sense of motion.

- An accurate description of the patient's dizziness is the first step to narrowing down their differential diagnosis.

- Vestibular migraine is diagnosed by clinical history and exclusion of other causes of dizziness, with no single feature or laboratory test that is pathognomonic.

- The implementation of formal diagnostic criteria may lead to better identification and understanding of vestibular migraine, allowing for more formal treatment algorithms.

- Current treatment of vestibular migraine resembles treatment for migraine headache, with similar preventive and acute therapies.

REFERENCES

1. Huang TC, Wang SJ, Kheradmand A. Vestibular migraine: an update on current understanding and future directions. *Cephalalgia.* 2020;40(1):107-121.
2. Headache Classification Committee of the International Headache Society (IHS). *The International Classification of Headache Disorders*, 3rd edition. *Cephalalgia.* 2018;38(1):1-211.
3. Tamber AL, Wilhelmsen KT, Strand LI. Measurement properties of the dizziness handicap inventory by cross-sectional and longitudinal designs. *Health Qual Life Outcomes.* 2009;7:101.
4. Wiltink J, Tschan R, Michal M, et al. Dizziness: anxiety, health care utilization and health behavior—results from a representative German community survey. *J Psychosom Res.* 2009;66(5):417-424.

Primary Headaches

5. Neuhauser HK. The epidemiology of dizziness and vertigo. *Handb Clin Neurol.* 2016;137:67-82.

6. Lempert T, Olesen J, Furman J, et al. Vestibular migraine: diagnostic criteria. *J Vestib Res.* 2012; 22(4):167-72.

7. Lempert T, Neuhauser H. Epidemiology of vertigo, migraine and vestibular migraine. *J Neurol.* 2009;256(3):333-8.

8. Bednarczuk NF, Bonsu A, Ortega MC, et al. Abnormal visuo-vestibular interactions in vestibular migraine: a cross sectional study. *Brain.* 2019; 142(3):606-16.

9. Baloh RW. Vestibular migraine I: Mechanisms, diagnosis, and clinical features. *Semin Neurol.* 2020;40(1):76-82.

10. Axer H, Finn S, Wassermann A, Guntinas-Lichius O, Klingner CM, Witte OW. Multimodal treatment of persistent postural-perceptual dizziness. *Brain Behav.* 2020;10(12):e01864.

11. von Brevern M, Lempert T. Vestibular migraine: treatment and prognosis. *Semin Neurol.* 2020; 40(1):83-6.

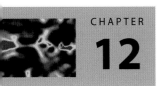

Migraine and Episodic Syndromes

Sara Pavitt and Cynthia Morris

Abdominal migraine and cyclic vomiting syndrome (CVS) are considered two main episodic syndromes and migraine variants that tend to start in childhood.[1] Both syndromes include recurrent episodes of gastrointestinal dysfunction with symptom-free periods between attacks. It is important to recognize and diagnose these syndromes as symptoms can be moderate to severe and impact daily functioning. The majority of children with these syndromes will develop migraine in their lifetime. There have been proposed diagnostic criteria for both disorders by multiple organizations. This chapter refers to the criteria proposed by the third edition of *International Classification of Headache Disorders*.[1]

Epidemiology

The prevalence of abdominal migraine varies based on the diagnostic criteria used, but has been reported between 2.4% and 4.2% of children with peak prevalence at the age of 12.[2] CVS is less common with a prevalence of 1.9% to 2.3% in the pediatric population.[3] Both disorders are more common in females, and 72% to 82% in patients with CVS and 65% to 90% of patients with abdominal migraine have family history of migraine.[2,3]

Pathophysiology

The pathophysiology of CVS remains greatly hypothetical. Underlying mechanisms that have been considered include autonomic abnormalities, hypothalamic-pituitary-adrenal activation, genetic abnormalities, neuronal excitability in the central nervous system throughout the brain stem and peripherally in the enteric nervous system, and gastric dysmotility.[3] Abdominal migraine is similarly poorly understood, but may be due to changes to the gut-brain axis, vascular dysregulation, changes to the central nervous system, and genetic factors.

Clinical Presentation and Diagnosis

Abdominal Migraine

Abdominal migraine typically starts in childhood between the ages of 2 and 12 years old. While it can continue into adulthood, the vast majority of children will have resolution by adolescence and/or transformation into migraine.[4] It is a clinical diagnosis characterized by recurrent episodes of midline or poorly localized abdominal pain that lasts 2 to 72 hours and is associated with at least two of the following symptoms: pallor, anorexia, nausea, and/or vomiting. In between attacks, patients return to their baseline state of health. A detailed history needs to be conducted to evaluate for gastrointestinal red flags that would warrant further investigations (Box 12-1) and the physical exam should be normal between attacks. Children with abdominal migraine experience on average 14 attacks per year.

Box 12-1. Red Flag Symptoms That May Indicate a Secondary Cause to Gastrointestinal Symptoms

Polyuria/polydipsia	Weight loss
Localized pain with guarding	Change in bowel habits
Bilious or bloody vomiting	Growth failure/delayed puberty
Bloody stool	Persistent vomiting
Dysuria/hematuria	Perianal abnormalities
Pain that radiates to the groin	Arthritis or family history of inflammatory bowel disease
Dysphagia	

Cyclic Vomiting Syndrome

CVS is a childhood disorder with an average age of onset of 5 years.[5] A child with this syndrome can experience discrete episodes of frequent nausea and vomiting (at least four times an hour) which lasts for 1 hour to 10 days. These episodes are stereotyped and occur in a predictable pattern. Each attack is followed by symptom-free interval lasting at least 1 week. The most frequent time for the onset of an attack is late night to early morning, typically 2 to 7 AM.

The differential diagnosis is broad and includes gastrointestinal anatomic abnormalities, metabolic disorders, renal disorders, neurologic disorders including certain epilepsy syndromes, such as self limited epilepsy with autonomic seizures or epilepsy with prominent autonomic features, and hormonal dysfunction.[2] It is recommended that all patients have a screening comprehensive metabolic panel and upper gastrointestinal series after initial evaluation. If patients fail to respond to treatment, further workup should be pursued and targeted, considering additional symptoms. This may include evaluations such as an abdominal ultrasound and/or CT, porphyria evaluation, EEG, brain MRI, expanded gastrointestinal serum testing, and metabolic screen. A stepwise approach to workup can be found in the referenced articles.

Treatment

Nonpharmacological Treatments

Lifestyle regularity and trigger avoidance are recommended preventive strategies for both disorders.[6,7] This includes maintaining consistent sleep schedules to promote adequate total sleep time, maintaining sufficient hydration, regular physical activity, and maintaining consistent mealtimes throughout the day. Patients often have a variety of potentially modifiable triggers such as associations with specific foods which should be investigated. While lifestyle regularity and trigger avoidance are an important part of treatment, it is imperative to create a feasible plan to target achievable goals with the patient. Behavioral treatment with cognitive behavioral therapy and/or biofeedback may be helpful as nonpharmacological preventive treatment strategies in both CVS and abdominal migraine.

Pharmacological Treatments

Below are discussions on both acute and preventive medication options in abdominal migraine and CVS. The doses of recommended medications are based on case reports, small studies, or clinical expertise based on dosing in migraine.

Cyclic Vomiting Syndrome

Acute Treatment

First-line acute therapy is often supportive including placing patients in a dark, relaxing environment with oral or intravenous hydration (often dextrose-containing fluid to treat the developed catabolic state) and possible electrolyte correction.[6] Symptomatic care is often offered which includes antiemetics, analgesics, and migraine-specific medications. Sumatriptan is often used intranasally (5-20 mg/dose) or subcutaneously (3-6 mg/dose) at the onset of an attack (see also Chapter 7). This may be paired with antiemetics including ondansetron, aprepitant, or prochlorperazine. Aprepitant (3 mg/kg with max of 125 mg on day followed by 2 mg/kg with max of 80 mg on subsequent days) is a neurokinin receptor antagonist and has found to be particularly helpful to treating attacks early during the prodromal phase. Generalized pain is often treated with ketorolac and epigastric pain with H2 blockers, such as famotidine or ranitidine. If typical treatment fails to provide symptomatic relief, the use of sedating medications has been reported including repetitive doses of lorazepam (0.05 mg/kg every 6 hours with max dose 2 mg) or chlorpromazine (0.5-1.0 mg/kg/dose every 6-8 hours with max 25 mg/dose) with diphenhydramine (1 mg/kg with max 50 mg/dose) has been reported.

Preventive Treatment

If attacks occur more than every 1 to 2 months, tend to be particularly long or severe, or are interfering with quality of life, preventive treatment should be considered.[6] The goal of this treatment is overall reduction of attack frequency. Medications should be started at low dose and titrated slowly for effect. Typically, specific treatment options are chosen based on the patient's age, ability to swallow pills, and side-effect profile. Cyproheptadine (0.25-0.5 mg/kg/day with max of 16 mg/day as a single dose or divided two to three times a day), an antihistamine and calcium channel blocker, is considered first line for patients under 5 years old. For patients over 5 years old, first-line options include propranolol (0.5-3.0 mg/kg/day divided twice a day with max of 120 mg/day) and amitriptyline (titrated from 0.25 mg/kg/day to 1 mg/kg/day with max of 125 mg/day). It may be beneficial to pair these prescription medications with supplements that support mitochondrial function which include coenzyme Q10 (10 mg/kg/day with max of 400 mg/day), L-carnitine (50-100 mg/kg/day with max of 1000 mg twice a day), and riboflavin (5 mg/kg twice a day with max of 200 mg/dose). If these first-line preventive treatment options are unsuccessful, aprepitant (40-125 mg twice weekly) can be considered.

Abdominal Migraine

Acute Treatment

There is limited available evidence evaluating treatment options for abdominal migraine and it is often adapted from treatment options for migraine.[7] During an acute attack, patients may benefit from being in a dark, quiet environment. Intranasal sumatriptan (5-20 mg/dose) is recommended for abortive therapy, often paired with ibuprofen or acetaminophen at attack onset (see Chapter 7). Antiemetics such as ondansetron (0.15-0.4 mg/kg q 8 hours with max of 16 mg/dose) should be offered if the patient has prominent nausea and/or vomiting. Furthermore, repetitive doses of intravenous valproic acid (500-1000 mg every 6 hours) or dihydroergotamine (0.5-1 mg/dose every 8 hours) may be considered for refractory, severe, or prolonged attacks.

Preventive Treatments

Similar to CVS, if attacks are frequent or interfere with quality of life, preventive treatment options should be explored. Daily pizotifen (0.5-1.5 mg/day), a serotonin and antihistamine antagonist, has the strongest evidence to support its use,[2] but is not available in the United States. Small studies exist suggesting propranolol (0.5-3.0 mg/kg/day divided twice a day with max of 120 mg/day) and cyproheptadine (0.25-0.5 mg/kg/day with max 16 mg/day as a single dose or divided two to three times a day) as first-line medications.[2,7] Additional options come from expert opinion and include amitriptyline, topiramate, and supplements including coenzyme Q10 and riboflavin (see Chapter 8).

Primary Headaches

Prognosis

In 50% to 70% of children, CVS resolves in late childhood or early adolescence.[3] However, patients frequently go on to develop a primary headache disorder such as migraine (56%) or tension-type headache (23%). Abdominal migraine follows a similar pattern, with about 60% of cases resolving by adulthood, but about 70% going on to develop migraine.

Summary

- Abdominal migraine and CVS are migraine variants that start in childhood and can cause significant disability.
- Abdominal migraine is characterized by recurrent attacks of abdominal pain with associated symptoms that last several hours.
- CVS features stereotyped episodes of frequent, recurrent vomiting with at least a week between episodes.
- Treatment of both disorders can involve sumatriptan, antiemetics, and analgesics for acute treatment and more traditional migraine medications for preventive treatment.
- Most children outgrow both disorders, but are likely to develop migraine in the future.

REFERENCES

1. Headache Classification Committee of the International Headache Society (IHS). The International Classification of Headache Disorders, 3rd edition. *Cephalalgia.* 2018;38(1):1-211.
2. Angus-Leppan H, Saatci D, Sutcliffe A, Guiloff R J. Abdominal migraine. *BMJ.* 2018;360:k179.
3. Raucci U, Borrelli O, Di Nardo G, et al. Cyclic vomiting syndrome in children. *Front Neurol.* 2020;11:583425.
4. Abu-Arafeh I, Russell G. Prevalence and clinical features of abdominal migraine compared with those of migraine headache. *Arch Dis Child.* 1995; 72:413-417.
5. Li BU, Balint JP. Cyclic vomiting syndrome: evolution in our understanding of a brain-gut disorder. *Adv Pediatr.* 2000;47:117-160.
6. Kovacic K, Li BUK. Cyclic vomiting syndrome: a narrative review and guide to management. *Headache.* 2021;61(2):231-243.
7. Azmy DJ, Qualia CM. Review of abdominal migraine in children. *Gastroenterol Hepatol (N Y).* 2020;16(12):632-639.

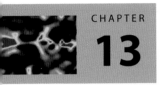

Tension-Type Headache

Sait Ashina, Rigmor Jensen, and Robert Kaniecki

Tension-type headache (TTH) is a common neurological disorder.[1] It is the most common primary headache in the general population.[2] It is frequently seen by general practitioners, but neurologists also encounter this condition. Although TTH is not life-threatening, it can be disabling and interfere with daily activities, work, and social functioning. Unfortunately, TTH is often undertreated and underrecognized, despite its high prevalence. TTH is commonly associated and comorbid with migraine, which can make diagnosis and treatment challenging.[3,4]

Epidemiology

Incidence and prevalence rates of TTH vary across studies. One 2017 study estimated a global incidence rate of 882.4 million new cases.[2] The incidence of frequent episodic TTH (ETTH) and chronic TTH (CTTH) was found to be 14.2 per 1000 person–years, with incidence 2.6 times higher in women than in men. Incidence of 3.9 per 1000 person–years has been reported in adolescents aged 13 to 14 years, with 4.6 times higher incidence in females than in males.

The same 2017 study reported an estimated global prevalence of 2.33 billion people with TTH.[2] The estimated 1-year prevalence of TTH varies widely across countries ranging from 10.8% to 86.6%.[2] Prevalence increased by 31.7% in the United States from 1990 to 2017.[5] TTH has a female preponderance with a sex prevalence ratio of 1.2:1, far lower than the 3:1 ratio that is typical for migraine. The prevalence of CTTH is 2% to 3% in most population studies, with higher prevalence in females than in males. The prevalence of CTTH is rare in young adolescents and increases until age 39 and then declines. Risk factors for the development of TTH include educational level, fatigue, lack of ability to relax after work, and sleep disturbances. Comorbidities that have been associated with TTH include anxiety, depression, sleep disturbances, neck pain, and low back pain.

Epidemiological studies of TTH have several limitations including differences in case definitions and study methods, coexistence with migraine, and the challenge of accurately recalling and reporting infrequent TTH. Available data suggests consequences of TTH include impaired HRQOL and reduced functioning, which may worsen with headache frequency. Development of psychological comorbidities, loss of work productivity, and significant economic costs have also been associated with the condition.

Pathophysiology

Pathophysiological mechanisms of TTH involve genetic factors, peripheral myofascial and nociceptive mechanisms, and central factors.[2] Genetic studies suggest that TTH is a polygenic disorder with greater genetic contributions in frequent ETTH and CTTH compared to infrequent TTH. Potential peripheral myofascial mechanisms behind TTH include involvement of tender pericranial muscles and myofascial trigger points. Peripheral nociceptive mechanisms contributing to TTH may include activation of muscle nociceptors by several inflammatory mediators, leading to the sensitization of peripheral sensory afferents. Intracranial and extracranial vascular factors may play a minor role in TTH. Potential central factors leading to TTH include sensitization of central pain processing regions leading to hyperalgesia and allodynia. Dysfunction of the descending pain modulatory system may also contribute to increased pain sensitivity and central sensitization in TTH.

Serotonin, a monoamine neurotransmitter, has been studied in TTH.[6] Patients with ETTH have increased platelet and plasma levels of serotonin, while those with CTTH have normal or decreased levels. Differences in serotonin metabolism may predispose CTTH patients to dysfunctional pain processing or modulation. Serotonin acts with other neurotransmitters to modulate pain, but selective serotonin reuptake inhibitors have not shown better outcomes compared to nonselective agents. Endogenous opioids and neuropeptides, such as calcitonin gene-related peptide (CGRP), have been investigated in TTH but research has been inconclusive.

The underlying mechanisms of pain and the roles of various structures and chemical mediators in TTH are complex, and further research is needed.

Diagnosis and Clinical Presentation

TTH is diagnosed based on medical history referencing specific criteria published in the *International Classification of Headache Disorders*, Third Edition (ICHD-3).[7] These criteria outline the diagnostic features for infrequent ETTH, frequent ETTH, and CTTH, which are differentiated based on headache frequency and presence of pericranial tenderness (Box 13-1). A thorough medical history should address headache onset, duration, frequency, pain features, and accompanying symptoms. Clinical features of ETTH include bilateral headache, pressing or tightening pain, mild or moderate intensity, and little aggravation by routine physical activity. Frequent ETTH may also be accompanied by photophobia or phonophobia but these symptoms are typically less intense when compared to migraine headache.[3] Unlike migraine, TTH is not usually worsened by physical activity and is rarely accompanied by nausea and never linked to vomiting. Physical examination may include manual palpation for pericranial tenderness, which is more common in individuals with CTTH. CTTH is characterized by more severe pain intensity and higher frequency than ETTH, with pericranial tenderness being a common finding. Diagnostic headache diaries can help differentiate TTH from other headache disorders and help inform clinical decision-making. Red flags in medical history and physical examination can alert clinicians to consider other diagnoses, including structural conditions involving the head and neck (mass lesion, temporomandibular disorders), migraine, medication-overuse headache, and new daily persistent headache (see Chapter 1). Comorbidities such as anxiety, depression, sleep disturbances, and other pain conditions should also be assessed at the initial evaluation. Imaging for typical presentations of ETTH is not indicated in the presence of a normal exam. Certain clinical concerns, progressive CTTH, and abnormal exam findings may be indications for imaging.

Treatment

TTH management includes a range of pharmacological and nonpharmacological interventions, with patient education and a shared decision-making approach being critical for successful treatment outcomes.[2] Patient education should emphasize the patient's understanding of their medical condition, therapeutic goals, and their own role in achieving treatment success. Patients should initially be

Box 13-1. Diagnostic Criteria of Infrequent Episodic Tension-Type Headache, Frequent Episodic Tension-Type Headache, Chronic Tension-Type Headache According to the *International Classification of Headache Disorders*, Third Edition (ICHD-3)

Infrequent Episodic Tension-Type Headache

A. At least 10 episodes of headache occurring on <1 day/month on average (<12 days/year) and fulfilling criteria B-D

B. Lasting from 30 minutes to 7 days

C. At least two of the following four characteristics:
   1. Bilateral location
   2. Pressing or tightening (nonpulsating) quality
   3. Mild or moderate intensity
   4. Not aggravated by routine physical activity such as walking or climbing stairs

D. Both of the following:
   1. No nausea or vomiting
   2. No more than one of photophobia or phonophobia

E. Not better accounted for by another ICHD-3 diagnosis

Frequent Episodic Tension-Type Headache

A. At least 10 episodes of headache occurring on 1-14 days/month on average for >3 months (≥12 and <180 days/year) and fulfilling criteria B-D

B. Lasting from 30 minutes to 7 days

C. At least two of the following four characteristics:
   1. Bilateral location
   2. Pressing or tightening (nonpulsating) quality
   3. Mild or moderate intensity
   4. Not aggravated by routine physical activity such as walking or climbing stairs

D. Both of the following:
   1. No nausea or vomiting
   2. No more than one of photophobia or phonophobia

E. Not better accounted for by another ICHD-3 diagnosis

Chronic Tension-Type Headache

A. Headache occurring on ≥15 days/month on average for >3 months (≥180 days/year), fulfilling criteria B-D

B. Lasting hours to days, or unremitting

C. At least two of the following four characteristics:
   1. Bilateral location
   2. Pressing or tightening (nonpulsating) quality
   3. Mild or moderate intensity
   4. Not aggravated by routine physical activity such as walking or climbing stairs

D. Both of the following:
   1. No more than one of photophobia, phonophobia, or mild nausea
   2. Neither moderate or severe nausea nor vomiting

E. Not better accounted for by another ICHD-3 diagnosis

Primary Headaches

offered nonpharmacologic options. These may be helpful for headache prevention and sometimes are successful in alleviating acute attacks. Recommendations for adequate nutrition, hydration, sleep, and physical activity should be provided. There is reasonable scientific support for the effectiveness of relaxation training and cognitive behavioral therapies and some evidence suggesting benefit from acupuncture in prevention of chronic tension-type headache. Massage, physical therapy, and chiropractic care have no established efficacy.

Pharmacologic therapy may be selected based on established efficacy and safety as well as patient preference. Clinical experience plays a large role in making treatment choices for TTH since evidence from well-designed studies is limited. Individual patient characteristics and comorbidities, such as psychiatric, neurologic, and medical conditions, should be considerations in treatment planning.

Medical management of acute attacks of TTH often begins with over-the-counter analgesics. Acetaminophen, aspirin, and nonsteroidal anti-inflammatory drugs (NSAIDs) are effective in treating most TTH attacks. Caffeine when combined with analgesics can improve efficacy, but may produce adverse events such as palpitations and insomnia. The available evidence covering the acute treatment of TTH is limited compared to the clinical needs. According to the European Federation of Neurological Societies Task Force (EFNS-TF),[8] the acute treatment of TTH can include oral doses of ibuprofen (200-800 mg), ketoprofen (25 mg), aspirin (500-1000 mg), naproxen (375-500 mg), diclofenac (12.5-100 mg), and paracetamol (1000 mg), all of which have a level A labeling. Caffeine (65-200 mg) combinations are also an option with a B-level labeling.

Preventive treatment aims to reduce the frequency and severity of attacks. For infrequent TTH, there is no need for prophylactic treatment, but frequent TTH may require prevention. There is only one evidence-based guideline for the pharmaceutical prophylaxis of TTH, the EFNS-TF.[7] Guidelines recommend three agents for the preventive treatment of TTH:

- Amitriptyline (30-75 mg/day) with A labeling as first line. Tolerability issues may include drowsiness, weight gain, dry mouth, dizziness, sweating, and constipation.
- Venlafaxine (150 mg/day) and mirtazapine (30 mg/day) with B labeling as second-line treatments. Venlafaxine may cause tachycardia and diaphoresis, mirtazapine sedation, and both can provoke weight gain.
- Clomipramine (75-100 mg/day), maprotiline (75 mg/day), and mianserin (30-60 mg/day) with B labeling as third-line treatments. Palpitations, sedation, constipation, and weight gain are possible with each of these agents.

A systematic meta-analysis revealed limited scientific evidence for the use of selective serotonin reuptake inhibitors (SSRIs) and venlafaxine for the prevention of TTH in adults.[2] Tizanidine (12-18 mg per day) might be useful in practice for the prevention of CTTH. Another systematic meta-analysis found that botulinum toxin A is associated with significant improvements in headache intensity, frequency, duration, and acute pain medication use in patients with CTTH, exceeding minimal clinically important differences, although further high-quality controlled trials are needed to confirm these findings.[9]

The duration of prophylaxis remains an active challenge. All studies lasted from 2 to 6 months, but there may be a need for longer treatment in many cases. Comorbidity, response to prior treatment, personal patient characteristics, previous headache history, patients' preferences, and lifestyle choices should be considered in decisions regarding medication selection and duration of use. In the setting of an excellent response, pausing the treatment after 3 or 6 months and monitoring for any recurrence of the headache is a widely used approach. Certain patients with comorbid anxiety, depression, or insomnia may require longer periods of treatment despite an achievement of headache response.

Evidence for managing TTH in children and adolescents is limited with high placebo responses (see Chapter 49). Nonpharmaceutical interventions are preferred. Acetaminophen may be considered for TTH attacks, while amitriptyline shows promise for TTH prevention. Nonpharmacological interventions are the first choice for treating TTH in elderly patients, followed by acetaminophen for acute treatment (see Chapter 50). In this population, amitriptyline is the preferred drug for TTH prevention, but venlafaxine and mirtazapine are additional favorable options with fewer adverse events. Monitoring adverse effects and comorbidities is necessary in elderly patients. Nonpharmaceutical treatments are also preferred for TTH during pregnancy and breastfeeding (see Chapter 48). Acetaminophen is the first choice for symptomatic treatment in these patients. Amitriptyline may be preferred for prevention, while venlafaxine or mirtazapine may be used with caution. Guidelines published by the American College of Gynecology suggest weighing relative risks and benefits when prescribing any of these preventive agents, but none are considered high risk. Low-dose aspirin may be helpful and appears to pose no risk to the pregnancy or fetus.

Prognosis

The prognosis of TTH varies depending on several factors, including the type of TTH, the presence of comorbidities, and the efficacy of treatment.[2] ETTH patients typically have a good prognosis, with many patients experiencing remission or reduction in headache frequency over time. CTTH appears to carry a poorer prognosis. In cross-sectional and longitudinal studies, young age, female sex, poor self-rated health, and insufficient sleep have been identified as risk factors for incident TTH.[2] In addition, acute headache medication overuse (Chapter 28), a history of migraine, and depression severity have been associated with a higher prevalence of CTTH and poorer outcomes. Effective treatment is essential for improving the prognosis of TTH. Nonpharmacological therapies, such as biobehavioral and physical therapies, have strong evidence for reducing headache frequency and related disability in TTH patients.

Summary

- TTH is highly prevalent primary headache in the population, predominantly affects females and is associated with impaired quality of life and disability.
- The diagnosis of TTH is clinical and involves medical history and ICHD-3 criteria, with physical examination for potential pericranial tenderness.
- Pathophysiology of TTH involves genetic, peripheral, and central mechanisms, with myofascial trigger points and peripheral nociceptive mechanisms contributing to TTH attacks and central sensitization leading to chronification of TTH.
- Acute treatment of TTH includes over-the-counter drugs with ibuprofen, ketoprofen, aspirin, naproxen, diclofenac, and acetaminophen being effective, and nonpharmacologic strategies.
- For preventive treatment of TTH, amitriptyline, venlafaxine, and mirtazapine are recommended.

REFERENCES

1. Jensen RH. Tension-type headache—the normal and most prevalent headache. *Headache.* 2018;58(2):339-345.
2. Ashina S, Mitsikostas DD, Lee MJ, et al. Tension-type headache. *Nat Rev Dis Primers.* 2021;7(1):24.
3. Kaniecki RG. Migraine and tension-type headache: an assessment of challenges in diagnosis. *Neurology.* 2002;58(9 Suppl 6):S15-S20.
4. Onan D, Younis S, Wellsgatnik WD, et al. Debate: differences and similarities between tension-type headache and migraine. *J Headache Pain.* 2023;24(1):92.
5. GBD 2017 US Neurological Disorders Collaborators; Feigin VL, Vos T, et al. Burden of neurological disorders across the US from 1990-2017: a global burden of disease study. *JAMA Neurol.* 2021;78(2):165-176.
6. Ashina S, Bendtsen L, Ashina M. Pathophysiology of tension-type headache. *Curr Pain Headache Rep.* 2005;9(6):415-422.
7. Headache Classification Committee of the International Headache Society (IHS). *The International Classification of Headache Disorders,* 3rd edition. *Cephalalgia.* 2018;38(1):1-211.
8. Bendtsen L, Evers S, Linde M, Mitsikostas DD, Sandrini G, Schoenen J. EFNS guideline on the treatment of tension-type headache—report of an EFNS task force. *Eur J Neurol.* 2010;17(11):1318-1325.
9. Dhanasekara CS, Payberah D, Chyu JY, Shen CL, Kahathuduwa CN. The effectiveness of botulinum toxin for chronic tension-type headache prophylaxis: a systematic review and meta-analysis. *Cephalalgia.* 2023;43(3):3331024221150231.

SECTION C: CLUSTER HEADACHE AND OTHER TRIGEMINAL AUTONOMIC CEPHALALGIAS

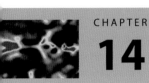

CHAPTER

14

Cluster Headache

Maria Dolores Villar-Martinez and Peter J. Goadsby

Cluster headache is the third most common primary headache disorder. It is classified as a trigeminal autonomic cephalgia in the third edition of *International Classification of Headache Disorders* (ICHD-3). It is typically one-sided headache accompanied by ipsilateral cranial autonomic symptoms.

Epidemiology

The prevalence of cluster headache is low compared to migraine. The prevalence rates range between 0% and 1.3% and one meta-analysis calculated a lifetime prevalence of around 0.12%.[1] The 1-year incidence has been reported to be 2 to 10 per 100,000. Age of onset is around 30 years in both men and women, although it is not infrequent to encounter adult patients, referred for suspicion of cluster headache, who have had severe headaches also in their childhood. Recent survey studies show that pediatric onset was found in about 27.5%, with the majority diagnosed during their adulthood.[2] Cluster headache has always been considered a predominantly male disorder, although reports in recent decades indicate an increase in prevalence among females.

As an extremely disabling condition, cluster headache can have much higher rates of sickness absence and disability pension compared to unaffected individuals.[3] Given the rarity of this headache, finding empathy from surrounding colleagues and family/friends can be difficult for the patients, who can feel less understood when the number of sick leave days is neither very low nor very high. Cluster headache patients are at higher risk of lifetime active suicidal ideation, which may be related to being demoralized, rather than being depressed.

Pathophysiology

Genetics

The genetic component of cluster headache has been estimated to be around 6% to 8%,[4] but the heritability pattern seems a likely underestimate. There is a higher likelihood of cluster headache among first- and second-degree relatives,[5] with the risk for first degree being as high as 35- to 45-fold. Inheritance patterns seem complex, and an anticipation phenomenon has been suggested, which could also be attributed to memory bias. One genome-wide association study[6] found four loci of interest, namely rs11579212, rs6541998, rs10184573, and rs2499799. Interestingly, it has been proposed that genetic variants involved in circadian regulation may be related to specific phenotypes of cluster headache with particular circadian patterns,[7] whereas other variants may not be.[8]

Risk Factors

A recent meta-analysis[9] suggested certain risk factors to be linked with cluster headache, such as smoking habit, alcohol consumption, or head trauma, although causality remains to be demonstrated.

Trigeminal Nociceptive Pathways

The mechanisms behind cluster headache consist of a network involving several craniofacial and brain structures, as well as signaling molecules, without a clear understanding of the mechanism of individual attack onset.[10] The distinctive referred pain areas are innervated by the trigeminal nerve, through which afferent signals are conveyed to the trigeminocervical complex from the dura mater, cerebral vessels, and facial regions, especially the periorbital area.[9,11] The trigeminocervical complex represents a region of confluence for the occipital and trigeminal afferents.

Cranial Parasympathetic Efferents

The characteristic cranial autonomic symptoms accompanying the headache may be generated by activation of the processes comprising the trigeminal-autonomic reflex. This reflex is mediated by parasympathetic neurons of the sphenopalatine ganglion (SPG), and it originates in the pons in the superior salivatory nucleus. The efferents project through the facial nerve bypassing the geniculate ganglion and synapsing in the SPG, situated in the pterygopalatine fossa, and project to cranial structures such as the lacrimal gland, nasal, palatine mucosa, and cerebral vessels.[12]

Hypothalamus

The hypothalamus, given its involvement in the circadian regulation, has been considered one of the main candidate brain areas to play a major role in the appearance or disappearance of the spontaneous attacks of cluster headache.[13] The hypothalamic suprachiasmatic nucleus, in particular, presents seasonal variation in the number of cells, being maximum at spring and autumn. This fluctuation agrees with the attack frequency reported by patients.[14] Positron emission tomography (PET) studies showed a hypothalamic region activation strictly during the bout in participants with the episodic form of cluster headache, in patients triggered with nitroglycerin, as well as diencephalic, cingulate, and insulae cortex activation. Independently of the bout, episodic participants had decreased regional brain metabolism in structures involved in descending pain mechanisms.

In structural MRI imaging studies, patients with chronic cluster headache have also shown hypothalamic abnormalities using voxel-based morphometry.[15] A slightly different neuroanatomical hypothalamic architecture in patients with episodic cluster headache has also been suggested. Other diencephalic systems display structural variations, as is the case of thalamic alterations that have also been found in bilateral medial geniculate nuclei volumes, as well as reduced cortical thickness in the left posterior insula, and other areas involved in nociception, sensory-motor, autonomic and social cognition. Recently, a glymphatic system dysfunction has also been suggested given differences in brain perivascular spaces, and no neurovascular inflammation was appreciated either during or in between attacks of cluster headache using vessel-wall magnetic resonance imaging (MRI) techniques.[16] Functional MRI has shown that chronic cluster headache patients may have a reduced connectivity between the frontal pole and the right amygdala, and increased cerebral blood flow in several cortical areas ipsilateral to the side of pain, as well as in the hypothalamus and ventral pons.

Participants who respond to treatment with occipital nerve block presented relative regional cerebral blood flow increases at baseline in medial prefrontal cortex and lateral occipital cortex, but relative reductions in middle temporal and cingulate cortices. This provides further support for altered connectivity between rhombencephalic areas of the trigeminocervical complex with higher diencephalic and telencephalic structures in individuals with cluster headache.

Neuropeptides

Among the molecules potentially involved in the pathogenesis of cluster headache, some require highlighting: calcitonin gene-related peptide (CGRP), pituitary adenylate-cyclase-activating polypeptide 38 (PACAP-38), and vasoactive intestinal peptide (VIP).[17] CGRP seems to be of importance in the pathophysiology of cluster headache. Infusion of CGRP can trigger a cluster headache attack in most patients with episodic cluster headache during the active bout, in comparison with those out of the bout. The chronic form of cluster headache, however, presents much lower plasma levels of CGRP, in comparison with episodic cluster headache. Sumatriptan and oxygen have been shown to reduce the levels of this molecule during an attack.

Plasma levels of PACAP-38 are also higher during the episodic bout of cluster headache. VIP and PACAP-38, along with nitric oxide synthase, may be fundamental in the activation of the parasympathetic outflow of cranial autonomic symptoms during the attacks, orchestrated through the SPG. Recent research suggests that VIP and PACAP-38 can also trigger attacks in participants with the episodic form, during the active bout, although at a much lower rate than CGRP is capable of, and about 50% of patients with chronic cluster headache can have a headache attack triggered by CGRP, VIP, and PACAP-38.

Given the evident implication of diencephalic structures, hormones and neuropeptides synthesized in the hypothalamus have also been proposed to participate in the mechanisms of cluster headache. Melatonin and cortisol levels seem to lose their secretion rhythmicity in participants with cluster headache, in comparison with controls. The orexinergic neuron network also plays a role in the processing of nociceptive information and modulation. Cerebrospinal levels of orexin A are reduced in patients with episodic and chronic cluster headache, in comparison with controls.

Clinical Presentation and Diagnosis

Symptoms

Perhaps the characteristic feature that distinguishes cluster headache from other primary headache disorders is the grouping of the attacks in "clusters" or bouts, that have a duration of weeks to months, followed by a remission period. When these breaks are longer than 3 months in a year, the condition can be classified as episodic, and otherwise, is described as chronic. Cluster headache consists of headache attacks, typically with a duration between 15 minutes to 3 hours, if untreated, occurring with a frequency from once every second day to 8 attacks per day (Box 14-1). The pain has an excruciating quality, said by patients to be the worse pain they have experienced, and is usually unilateral, characteristically involving distribution of the first branch of the trigeminal nerve. Headache is associated with a sensation of restlessness or agitation, or ipsilateral cranial autonomic symptoms, such as conjunctival injection, lacrimation, rhinorrhea, or aural fullness. Differences in the clinical phenotype are many, regarding either headache frequency, location, laterality, or cranial autonomic symptoms. Although the trigeminal, and particularly, the periorbital region is still the most frequently reported area of maximum pain, presentations outside the orbito-temporal area, such as the occipital, nuchal or dorsal areas are not uncommon, especially during the headache onset and as a radiation phenomenon.

Other symptoms occurring with the headache may vary between individuals. Parasympathetic cranial autonomic symptoms, for example, may not be just limited to the cranial area externally such as laryngeal symptoms, which have been recently reported. Cranial autonomic symptoms may vary

> **Box 14-1.** ICHD-3 Diagnostic Criteria for Cluster Headache
>
> Attacks of severe, strictly unilateral pain which is orbital, supraorbital, temporal, or in any combination of these sites, lasting 15-180 minutes and occurring from once every other day to eight times a day. The pain is associated with ipsilateral conjunctival injection, lacrimation, nasal congestion, rhinorrhea, forehead and facial sweating, miosis, ptosis and/or eyelid edema, and/or with restlessness or agitation:
>
> A. At least five attacks fulfilling criteria B-D
>
> B. Severe or very severe unilateral orbital, supraorbital, and/or temporal pain lasting 15-180 minutes (when untreated)
>
> C. Either or both of the following:
>
> 1. At least one of the following symptoms or signs, ipsilateral to the headache:
>   – conjunctival injection and/or lacrimation
>   – nasal congestion and/or rhinorrhea
>   – eyelid edema
>   – forehead and facial sweating
>   – miosis and/or ptosis
> 2. A sense of restlessness or agitation
>
> D. Occurring with a frequency between one every other day and eight per day
>
> E. Not better accounted for by another ICHD-3 diagnosis

Headache Classification Committee of the International Headache Society (IHS). The International Classification of Headache Disorders, 3rd edition, (38(1)) 1–211. Copyright © 2018 by (International Headache Society). Reprinted by Permission of SAGE Publications.

slightly between sexes. Ethnic or geographical clinical variations also exist. Asian populations have reported less chronic forms and a low presence of restlessness.

Other associated symptoms may help in the differential diagnosis. Photosensitivity is characterized by being usually unilateral, ipsilateral to the side of pain, and can also be increased interictally in chronic and episodic cluster headache. In the latter, it reverts back to a similar photosensitivity to controls during the interictal period. Osmophobia is not typical of isolated cluster headache, and its presence should alert the clinician to migraine or a differential diagnosis. The presence of complicating habits, such as tobacco smoking, and the triptan response could distinguish different phenotypes of cluster headache that could be relevant for therapeutic management. Clinical features were generally similar between smokers and nonsmokers, although there may be a higher seasonal rhythmicity and triptan responsiveness in nonsmokers.

Aura has been rarely reported in patients with cluster headache. More than one-third of the patients are able to predict the next bout, with symptoms starting up to 1 week before the full-blown attack, including sensory changes, cranial autonomic symptoms, or hypothalamically mediated symptoms, such as yawning or appetite changes.

Presentation in Children

Pediatric patients with cluster headache can present milder features, with fewer cranial autonomic symptoms that may lead the physician toward a diagnosis of migraine, although it is the authors' experience that cluster headache in pediatric and adolescent populations can be just as awful as that seen in adults. The number of daily headache attacks in children can be lower than in adults. The pediatric population could develop longer remission periods, which may influence the late diagnosis. Familial cases of cluster headache do not present a remarkably different phenotype in comparison with the sporadic cases, apart from reports of a higher presence of nasal congestion.

Diagnosis

A thorough history remains essential for the diagnosis of cluster headache. Certain close-ended questions may help increase diagnostic certainty. Our experience is close-ended questions are an optimal way to establish the broad issues, with open-ended questions being less useful for most aspects of the phenotype to establish the diagnosis and options for treatment. The diagnosis of cluster headache is based on ICHD-3.[18] MRI of the brain will typically be normal. Given the lack of formal guidelines regarding the workup, and the existence of a considerable case series literature reporting serious causes of secondary cluster headache that fulfilled the ICHD-3 criteria, neuroimaging in a condition that will last decades is not unreasonable. Secondary causes include different pathologies, the most frequently reported being vascular, especially carotid dissection or cerebral venous thrombosis, tumors, especially of the pituitary, or treatable inflammatory sources like sinusitis. Therefore, a careful differential diagnosis must be considered in new onset cluster headache, and MRI brain with contrast and MRA of neck/cervical vascular structures, as well as pituitary profile has been recommended as part of the initial management of a recently developed cluster headache (Chapters 1-2).

Treatment

Treatment of cluster headache should include early access to therapeutic counselling and prescriptions, and adequate treatment of both the acute attack and preventive strategies (Table 14-1).[19]

Patient Education

The information provided to a patient with cluster headache can be crucial for a successful therapeutic management. Understanding basic mechanisms, the concept of bouts, attacks, remission periods, abortive, and preventive medication is especially necessary if other resources are not available. Otherwise, having access to an advice line or contact with multidisciplinary teams could prevent visits to emergency departments. Digital platforms, such as online support groups, can be extremely helpful.

Acute Treatment

Goal of acute treatment is to stop the individual headache attack or reduce its duration, severity, or both.

Oxygen

It can be considered one of the safest treatments due to the low risk of adverse events. The mechanism of action of oxygen in cluster headache is not fully clarified but may include altered neuropeptide release or the inhibition of the trigeminocervical complex. High-flow oxygen can be applied repeatedly throughout the day and can also be combined with other treatments. As drawbacks, oxygen cylinders are not widely available or reimbursed, and cumbersome to transport. One of the known possible adverse events associated with oxygen is rebound headache. Before abandoning this treatment, several strategies are recommended, such as starting the treatment inhalation at the beginning of the attack, increasing the duration of inhalation, or substituting the delivery system for a different one, such as the demand-valve systems.

Triptans: Serotonin 5-HT$_{1B/1D}$ Receptor Agonists

Subcutaneous injections of sumatriptan 6 mg are portable and have proven efficacy and tolerability. However, the safety recommendations for the total daily dose are troublesome in patients with a high number of attacks per 24 hours. In those cases, lower subcutaneous doses could be considered. Triptans should be avoided in patients with vascular conditions, such as uncontrolled hypertension,

Table 14-1. Treatment of Cluster Headache

	Route	Dose	Posology	Max Recommended Dose
Acute				
Oxygen	Inhaled, demand valve or nonre-breathable mask	High-flow, >12 L/min	PRN for at least 15 minutes	NA
Sumatriptan	Subcutaneous	3-6 mg	PRN	12 mg/day
Sumatriptan	Nasal Spray	20 mg	PRN	40 mg/day
Zolmitriptan	Nasal Spray	5-10 mg	PRN	10 mg/day
n-VNS	Transcutaneous	3 × 2-min stimulations	PRN	NA
Transitional				
Occipital nerve block	Intramuscular	MTP 80 mg and 2 mL of 2% Lidocaine 2%	PRN	4/year
Prednisolone	Oral	1 mg/kg	5-7 days + tapering	100 mg/day
Naratriptan	Oral	2.5 mg	Every 24 hours	5 mg/day
Frovatriptan	Oral	5 mg	Every 24 hours	7.5 mg/day
Preventive				
Verapamil	Oral	80-320 mg	TDS	960 mg/day
Galcanezumab	Subcutaneous	300 mg	Monthly	300 mg/month
Melatonin	Oral	10 mg	At night every 24 hours	25 mg/day
Topiramate	Oral	100 mg	2 divided doses/day	400 mg/day
Lithium carbonate	Oral	Adjusted for serum levels 0.8-1.2 mEq/L	2-3 divided doses/day	1200 mg/day
n-VNS	Transcutaneous	2-min stimulations	Once a day to three times a day, with progressive intensity	NA

MTP, methylprednisolone; NA, not applicable; n-VNS, noninvasive vagal nerve stimulation; PRN, pro re nata (as needed).

coronary disease, or stroke. Side effects include injection-site reactions, nausea, paresthesia, or chest tightness. Intranasal delivery options, including sumatriptan 20 mg and zolmitriptan 5 mg nasal sprays, should be considered, if the subcutaneous formulation is not well tolerated, or the patient has needle phobia.

Ergots

Intranasal dihydroergotamine (DHE) at 0.5 mg on each nostril could relieve pain severity during the acute attack. Intravenous DHE is administered as a 0.5 to 1 mg intravenous bolus that can be repeated every 8 hours over 3 to 5 days to induce bout remission or provide a "holiday" in chronic cluster headache. ECG should be performed and an intense antiemetic regimen provided, if needed, as nausea is the most frequent side effect.

Intranasal Lidocaine

Although the degree of benefit is low, small trials indicate that at least one-third of patients may benefit from intranasal lidocaine, which aims at blocking the SPG. Following the Barre method (head extended 45 degrees and turned 30-40 degrees toward the painful side), 1 mL of a 4% to 10% solution of lidocaine is instilled in the nostril ipsilateral to the cluster headache.

Octreotide

Subcutaneous octreotide at 100 μg may be effective in treating acute cluster headache at 30 min, with mild dyspepsia as main adverse event. Although not compared directly, octreotide may perform worse than triptans in terms of response rate and latency to relief in acute cluster headache. It is not a practical median term option.

Noninvasive Vagal Nerve Stimulation

Noninvasive vagal nerve stimulation (nVNS) can be achieved through the application of repetitive, high-frequency electrical stimuli at low intensity on the anterolateral cervical region (Chapter 46). Stimulations last for 2 minutes and can be repeated several times per day. A nVNS device, gammaCore™, is approved by United States Food and Drug Administration (FDA) and is one of the safest therapeutic options for acute treatment of episodic cluster headache. Efficacy has been proven by pain relief and attack termination in patients with episodic cluster headache, applying three consecutive 2-minute stimulation, ipsilateral to the headache. It can be effective in patients with chronic cluster headache when added to standard-of-care. Its therapeutic action might be exerted through vagus nerve connections in the brainstem either by modulation of trigeminocervical neurons, or by connections directly with areas pertaining to the pain matrix. Skin irritation and muscle contraction can happen as side effects of treatment with gammaCore™.

Transitional Treatment

Effective preventive treatment may take up to several weeks to achieve therapeutic doses. Transitional treatment can result in temporary relief or even remission while the titration of the preventive takes place. There is some evidence for recommending short periods of systemic corticosteroids as transitional treatment. To avoid long-term side effects, a short-term treatment with stable dose of oral prednisone for 5 days, followed by a tapering or intravenous methylprednisolone has been recommended. Limited evidence suggests that triptans with a long semi-life, such as frovatriptan up to 5 mg, could be effective as transitional treatment.

Preventive Treatment

Preventive treatment should always be considered in individuals with cluster headache. Patients with chronic forms may benefit from continuous treatment to reduce either the frequency or intensity of the attacks. Preventive options should be started in the early stages of a bout in episodic patients with suitable length bouts, with the aim of finishing the bout earlier or reducing its severity.

Primary Headaches

Verapamil

This medication represents the first-line preventive treatment for cluster headache, even though it has not been approved by the FDA or EMA[20] regulatory agencies. Doses range between 80 and 320 mg three times a day, with slow increments and ECG control after each titration. In patients with episodic cluster headache, once the bout is finished, verapamil should be gradually withdrawn to stop. There is no consensus on the exact withdrawal duration, but the absence of "shadows" or headaches generated by usual triggers is desirable. The mechanism of action of verapamil is not clear but could be related to the prevention of CGRP release, by inhibition calcium influx presynaptically. Verapamil could also have a modulatory effect on the circadian rhythm. Its efficacy has been demonstrated in small trials, with a reduction in the number of attacks in episodic and chronic forms of cluster headache. Apart from ankle edema or gingival hyperplasia, verapamil is overall well tolerated. Preventive treatment with verapamil requires regular electrocardiograms. The most critical side effects are cardiac rhythm and atrioventricular abnormalities seen in about 20% of patients, which is marked by PR interval prolongation.

Galcanezumab

At a dose of 300 mg, a subcutaneous humanized CGRP monoclonal has shown long-term safety and tolerability in patients with chronic and episodic cluster headaches. It has FDA approval for prevention of episodic cluster headache. In addition, patients with concomitant migraine may also benefit from galcanezumab.

Topiramate

The evidence for recommending the antiepileptic drug topiramate for cluster headache is scarce. The recommended starting dose of topiramate is 25 mg per day. Typically, it is titrated every week in 25-mg increments according to response and tolerance. The usual total recommended dose is 100 mg per day which can be divided into two doses. Side effects such as cognitive troubles or suicidal tendencies make this preventive to be chosen with caution, considering at-risk subjects. Other side effects include paresthesia and weight loss. It must be avoided during pregnancy and in patients with a history of nephrolithiasis.

Lithium

The initial dose of lithium carbonate is usually 300 mg once daily, but the dose increased every 4 to 5 days with close monitoring to 900 to 1200 mg per day divided into two to four divided doses depending on formulations. Lithium may modulate excitatory neurotransmission by reducing its activity. Preventive treatment with lithium requires careful monitoring, including serum levels every 1 to 2 months, as well as renal, liver, and thyroid function. Its latency for efficacy is longer than that of verapamil, and is not exempt from a large array of adverse effects, extrapyramidal side effects, or gastrointestinal disturbances.

Melatonin

Melatonin at high doses, 10 to 25 mg, has shown promising results in episodic cluster headache, in reducing the frequency of the attacks during the early days of the bout. This could be especially useful in patients with tolerability issues or contraindications for other preventive treatments, as it is usually well tolerated and has a low interaction profile. The evidence supporting the use of melatonin for cluster headache is still limited, and larger trials are needed.

Noninvasive Vagal Nerve Stimulation

Approved by FDA, nVNS (gammaCore™) can be used as a preventive treatment of episodic cluster headache (Chapter 46). Efficacy has been proven by reduced attack frequency and reduction of acute medication in patients with episodic cluster headache.

Greater Occipital Nerve Blocks

Modulating the trigeminocervical complex, where trigeminal and occipital afferents converge, is likely the basis of the efficacy of the occipital nerve block, described below. Greater occipital nerve block consists of a safe procedure involving an injection of corticosteroids mixed with local anesthetics in the suboccipital region, and has demonstrated clinical efficacy. Repetitive nerve blocks have been reported to be safe in episodic and chronic cluster headache, with a median interval of 100 days between procedures. In a study performing three injections every other day, side effects including neck stiffness and pain at the site of injection were reported by almost 40%, and relief to patients with chronic cluster headache of a median of 3 months. Treatment response has been correlated with a shorter duration of the cluster headache attack since the first bout, with a negative response in those having had cluster headache for more years. See also Chapter 44.

Complementary/Alternative Treatments

There is not enough evidence to recommend complementary and alternative therapeutic strategies in cluster headache, although small studies including specific diet modifications, supplements or plant extracts, and topical components, among others, have been conducted.

Interventional and Surgical Treatments

Treatment can be challenging in some cluster headache patients who have exhausted all lines of oral and noninvasive procedures and remain refractory to treatment. A careful assessment of the case, including medication posology, compliance, and eventual interactions with other treatments should be reviewed, before considering more invasive, nonreversible techniques that are not exempt from the possibility of adverse events.

Occipital Nerve Stimulation

The occipital nerve has also been objective of study in noninvasive modalities of treatment, and has been mainly studied in chronic forms or patients not responding to treatment. Occipital nerve stimulation may be effective in reducing the weekly number of attacks in patients with chronic cluster headache; however, it is not exempt from serious adverse events.

Percutaneous pulsed radiofrequency directed toward nerve roots and ganglions of C1 and C2 levels showed mild improvement without serious adverse events.

A cohort of patients with chronic cluster headache may be responders to percutaneous electric current stimulation in the craniofacial areas involved: more research is needed in this field.

Surgery and Deep Brain Stimulation

Regarding more invasive treatments requiring higher-risk procedures, gamma knife radiosurgery was recently evaluated in a systematic review identifying five small, open-label studies.[21] Studies used different approaches, with persistent pain reduction in 42% of the patients, but 58% reported side effects in the form of trigeminal sensory disturbances; we do not recommend its use. Deep brain stimulation has been tried in the ventral tegmental area, unilateral or bilateral posterior hypothalamic regions. The only sham-controlled trial did not find any significant outcome changes, although the open-label studies show promising results. Infrequent adverse events with high mortality imply the need for a careful selection of patients with a chronic, unilateral cluster headache, who have exhausted every other conceivable option.

Pregnancy and Lactation Treatment Considerations

The management of cluster headache in pregnant and lactating women can be challenging. Cluster headache is clinically complex enough, which added to the ethical implications surrounding pregnancy, makes the quality of the evidence supporting the use of acute and preventive treatment suboptimal. Therefore, treatment recommendations have been based on safety for mother and fetus. When possible, a careful therapeutic plan should be anticipated and agreed upon with the patient, considering the different options, and support should be provided throughout the pregnancy and postpartum process. Triptans may possibly be safe to use, given the low rate of adverse events reported. Antiepileptics and oral corticosteroids may increase the risk of congenital malformations. Oxygen, topical anesthetics such as intranasal lidocaine, and injection of the occipital nerve, either alone or accompanied by corticosteroids, do not seem to increase risk for mother or child. There is not sufficient evidence to recommend botulinum toxin, galcanezumab, nVNS, or melatonin in pregnancy.

Prognosis

Longitudinal data from individuals with cluster headaches reveal a decreasing frequency of bouts over time. Observations suggest that as these individuals age, the intervals between these bouts tend to lengthen. It remains uncertain whether this represents a true remission or is merely an approach to mortality. Notably, some patients in their nineties have been observed to experience intervals of nearly 20 years between bouts.

Summary

- Cluster headache is a primary headache disorder with a high impact on quality of life, characterized by severe, unilateral headache attacks with a duration from 15 to 180 minutes, with associated cranial autonomic symptoms, and appearing in "bouts."

- Pathophysiology of cluster headache involves neuropeptides like CGRP, VIP, PACAP-38, and brain structures such as the hypothalamus, resulting in the activation of the trigeminal autonomic reflex.

- The clinical history remains crucial for the diagnosis of cluster headache, and secondary headaches should be excluded by neuroimaging including vascular sequences and pituitary function.

- Treatment should be based on patient education, an effective abortive and preventive treatment, with the aim to reduce the frequency, duration, or severity of the attack, that should be individualized and withdrawn once the bout has finished.

- Transitional treatment, especially occipital nerve block, should be considered in individual with cluster headache.

REFERENCES

1. Fischera M, Marziniak M, Gralow I, Evers S. The incidence and prevalence of cluster headache: a meta-analysis of population-based studies. *Cephalalgia.* 2008;28(6):614-618.

2. Schor LI, Pearson SM, Shapiro RE, Zhang W, Miao H, Burish MJ. Cluster headache epidemiology including pediatric onset, sex, and ICHD criteria: results from the International Cluster Headache Questionnaire. *Headache.* 2021;61(10):1511-1120.

3. Steinberg A, Josefsson P, Alexanderson K, Sjöstrand C. Cluster headache: prevalence, sickness absence, and disability pension in working ages in Sweden. *Neurology.* 2019;93(4):e404-e413.

4. Waung MW, Taylor A, Qualmann KJ, Burish MJ. Family history of cluster headache: a systematic review. *JAMA Neurol.* 2020;77(7):887-896.

5. Russell MB. Epidemiology and genetics of cluster headache. *Lancet Neurol.* 2004;3(5):279-283.

6. Harder AVE, Winsvold BS, Noordam R, et al. Genetic susceptibility loci in genomewide association study of cluster headache. *Ann Neurol.* 2021;90(2):203-216.

7. Fourier C, Ran C, Sjöstrand C, Waldenlind E, Steinberg A, Belin AC. The molecular clock gene cryptochrome 1 (CRY1) and its role in cluster headache. *Cephalalgia.* 2021;41(13):1374-1381.

8. Jennysdotter Olofsgård F, Ran C, Fourier C, et al. PER gene family polymorphisms in relation to cluster headache and circadian rhythm in Sweden. *Brain Sci.* 2021;11(8):1108.

9. Elbadawi ASA, Albalawi AFA, Alghannami AK, et al. Cluster headache and associated risk factors: a systemic review and meta-analysis. *Cureus.* 2021;13(11):e19294.

10. Hoffmann J, May A. Diagnosis, pathophysiology, and management of cluster headache. *Lancet Neurol.* 2018;17(1):75-83.

11. May A, Goadsby PJ. The trigeminovascular system in humans: pathophysiologic implications for primary headache syndromes of the neural influences on the cerebral circulation. *J Cereb Blood Flow Metab.* 1999;19(2):115-127.

12. Spencer SE, Sawyer WB, Wada H, Platt KB, Loewy AD. CNS projections to the pterygopalatine parasympathetic preganglionic neurons in the rat: a retrograde transneuronal viral cell body labeling study. *Brain Res.* 1990;534(1-2):149-169.

13. Holland PR, Goadsby PJ. Cluster headache, hypothalamus, and orexin. *Curr Pain Headache Rep.* 2009;13(2):147-154.

14. Radziwon J, Waszak P. Seasonal changes of internet searching suggest circannual rhythmicity of primary headache disorders. *Headache.* 2022;7(10):14329.

15. May A, Ashburner J, Buchel C, et al. Correlation between structural and functional changes in brain in an idiopathic headache syndrome. *Nat Med.* 1999;5(7):836-838.

16. Merli E, Rustici A, Gramegna LL, et al. Vessel-wall MRI in primary headaches: the role of neurogenic inflammation. *Headache.* 2022;8(10):14253.

17. Joshi S. Peptides, MAbs, molecules, mechanisms, and more: taking a stab at cluster headache. *Headache.* 2020;60(8):1871-1877.

18. Headache Classification Committee of the International Headache Society (IHS). *The International Classification of Headache Disorders*, 3rd edition. *Cephalalgia.* 2018;38(1):1-211.

19. Medrea I, Christie S, Tepper SJ, Thavorn K, Hutton B. Effects of acute and preventive therapies for episodic and chronic cluster headache: a scoping review of the literature. *Headache.* 2022;62(3):329-362.

20. Petersen AS, Barloese MCJ, Snoer A, Soerensen AMS, Jensen RH. Verapamil and cluster headache: still a mystery. A narrative review of efficacy, mechanisms and perspectives. *Headache.* 2019;59(8):1198-1211.

21. Franzini A, Clerici E, Navarria P, et al. Gamma Knife radiosurgery for the treatment of cluster headache: a systematic review. *Neurosurg Rev.* 2022;45(3):1923-1931.

Primary Headaches

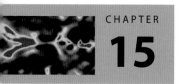

Other Trigeminal Autonomic Cephalalgias

Soma Sahai-Srivastava and Maksym S. Marek

Trigeminal autonomic cephalalgias (TACs) are primary headache disorders characterized by unilateral and usually side-locked headaches associated with ipsilateral cranial autonomic features. Cluster headache, a form of TAC, is discussed in Chapter 14. In this chapter, three other rare TACs, two of which, paroxysmal hemicrania (PH) and hemicrania continua (HC), are indomethacin-responsive headaches, are discussed. A comprehensive history and neurological examination, followed by brain imaging to exclude mimickers and structural pathology, are essential parts of the management of these patients. Imaging should include magnetic resonance imaging (MRI) of brain with emphasis on screening of the pituitary area, orbits, and trigeminal structures. In addition, MR angiogram or computed tomography (CT) angiogram of the head and neck vessels to exclude pathologies, such as dissection and aneurysm, are also essential parts of workup for these headaches.

Paroxysmal Hemicrania

Epidemiology

PH is a rare type of unilateral headache with a handful of case series reported in literature and with a poorly known prevalence and incidence. It is estimated that PH accounts for about 5% of all TACs. PH is an adult-onset disorder, with a slight female predominance. The estimated prevalence of PH is 1 per 50,000, with a female:male ratio of 2.36:1, mean age of onset of 34.1 ± 16.7 years (range 11-81 years), mean age at diagnosis at 47.4 ± 14.4 years (22-82 years).[1]

Pathophysiology

The pathophysiology of TACs, including PH, has not been completely elucidated. PH and other TAC syndromes such as cluster headache, short-lasting unilateral neuralgiform headache with conjunctival injection and tearing (SUNCT) and short-lasting unilateral neuralgiform headache attacks with cranial autonomic symptoms (SUNA), and HC are presumed to have similar mechanisms, centered around hypothalamic dysfunction and its downstream effects. Most of the studies have been done specifically with cluster headache (CH), demonstrating alterations in the trigeminal vascular, trigeminocervical, and trigemino-autonomic reflex systems along with dysfunction of the hypothalamic, pituitary, and nociceptive systems. Specific to PH, various clinical, genetic, biochemical, electrophysiological, and functional imaging studies have clarified components of its nebulous pathophysiology. There are limited genetic studies on PH and specific genetic markers have not been yet identified, though there are published case reports of family members who have PH.

Like other TACs, electrophysiological studies suggest that during PH attacks there is parasympathetic activation. The levels of both calcitonin gene-related peptide (CGRP), a vasodilator and neurotransmitter of trigeminal nociception, and vasoactive intestinal polypeptide (VIP), a substance associated with parasympathetic activation, were elevated in the cranial circulation during acute PH attacks and normalize after treatment with indomethacin.[2] In addition, positron emission tomography (PET) imaging studies demonstrated posterior hypothalamic activation on contralateral side in PH patients, a unique feature of PH compared to CH, which resolved in treated patients with indomethacin.[3]

Diagnosis and Clinical Presentation

The headache lasts 10 to 30 minutes but can range from 2 to 45 minutes. PH attacks occur at a high frequency, with more than five attacks per day. There is no clustering or preponderance of nocturnal attacks. There is a higher frequency and shorter duration of individual attacks compared to cluster headaches. Attacks are spontaneous, but on occasion can be precipitated by bending or movement of the head, or external pressure on the greater occipital nerve. Interictal discomfort or pain is present in up to 1/3 of patients. There are no reliable biomarkers for PH. The diagnosis of PH is based on the ICHD-3 (International Classification of Headache Disorders) criteria that include absolute response to indomethacin, either one or more of five autonomic symptoms or a sense of agitation and restlessness (Box 15-1). There is some overlap between PH and cluster headaches as in some cases of PH there is a circadian periodicity; however, unlike cluster headaches, 80% of PH is chronic. In addition, PH does not respond to oxygen as seen with cluster headache attacks, and cluster attacks do not respond to indomethacin. Although PH is considered an adult-onset disease, a recent study reported 35 children or adolescents with PH, with onset at age 1 to 14 years old and mean age of onset at 6.5 years. Attacks of pain were spontaneous with a complete response to indomethacin treatment. Pain was severe in intensity and left-sided attacks were more frequently reported than right-sided attacks.[4]

PH is further subdivided into episodic PH (EPH) and chronic PH (CPH), depending on the length of remission periods. Remission periods of at least 3 months in a year would classify the headache disorder as episodic. CPH is a rare, debilitating headache, with an estimated prevalence of 1%, occurring more often in females.

Treatment

Indomethacin

Response to indomethacin treatment is the *sine-qua-non* of PH and should be tried on all patients for diagnostic purposes. Initial dose of indomethacin is 25 mg three times a day for a week, followed

---

Box 15-1. ICHD-3 Diagnostic Criteria for Paroxysmal Hemicrania

Attacks of severe, strictly unilateral pain which is orbital, supraorbital, temporal, or in any combination of these sites, lasting 2-30 minutes and occurring several or many times a day. The attacks are usually associated with ipsilateral conjunctival injection, lacrimation, nasal congestion, rhinorrhea, forehead and facial sweating, miosis, ptosis, and/or eyelid edema. They respond absolutely to indomethacin:

A. At least 20 attacks fulfilling criteria B-E

B. Severe unilateral orbital, supraorbital, and/or temporal pain lasting 2-30 minutes

C. Either or both of the following: (1) at least one of the following symptoms or signs, ipsilateral to the headache: (a) conjunctival injection and/or lacrimation, (b) nasal congestion and/or rhinorrhea, (c) eyelid edema, (d) forehead and facial sweating, and (e) miosis and/or ptosis; (2) a sense of restlessness or agitation

D. Occurring with a frequency of >5 per day

E. Prevented absolutely by therapeutic doses of indomethacin

Primary Headaches

by 50 mg three times a day. Then dosing can be converted to once daily indomethacin of 75-mg control release for ease of use if the initial treatment trial is effective and tolerable. Response to treatment is seen quickly and provides dramatic relief. Complete resolution of the headache is expected within 1 to 3 days of initiating the effective dose. Stopping the medication results in reoccurrence of the headache. The maximum recommended dose of indomethacin is 200 mg per day. Intramuscular injections can also be given at the same doses and are the basis for the historical description of the INDOTEST which could provide a diagnosis in a single office visit. Indomethacin can cause gastric irritation, hemorrhage, or bleeding and should be taken with food. A proton pump inhibitor is routinely prescribed with the medication to prevent gastritis/ulcer formation. However, H2 blockers, misoprostol, and antacids can also be considered. Indomethacin should be avoided in patients with renal insufficiency, prior stroke, or myocardial infarction. If indomethacin use is contraindicated, unfortunately the diagnosis of PH cannot be firmly established. In patients with EPH, indomethacin should be given for longer than the typical headache episode and then gradually reduced over 1 to 3 months. In patients with CPH, long-term treatment is usually necessary but long-lasting remissions have been reported in some patients following cessation of indomethacin, and hence drug withdrawal is advised once every 6 months. In most pediatric patients with CPH, successful discontinuation of indomethacin can be achieved, though it may take multiple attempts to do so. The mechanism behind the absolute responsiveness to indomethacin is unknown and is a unique characteristic of this NSAID (nonsteroidal anti-inflammatory drug) since other medications in the same class do not have the same treatment effect. It is believed that indomethacin reduces the cerebral blood flow, thereby decreasing the load on the presumed phlebotic cavernous sinus, which results in a decline in cerebral permeability and cerebrospinal pressure. The anti-inflammatory effect of indomethacin on these vessels also has a role in aborting pain in CPH.[5]

Alternative Treatments

If indomethacin is not feasible treatment due to tolerability or contraindications, there is anecdotal evidence for other options. The evidence for these treatments is limited. There is some evidence for the use of Gliacin, a derivative of *Boswellia serrata* extract, in indomethacin-responsive headache syndromes. Other treatment options include verapamil, topiramate, celecoxib, gabapentin, acetazolamide, onabotulinumtoxin A, and dihydroergotamine (subcutaneous or intranasal). It has been reported that a patient with PH may respond to treatment with sumatriptan. In rare cases, a response to calcium-channel blockers such as nicardipine and flunarizine in patients with EPH has been demonstrated. Acetylsalicylic acid (and naproxen and diclofenac) and verapamil are the most effective drugs of second choice in CPH. More recently, response to noninvasive vagus nerve stimulation has been described.[6]

Hemicrania Continua

Epidemiology

Hemicrania continua (HC) is a rare type of TAC characterized by a continuous side-locked headache with absolute indomethacin-responsiveness. Like PH, a "complete" response to indomethacin is as *sine-qua-non* for HC. It is estimated that HC constitutes 1% to 2% of total headache patients in the clinical settings. HC is an adult-onset disorder typically in the fourth decade of life, with a slight female preponderance (1.8:1).[7]

Pathophysiology

The pathophysiology of this disease is thought to overlap with other TAC syndromes. The indomethacin-responsive nature of HC also raises the possibility that it has more in common from a biological basis with PH. On the other hand, since there is significant overlap of migraine-like symptoms, some have suggested that HC is a migraine variant. From a genetic standpoint, further overlap between migraine and HC has been suggested, where 74.5% of patients had episodic migraine or a migraine disorder prior to developing HC. A total of 67.5% of these patients also reported a family history notable for migraine.[8] Cases of PH evolving to CH, as well as CH cases reverting to PH have been described. PET imaging showed significant activation of the contralateral posterior hypothalamus and ipsilateral dorsal rostral pons in association with a flare of pain.[9] Activation of the posterior hypothalamus in these patients mirrors the clinical phenotype seen in other TAC disorders such as cluster headache and SUNCT. With the lack of robust biochemical, electrophysiologic, and clinical studies on HC pathophysiology, it is difficult to say whether activation of this hypothalamic nucleus is central to or a consequence of the underlying disease process. Activation of the dorsal rostral pons further points to an overlap with migraine pathophysiology as prior functional imaging demonstrated activation of the same brain stem area in patients with episodic and chronic migraine. The major distinction seen between HC and migraine was that in HC brainstem activation was seen on the ipsilateral side of attacks as opposed to migraine where it was seen on the contralateral side of attacks. Lastly, initial functional imaging done on HC patients also showed activation of the ipsilateral ventrolateral midbrain, demonstrating activation of the spinal trigeminal nucleus.[10] In general, various subcortical regions are implicated in HC pathophysiology, both overlapping with the processes seen in other TAC syndromes such as CH and migraine.

Diagnosis and Clinical Presentation

A continuous, background, dull side-locked pain is the hallmark of HC and pain is typically in the V1 distribution of trigeminal nerve, but V2/V3 and extra trigeminal areas have also been described. Rarely the pain of HC may shift sides. Toothache and jaw pain have also been described with the syndrome. Intermittent exacerbation of pain into sharp throbbing "jabs and jolts" is reported by most patients. The duration of exacerbations may last minutes to several weeks. Diurnal variations including nocturnal exacerbations have been reported. A foreign body sensation in the eye has also been reported during periods of exacerbation. Voice change and throat swelling have been proposed as additional parasympathetically mediated symptoms. The ICHD-3 diagnostic criteria add two more autonomic features to the previous list of five for PH—ipsilateral facial or forehead flushing and sensation of fullness in the ear (Box 15-2). Among the reported autonomic symptoms, the most common are conjunctival tearing and redness. Another interesting feature of the ICHD-3 diagnostic criteria is that in addition to a sense of restlessness or agitation, aggravation of pain by movement (a migraine diagnostic criterion) is part of the absolute diagnostic criteria. Migrainous features (nausea, vomiting, photophobia, and phonophobia) are quite common in patients with HC during exacerbations. The mean relative frequency of at least one migrainous feature has been reported to be as high as 60%. However, auras are not common.[10]

Treatment

Indomethacin

Response to indomethacin treatment is the *sine-qua-non* of HC and recommended to be tried on all patients for diagnostic purposes. The dosing and titration schedule is identical to the PH patients and side-effect concerns are therefore similar. Historically, injectable indomethacin of 50 to 100 mg, with a single intramuscular injection (the INDOTEST) has been used as a diagnostic test for HC. A complete response is usually noted within 2 hours of injection. Another important feature of HC is immediate reappearance of headache (within 6-24 hours) after skipping a dose.

Alternative Treatments

Various medications have been found effective in case reports and open-label studies. These include COX-2 inhibitors (celecoxib and rofecoxib) topiramate, melatonin, gabapentin, ibuprofen, piroxicam,

> ## Box 15-2. ICHD-3 Diagnostic Criteria for Hemicrania Continua
>
> Persistent, strictly unilateral headache, associated with ipsilateral conjunctival injection, lacrimation, nasal congestion, rhinorrhea, forehead and facial sweating, miosis, ptosis and/or eyelid edema, and/or with restlessness or agitation. The headache is absolutely sensitive to indomethacin:
>
> A. Unilateral headache fulfilling criteria B-D
>
> B. Present for >3 months, with exacerbations of moderate or greater intensity
>
> C. Either or both of the following:
>   1. at least one of the following symptoms or signs, ipsilateral to the headache:
>   - conjunctival injection and/or lacrimation
>   - nasal congestion and/or rhinorrhoea
>   - eyelid oedema
>   - forehead and facial sweating
>   - >miosis and/or ptosis
>   2. a sense of restlessness or agitation, or aggravation of the pain by movement
>
> D. Responds absolutely to therapeutic doses of indomethacin
>
> E. Not better accounted for by another ICHD-3 diagnosis.
>
> Unremitting subtype: continuous pain for at least 1 year, without remission periods of at least 24 hours. Unremitting HC can arise de novo (i.e., chronic from the onset) or may evolve from HC, remitting subtype. About 50-60% HC have the unremitting subtype from onset.
>
> Remitting subtype: the pain is not continuous but is interrupted by remission periods of at least 1 day. This constitutes 15-40% of total HC.

Headache Classification Committee of the International Headache Society (IHS). The International Classification of Headache Disorders, 3rd edition, (38(1)) 1–211. Copyright © 2018 by (International Headache Society). Reprinted by Permission of SAGE Publications.

naproxen, aspirin, verapamil, and steroids. Melatonin has also been reported to be effective in HC. More recently, there has been a report of HC responding to galcanezumab. Greater occipital or supraorbital nerve with anesthetic or steroids or a combination, done individually or in combination, may be effective in partial or total cessation of pain for 2 to 10 months. Other procedures that have been shown to be effective in individual cases include radiofrequency ablation of the superior optic nerve or the C2 ventral rami, sphenopalatine ganglion blocks or ablation, occipital nerve, or vagus nerve stimulation, and onabotulinumtoxinA.[6]

Short-Lasting Unilateral Neuralgiform Headache Attacks (SUNHA)

Epidemiology

The prevalence or incidence of SUNHA is not known. The extremely small number of reported cases suggests that it is an exceedingly rare syndrome. SUNHA has a male predominance with a sex ratio of 2:1 with the typical age of onset between 40 and 70 years.[11]

Pathophysiology

Research points to multiple theories regarding the pathophysiology of SUNCT/SUNA syndromes as the definite cause of these diseases has yet to be elucidated. Genetic, electrophysiologic, and biochemical studies are limited for SUNCT/SUNA, with most of the research being centered around clinical and functional neuroimaging studies. As is the case with other TAC syndromes, hypothalamic dysfunction is central to pathophysiology with an additional component of trigeminal nerve irritation playing a unique role in SUNCT/SUNA. Functional MRI (fMRI) imaging studies in SUNCT patients support the role of central disinhibition of the trigeminal-autonomic reflex that is also seen in other TAC syndromes such as CH. Using fMRI technology in a patient with SUNCT, the activation of the ipsilateral hypothalamic gray region during the pain state has been reported in patient with SUNCT.[12]

Secondary cases of SUNCT and SUNA have also been reported, suggesting that posterior fossa lesions could cause classical symptoms. Vascular malformations such as arteriovenous malformations, vascular loops, and cavernous hemangiomas have been implicated with SUNHA. Other causes include white matter lesions (such as those in neuromyelitis optica), infection (i.e., HSV/VZV), neoplasms (i.e., CNS multiple myeloma, meningioma), and bone abnormalities. Facial nerve compression has also been implicated with the disorder. Specifically, there are case reports of patients with SUNCT/SUNA having vascular loop compression of the ipsilateral trigeminal nerve that demonstrate improvement in symptomology after surgical decompression or nerve ablation. This theory has been further supported by cross-sectional MRI studies demonstrating the presence of neurovascular contact with morphological changes that correlate highly with the laterality of symptoms. Specific to this disease, high rates of both vascular loop compression and pituitary abnormalities have been reported, and as a result, it is recommended patients with this syndrome are to be investigated with brain MRI.

Diagnosis and Clinical Presentation

SUNHA is unique due to the noticeably short, severe unilateral orbital/periorbital pain attacks, lasting seconds with dramatically intense conjunctival injection and/or tearing (Boxes 15-3a, 3b, and 3c). Pain is maximal in the distribution of the trigeminal nerve; individual attacks are very brief lasting 5 to 250 seconds and start and stop abruptly. These attacks are very frequent often hundreds of times in a day, and are extremely painful and debilitating, and can lead to depression, anticipation anxiety, and even suicidal ideation. Attacks can be precipitated by triggers including touching the face, eating, chewing, brushing teeth, talking, and coughing. Neck movements can also precipitate attacks.

Features that distinguish this syndrome from others in the category are very brief duration of attacks that can occur very frequently with the presence of prominent conjunctival injection and lacrimation. Patients are completely pain free between attacks. Most attacks occur throughout the day with some morning and afternoon predominance, but nighttime attacks are not reported. Unlike PH and HC, restlessness is not a feature of SUNHA. Migraine-like symptoms including nausea, vomiting, photophobia, and phonophobia are not associated with SUNHA. SUNHA can be confused with primary stabbing headache in which there is a female preponderance, and the site and radiation of pain varies between attacks. In primary stabbing headache, cranial autonomic features are absent, and it is an indomethacin-responsive headache, which distinguishes it from SUNHA. Trigeminal neuralgia shares significant demographic and clinical characteristics with SUNHA making the two conditions difficult to distinguish from one another; yet it also suggests a possible unifying pathophysiologic mechanism. Differentiating features of SUNHA from trigeminal neuralgia include maximal pain in the ophthalmic division of the trigeminal nerve (V1), association of autonomic features (particularly lacrimation) with pain attacks, absence of a refractory period after attacks, and the presence of a constant, background of pain ipsilateral to attack.

Treatment

Treatment for SUNCT and SUNA is centered around preventative therapy as attacks seen in these diseases are too short to target with acute medications. Response to medical treatment often is variable and does not result in complete resolution of symptoms. Published data shows that lamotrigine as a prophylactic and parenteral lidocaine as transitional treatment are the therapies of choice for SUNHA. Lamotrigine 100 to 200 mg daily may induce complete remission of pain. Next line of

Box 15-3a. ICHD-3 Diagnostic Criteria for Short-Lasting Unilateral Neuralgiform Headache Attacks

Attacks of moderate or severe, strictly unilateral head pain lasting seconds to minutes, occurring at least once a day and usually associated with prominent lacrimation and redness of the ipsilateral eye:

A. At least 20 attacks fulfilling criteria B-D

B. Moderate or severe unilateral head pain, with orbital, supraorbital, temporal, and/or other trigeminal distribution, lasting for 1-600 seconds and occurring as single stabs, series of stabs, or in a saw-tooth pattern

C. At least one of the following five cranial autonomic symptoms or signs, ipsilateral to the pain:
   1. conjunctival injection and/or lacrimation
   2. nasal congestion and/or rhinorrhoea
   3. eyelid oedema
   4. forehead and facial sweating
   5. forehead and facial flushing
   6. sensation of fullness in the ear
   7. miosis and/or ptosis

D. Occurring with a frequency of at least once a day

E. Not better accounted for by another ICHD-3 diagnosis

Headache Classification Committee of the International Headache Society (IHS). The International Classification of Headache Disorders, 3rd edition, (38(1)) 1–211. Copyright © 2018 by (International Headache Society). Reprinted by Permission of SAGE Publications.

Box 15-3b. ICHD-3 Diagnostic Criteria for Short-Lasting Neuralgiform Pain with Conjunctival Injection and Tearing (SUNCT)

Attacks of moderate or severe, strictly unilateral head pain lasting seconds to minutes, occurring at least once a day, and usually associated with prominent lacrimation and redness of the ipsilateral eye:

A. Attacks fulfilling criteria for short-lasting unilateral neuralgiform headache attacks and criterion B below

B. Both of the following, ipsilateral to the pain:
   1. Conjunctival injection
   2. Lacrimation (tearing)

Chronic SUNCT: Attacks of SUNCT occurring for more than 1 year without remission, or with remission periods lasting less than 3 months

Headache Classification Committee of the International Headache Society (IHS). The International Classification of Headache Disorders, 3rd edition, (38(1)) 1–211. Copyright © 2018 by (International Headache Society). Reprinted by Permission of SAGE Publications.

medication are carbamazepine, oxcarbazepine, gabapentin, pregabalin, topiramate, duloxetine, and mexiletine. Gabapentin at high doses, 1800 to 2700 milligrams daily, has also been shown to be effective. The optimal dose of topiramate for the treatment of SUNHA is unknown, typical starting dose is 15 to 25 mg daily increased by 25 mg every 2 weeks to a target dose of 100 mg, increasing up to 400 mg total daily if needed.[13]

> **Box 15-3c.** ICHD-3 Diagnostic Criteria for Short-Lasting Unilateral Neuralgiform Headache Attacks with Cranial Autonomic Symptoms (SUNA)
>
> Attacks of moderate or severe, strictly unilateral head pain lasting seconds to minutes, occurring at least once a day, and usually associated with prominent lacrimation and redness of the ipsilateral eye:
>
> A. Attacks fulfilling criteria for short-lasting unilateral neuralgiform headache attacks and criterion B below
>
> B. Only one or neither of conjunctival injection and lacrimation (tearing)
>
> Chronic SUNA: Attacks occurring for more than 1 year without remission, or with remission periods lasting less than 3 months

Headache Classification Committee of the International Headache Society (IHS). The International Classification of Headache Disorders, 3rd edition, (38(1)) 1–211. Copyright © 2018 by (International Headache Society). Reprinted by Permission of SAGE Publications.

Primary Headaches

Refractory cases can be difficult to manage, and previous publications have reported that intravenous lidocaine could be useful for these patients. Safe administration of this medication requires continuous telemetry given the risk of cardiac arrhythmias with infusion. Additional treatments reported with some benefits include peripheral pericranial nerve blocks with local anesthetics and serial sphenopalatine ganglion blocks. Several surgical approaches including Janetta procedure, percutaneous trigeminal ganglion compression, and local opioid block of the superior cervical ganglion, may provide transient or temporary relief.[14]

Summary

- PH, a rare type of TAC, is an indomethacin-responsive, unilateral side-locked headache lasting 2 to 30 minutes.
- HC is a rare type of TAC, with a continuous, dull unilateral side-locked pain, that is exquisitely responsive to indomethacin, which can be considered in any migraine patients with side-locked pain; not responsive to usual treatment.
- SUNHA which includes SUNCT and SUNA is the rarest of the TACs, with unilateral sharp shooting pain lasting just seconds and with the maximum number of daily episodes of all TACs along with dramatic autonomic symptoms.
- Treatment of SUNHA is limited and migraine-related medication approaches can used.

REFERENCES

1. Osman C, Bahra A. Paroxysmal hemicrania. *Ann Indian Acad Neurol.* 2018;21(Suppl 1):S16-S22.
2. Goadsby PJ, Edvinsson L. Neuropeptide changes in a case of chronic paroxysmal hemicrania—evidence for trigemino-parasympathetic activation. *Cephalalgia.* 1996;16(6):448-450.
3. Matharu MS, Cohen AS, Frackowiak RS, Goadsby PJ. Posterior hypothalamic activation in paroxysmal hemicrania. *Ann Neurol.* 2006;59:535-545.
4. Matharu MS, Goadsby PJ. Trigeminal autonomic cephalgias. *J Neurol Neurosurg Psychiatry.* 2002;72(Suppl 2):ii19-ii26.
5. Antonaci F, Sjaastad O. Chronic paroxysmal hemicrania (CPH): a review of the clinical manifestations. *Headache.* 1989;29(10):648-656.
6. Baraldi C, Pellesi L, Guerzoni S, et al. Therapeutical approaches to paroxysmal hemicrania, hemicrania continua and short lasting unilateral neuralgiform headache attacks: a critical appraisal. *J Headache Pain.* 2017;18(1):71.
7. Prakash S, Adroja B. Hemicrania continua. *Ann Indian Acad Neurol.* 2018;21(Suppl 1):S23-S30.
8. Karsan N, Nagaraj K, Goadsby PJ. Cranial autonomic symptoms: prevalence, phenotype and

laterality in migraine and two potentially new symptoms. *J Headache Pain.* 2022;23(1):18.

9. Wheeler SD, Allen KF, Pusey T. Is hemicrania continua a migraine variant? *Cephalalgia.* 2001;21:508.

10. Matharu MS, Cohen AS, McGonigle DJ, et al. Posterior hypothalamic and brainstem activation in hemicrania continua. *Headache.* 2004;44(8):747-761.

11. Matharu MS, Cohen AS, Boes CJ, et al. Short-lasting unilateral neuralgiform headache with conjunctival injection and tearing syndrome: a review. *Curr Pain Headache Rep.* 2003;7(4):308-318.

12. May A, Bahra A, Buchel C, et al. Functional MRI in spontaneous attacks of SUNCT: short-lasting neuralgiform headache with conjunctival injection and tearing. *Ann Neurol.* 1999;46:791-793.

13. Lambru G, Stubberud A, Rantell K, Lagrata S, Tronvik E, Matharu MS. Medical treatment of SUNCT and SUNA: a prospective open-label study including single-arm meta-analysis. *J Neurol Neurosurg Psychiatry.* 2021;92(3):233-241.

14. Sahai-Srivastava S, Gjurgevich A, Lee P. Sphenopalatine ganglion block for the treatment of SUNCT syndrome in a geriatric patient. *Headache.* 2020;60(S1):157-207.

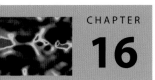

CHAPTER

16

New Daily Persistent Headache

Nada Hindiyeh

New daily persistent headache (NDPH) is a primary headache disorder which can be challenging for both the patient and the clinician. In some cases, it may be refractory to treatment. First described as a benign self-remitting daily headache, the defining criteria have since evolved to highlight its sudden onset and persistence.

Epidemiology

NDPH is considered a rare disorder. The 1-year prevalence of 0.1% using the original Silberstein-Lipton diagnostic criteria has been reported.[1] When using the *International Classification of Headache Disorders,* second edition (ICHD-2) criteria, the 1-year prevalence of 0.03% was estimated.[1] These numbers are expected to increase with the less restrictive ICHD-3 criteria. NDPH is slightly more common in women than men, with some studies reporting a female-to-male ratio of 1.3 to 2.5:1. The mean age of onset in adults is approximately 32 years in women and 36 years in men.

Pathophysiology

The exact pathophysiology of NDPH remains unknown, and few studies have elucidated the underlying biology of the disorder.[1] Nearly half of patients with NDPH report a precipitating flu-like illness and there is some evidence to suggest an association most commonly with Epstein-Barr virus (EBV) infection, but other infections such as recent herpes simplex virus (HSV) and cytomegalovirus (CMV) as well as others have been implicated. It is suggested that chronic central nervous system inflammation and release of proinflammatory cytokines, like tumor necrosis factor (TNF)-α, may be involved in NDPH pathogenesis.

Diagnosis and Clinical Presentation

The ICHD-3 characterizes NDPH as a daily and persistent headache within 24 hours from its clearly remembered onset for at least 3 months (Box 16-1).[1-3] The headache itself may resemble a migraine or tension-type headache (TTH). If persistent for less than 3 months, the diagnosis of probable NDPH is given. Two subtypes of NDPH are described, a self-limiting subtype that generally resolves within months without therapy, and a treatment-resistant, refractory subtype. People with NDPH are able to identify the month, week, and often exact day their headache started. The majority do not have a prior headache history,

> **Box 16-1.** ICHD-3 Diagnostic Criteria for New Daily Persistent Headache
>
> Persistent headache, daily from its onset, which is clearly remembered. The pain lacks characteristic features, and may be migraine-like or tension-type-like, or have elements of both.
>
> A. Persistent headache fulfilling criteria B and C.
>
> B. Distinct and clearly remembered onset, with pain becoming continuous and unremitting within 24 hours.
>
> C. Present for >3 months
>
> D. Not better accounted for by another ICHD-3 diagnosis

although a history of migraine, TTH, or other primary headache disorder does not exclude the development and diagnosis of NDPH. The headache is more commonly bilateral or biocciptal in location but can be temporal, ocular, or holocephalic. Intensity is generally moderate, although can range from mild to severe and can remain constant or fluctuate. Migrainous features such as photophobia, phonophobia, nausea, and vomiting are common in people with NDPH, especially in those with a family history of migraine. Approximately 47% may report a precipitating event with flu-like illness as the most common in 22%, stressful life events in 9%, surgical procedure with intubation in 9%, and 7% may report other events such as syncope, cervical massage, and hormones.[4] Comorbid mood disorders are common in people with NDPH, with 65% experiencing severe anxiety and 40% experiencing severe depression.[5] Other comorbid symptoms include insomnia, light-headedness, vertigo, paresthesias, and fatigue. NDPH is considered a diagnosis of exclusion, and most who reach a headache specialist have endured symptoms for over 3 months, with a prior workup to identify secondary causes of sudden onset headache (Chapters 1-3). A thorough evaluation for intracranial hypotension or hypertension as well as vascular disorders such as venous sinus thrombosis, reversible cerebral vasoconstrictive syndrome (RCVS), cranial artery dissection should be done. Other possible secondary causes of headache including cervicogenic headache, hemicrania continua, post-traumatic headache, meningitis, and sphenoid sinusitis should be excluded. All patients should undergo an MRI brain with contrast and MR venogram, and MR or CT angiography if warranted. Lumbar puncture can be considered in treatment-refractory cases and viral titers can be considered in select patients.

Treatment

There have been no randomized controlled prospective treatment studies in NDPH, and it is generally treated based on the primary headache phenotype it most closely resembles, migraine or TTH (Chapters 7, 8, and 13). Both acute and preventive strategies are used to try to stop the pain, and decrease the severity and possibly frequency of pain over time.

A small study of postinfectious NDPH patients found some benefit from 5 days of intravenous (IV) methylprednisolone followed by 2 to 3 weeks of oral steroids.[1] Another small study of NDPH patients reported improvement with IV lidocaine, while a small retrospective study reported benefit from subtherapeutic doses of IV ketamine.[1] Another study found a combination of IV methylprednisolone, IV sodium valproate an antidepressant (amitriptyline or dothiepin), and naproxen for 3 to 6 months to be helpful for some patients.[1] Nerve blocks with anesthetic and or steroid injected in painful areas have been reported to be helpful and beneficial as well.

As previously mentioned, no randomized controlled trials have been done on patients with NDPH, but a few small studies have reported benefits from certain medications. A small study reported doxycycline, a tetracycline derivative and a TNF-α receptor blocker, was beneficial in patients with elevated CSF levels.[1] Other case reports of therapeutic targets of inflammation and glial activation suggested the addition of montelukast to doxycycline or minocycline to have beneficial effects. There has also been a favorable outcome reported to either topiramate or gabapentin. Likewise, a few case reports have shown onabotulinumtoxinA to be helpful, ranging from partial to full relief. It is also important to consider behavioral interventions in combination with pharmacological treatment, especially in those with comorbid mood disorders.

Prognosis

In patients with the self-remitting subtype of NDPH, the headache resolves within months, with a median duration of 21 months.[6] In those with the refractory form of NDPH, the prognosis, although still not fully known, remains guarded, given its nature as a treatment-resistant headache disorder. For many this subtype of NDPH can persist over several years, or decades. There is some evidence to suggest that earlier treatment of NDPH, within 3 to 12 months, does confer a better response to treatment.[1]

Summary

- NDPH is a rare and refractory primary headache disorder known for its debilitating impact and resistance to treatment.

- NDPH presents as a daily and persistent headache within 24 hours of onset and can share phenotypic similarities with migraine or tension-type headache.

- The underlying pathophysiology of NDPH remains poorly understood, but it is suggested that viral illness and the release of proinflammatory cytokines could be potential contributing factors.

- Treatment of NDPH, both acute and preventive, is based on the specific phenotypic characteristics of the headache.

REFERENCES

1. Yamani N, Olesen J. New daily persistent headache: a systematic review on an enigmatic disorder. *J Headache Pain.* 2019;20:80.
2. Headache Classification Committee of the International Headache Society (IHS). *The International Classification of Headache Disorders,* 3rd edition. *Cephalalgia.* 2018;38:1-211.
3. Peng KP, Wang SJ. Update of new daily persistent headache. *Curr Pain Headache Rep.* 2022;26:79-84.
4. Rozen TD. Triggering events and new daily persistent headache: age and gender differences and insights on pathogenesis: a clinic-based study. *Headache.* 2016;56:164-173.
5. Uniyal R, Paliwal VK, Tripathi A. Psychiatric comorbidity in new daily persistent headache: a cross-sectional study. *Eur J Pain.* 2017;21:1031-1038.
6. Robbins MS, Grosberg BM, Napchan U, Crystal SC, Lipton RB. Clinical and prognostic subforms of new daily-persistent headache. *Neurology.* 2010;74:1358-1364.

Primary Headaches

Other Primary Headaches

Lauren R. Natbony

The category of other primary headache disorders encompasses a diverse group of highly recognizable headache disorders that require specific evaluation and management. These disorders can be classified into four categories:

1. Headaches associated with physical exertion, such as primary exercise headache and primary headache associated with sexual activity
2. Headaches attributed to direct physical stimuli
3. Epicranial headaches, including primary stabbing headache and nummular headache
4. Other miscellaneous headache disorders, including hypnic headache

The most prevalent disorders within this group are discussed in this chapter. The pathogenesis of these disorders remains poorly understood, and their treatments are often based on anecdotal reports or uncontrolled trials. Importantly, these headaches can be symptomatic of structural lesions or other underlying disorders, necessitating neuroimaging evaluation at the onset of symptoms.

Primary Exercise Headache

Primary exercise headache is characterized by the onset of headache during or after exercise, without the presence of an underlying intracranial disorder. Its presentation can be nonspecific, leading to confusion with other primary and secondary headache disorders, resulting in inadequate treatment.

Epidemiology

Primary exercise headache predominantly affects individuals aged 10 to 48 years, with estimated prevalence ranging from 1% to 26%.[1] Gender estimates vary, with a higher prevalence in females than males.[2] It is commonly observed in patients with a personal and/or family history of migraine.

Pathophysiology

The pathophysiological mechanisms responsible for primary exercise headache are not fully understood. It is suggested to have a vascular origin, with the hypothesis that pain is induced by venous or arterial distension secondary to physical exercise. Individuals with primary exercise headache exhibit a higher prevalence of internal jugular venous valve incompetence, suggesting a potential role of intracranial venous congestion due to retrograde jugular venous flow in the pathophysiology of this disorder.[2]

Diagnosis and Clinical Characteristics

The diagnosis of primary exercise headache requires the presence of at least two episodes, triggered by and occurring during or after intense physical activity, with pain lasting less than 48 hours.[3] Typically, any sustained, physically strenuous exercise can precipitate the headache, which commonly occurs at the peak of exercise (within 30 minutes of onset) and diminishes upon cessation of activity. The quality of pain is typically described as aching, pounding, or throbbing, and accompanying features like nausea, vomiting, photophobia, and phonophobia may be present but with lower frequencies than observed in migraine. Approximately 60% of cases manifest bilaterally.[1] Primary exercise headache is frequently observed in hot weather or at high altitudes.

It is important to recognize that primary exercise headache is a separate entity from exercise-induced migraine. In about 50% of patients, primary exercise headache is comorbid with migraine, which may also be triggered by exercise. Primary exercise headache is primarily precipitated by sustained strenuous exertion (e.g., weightlifting) and typically exhibits a shorter duration.[4] Moreover, it generally lacks the typical features associated with migraine except for the throbbing pain character. On the first occurrence of headache with these characteristics, excluding symptomatic causes of exercise headache, including subarachnoid hemorrhage, arterial dissection, and reversible cerebral vasoconstriction syndrome with neurovascular imaging is mandatory. In patients with multiple vascular risk factors, consideration should be given to cardiac cephalalgia.[2]

Treatment

Treatment of exercise-induced headaches typically focuses on prophylactic or preventative measures when the exercise is predictable. In cases of mild symptoms or infrequent occurrences, the initial recommendation may involve temporary exercise moderation or refraining from exercise altogether. Some reports suggest using pre-emptive ergotamine tartrate, which has shown success in certain cases.[5] Indomethacin has been found effective when administered 30 to 60 minutes before exercise.[2] For prevention, beta-blockers such as propranolol and nadolol have been found to be effective.[1]

Prognosis

For unknown reasons, primary exercise headache usually presents as a self-limited disorder in most patients.[2] Thus, preventative treatment can generally be discontinued after 3 to 12 months to assess if headaches reappear.

Headache Associated with Sexual Activity

Primary headache associated with sexual activity is often classified as a subtype of primary exercise headache due to the potential coexistence of these disorders and the similarity in their management approaches. In addition, both conditions commonly show comorbidity with migraine. It is worth noting that primary headache associated with sexual activity is relatively rare, representing an uncommon headache disorder overall.

Epidemiology

Primary headache associated with sexual activity has a prevalence of approximately 1% in the general population and can occur at any sexually active age.[2] It is observed to be more common in males, with male-to-female ratios ranging from 1.2:1 to 4:1. Typically, patients affected by this type of headache fall within the age range of 20 to 45 years.[6]

Pathophysiology

The exact pathophysiology of primary headache associated with sexual activity remains unknown, although hemodynamic factors are thought to be contributory. When compared to healthy individuals

Primary Headaches

and those with migraine, patients experiencing headaches associated with sexual activity demonstrate a more pronounced increase in systemic blood pressure during exercise. Administration of acetazolamide to these patients results in greater increases in cerebral blood flow velocity, indicating abnormal neurovascular coupling. These observations suggest that hemodynamic dysregulation may contribute to the development of this type of headache.[1]

Diagnosis and Clinical Characteristics

Headache triggered by sexual activity occurs specifically during sexual activity and can be associated with or independent of intercourse or orgasm. The frequency of headaches is typically correlated with the frequency of sexual activity. To meet the diagnostic criteria for this disorder, there should be an escalation in pain intensity with increased sexual activity and/or a sudden, intense headache occurring just before or after orgasm. The duration of severe pain can range from 1 minute to 24 hours, with the possibility of lingering mild pain for up to 72 hours. Most cases do not exhibit autonomic or migrainous symptoms. Two-thirds of patients experience bilateral headaches, with around 80% of cases located occipitally or presenting as a diffuse pattern.[3] If a patient presents with a new onset of headache associated with sexual activity, immediate evaluation should be considered to rule out subarachnoid hemorrhage using CT scan, followed by lumbar puncture if the CT is normal. Vascular imaging should be pursued to exclude conditions such as arterial dissection, intracranial aneurysm, and reversible cerebral vasoconstriction syndrome (RCVS). In cases where there are multiple explosive headaches during sexual activity, headache attributed to RCVS should be considered until proven otherwise.[2]

Treatment

The management approach for headache associated with sexual activity is similar to that of exertional headache. Once secondary causes are excluded, patients should be reassured of the benign and typically self-limited natural course. Nonpharmacologic management by assuming a more passive position during sexual activity may also reduce the incidence or severity of attacks. The preferred preventive option is indomethacin or triptans, such as sumatriptan, administered 30 to 60 minutes before sexual activity. In cases of frequent attacks, propranolol or indomethacin (or both) may be used daily for prevention.[5,7]

Prognosis

The prognosis of headache associated with sexual activity is relatively good. Like primary exercise headache, primary headache associated with sexual activity may have a self-limited course. In the majority, the headache appears in a bout and remits. Others may experience a relapsing-remitting course in which they are susceptible to headache for two or so months at a time. More studies have shown that up to 40% of all cases run a chronic course over more than a year.[7]

Primary Stabbing Headache

Primary stabbing headache, previously known as icepick headache or jabs and jolts syndrome, is characterized by brief, irregular stabs of pain that can last for a few seconds. The frequency of these episodes can vary. This type of headache is believed to be relatively common in the general population but often goes underestimated or undiagnosed.

Epidemiology

Estimating the prevalence of primary stabbing headache is challenging, as it has varied widely in different studies, ranging from 1% to 35% of the general population. It is more commonly observed in women, with a female-to-male ratio of 3:1, and it typically emerges after adolescence.[2] Primary stabbing headache often coexists with other primary headache disorders, with approximately 42% of individuals with migraine experiencing this type of headache.[8] In such cases, the stabbing pain is typically localized to the area habitually affected by migraines.

Pathophysiology

The exact pathophysiology of primary stabbing headache remains unknown. Various theories have been proposed, including the irritation of trigeminal and extratrigeminal nerves and intermittent impairment of central pain processing.[9] A vascular mechanism has been suggested due to the increased incidence of primary stabbing headache in individuals with migraines. In addition, associations have been observed between primary stabbing headache and autoimmune disorders in specific case series.[8]

Diagnosis and Clinical Characteristics

Clinically, patients with primary stabbing headache describe transient and localized stabs of pain in the head that occur spontaneously as singular stabs or in a series. Each stab typically lasts a few seconds, making it the shortest duration among known headache disorders. The frequency of stabs varies irregularly, ranging from one to multiple occurrences per day. Notably, there are no accompanying cranial autonomic symptoms or triggers on the skin.[3]

In 70% of cases, the pain extends beyond trigeminal regions and involves extratrigeminal areas. It may move from one area to another within the same or the opposite hemicranium. Only about one-third of patients experience pain in a fixed location.[9] However, when stabs are strictly localized to a particular area, structural changes in that region and the affected cranial nerve distribution must be ruled out through neuroimaging. While most cases of primary stabbing headache are idiopathic, adults experiencing new-onset primary stabbing headache should undergo a diagnostic evaluation to exclude secondary causes. The need for neuroimaging depends on the presence of headache red flags (Chapter 1). Short stabs of pain have been associated with intracranial lesions like pituitary tumors or meningiomas, the onset of herpes zoster, cranial trauma, and acute glaucoma.[2]

Treatment

Primary stabbing headache may show improvement when a coexisting primary headache disorder, such as migraine, is effectively treated. However, independent treatment specifically for primary stabbing headache is primarily based on anecdotal evidence from uncontrolled clinical series. Indomethacin has been reported as an effective option in some cases. Additionally, a few isolated cases have shown benefits with the use of melatonin, gabapentin, and celecoxib. It is important to note that the evidence for these treatments is limited, and individual responses may vary.

Prognosis

Primary stabbing headache typically has a benign course, characterized by short durations of pain and infrequent attacks that may remit with time. It usually doesn't require pharmacologic treatment.

Nummular Headache

Nummular headache, or coin-shaped headache, is a rare headache disorder that presents with continuous or intermittent head pain in a small, circumscribed area of the scalp without any underlying structural lesion.[3]

Epidemiology

The exact prevalence of nummular headache is uncertain. In one prospective study conducted at a neurology specialty clinic, 14 patients were diagnosed with nummular headache within a 1-year period.[10] In one hospital series, the estimated incidence of nummular headache was 6.4 per 100,000 per year.[2] Nummular headache appears more common in middle-aged women, with a mean onset of 45 years. About half of the patients have a preexisting headache diagnosis, most commonly migraine.[2]

Pathophysiology

The exact mechanism for nummular headache remains unclear. The sharply delineated borders of the painful area suggest a peripheral origin. Proposed mechanisms include neuropathy affecting a terminal branch of a cutaneous scalp nerve and localized nociceptive pain originating from epicranial tissues. However, a central mechanism cannot be ruled out.[11]

Diagnosis and Clinical Characteristics

Nummular headache is characterized by distinct clinical features. The painful area is sharply defined, maintaining a fixed size and shape, typically round or elliptical, with a 1 to 6 cm diameter. While the pain can occur anywhere on the scalp, it is commonly localized in the parietal region. The symptomatic area remains consistent in shape and size over time. Pain intensity is generally mild to moderate, occasionally reaching severe levels. The duration of pain can vary significantly, with most cases being chronic (lasting over 3 months). Exacerbations of pain can occur spontaneously or in response to triggers. The affected area may exhibit varying combinations of hypesthesia, dysesthesia, paresthesia, tenderness, and discomfort during both symptomatic and asymptomatic periods.[3,11] The differential diagnosis of nummular headache includes secondary headaches due to underlying structural lesions to the scalp, skull, or adjacent intracranial structures, such as those caused by metastatic cancer, multiple myeloma, Paget disease of the bone, or meningiomas.[2] Therefore, neuroimaging, such as a CT scan of the head or an MRI of the brain, should be performed.

Treatment

Treatment approaches for nummular headache lack consensus. Considering the potential neuropathic nature of the pain, medications such as gabapentin and other antiepileptic drugs, as well as amitriptyline, have been utilized. Case reports have shown positive outcomes with indomethacin and other nonsteroidal anti-inflammatory drugs (NSAIDs), transcutaneous electrical nerve stimulation (TENS), and onabotulinumtoxinA. Nerve blocks may also offer benefits for certain individuals.[2]

Prognosis

The prognosis of nummular headache varies among individuals. While some patients experience spontaneous remission of symptoms, the pain more often becomes resistant to preventive and pain-relieving treatments.

Hypnic Headache

Hypnic headache was initially described in 1988. It is a recurrent headache disorder occurring specifically during sleep and often starting at the same time of the night.[2] Aptly nicknamed "alarm clock headache," this recurrent and time-dependent pattern is truly pathognomonic.

Epidemiology

The exact prevalence of hypnic headache in the general population is unknown, although it is generally believed to be rare, even among patients at specialized headache centers, with estimates ranging from 0.07% to 0.35%. Hypnic headache appears to be more common in females, occurring about 1.5 times more frequently, and typically affects adults over the age of 50. However, it can also occur in younger individuals, including children.[2]

Pathophysiology

The underlying pathophysiology of hypnic headache has not been fully understood, although an MRI study with voxel-based morphometry (VBM) has reported a decrease in posterior hypothalamus gray matter.[12] The characteristic clinical picture of chronobiological abnormality in addition to pain suggests impairments of pain sensation and sleep rhythm at the trigeminal nerve in the hypothalamic-pituitary system.

Diagnosis and Clinical Characteristics

Hypnic headache is characterized by recurring attacks that specifically occur during sleep, leading to awakening. The duration of the headache can range from 15 minutes up to 4 hours after waking. While it typically arises at night during sleep, in some cases, it can also happen during a nap, although this is less common. The intensity of the headache is usually mild to moderate, but approximately 34% of cases may experience severe pain.[2] The location of the pain is not specific, with about two-thirds of cases reporting bilateral involvement, primarily in the frontotemporal or diffuse holocranial regions. To meet the diagnostic criteria, the attacks must occur on at least 10 days per month for more than 3 months. Some patients may experience multiple attacks per night.[3] Unlike cluster headache, hypnic headache does not present with cranial autonomic symptoms or restlessness. It is important to rule out other potential causes of headaches that develop during sleep and lead to awakening. This includes intracranial hypertension, nocturnal hypertension, sleep disorders like sleep apnea, hypoglycemia, medication-overuse headache (where analgesic withdrawal occurs during sleeping hours), and cervicogenic headache. To differentiate hypnic headache from cluster headache and hemicrania continua, it is important to assess for the presence of autonomic features and restlessness/agitation.

Treatment

There are no controlled trials for the treatment of hypnic headache. Caffeine is commonly used as an acute treatment and preventive measure. Consuming a cup of coffee when awakened by pain or before going to sleep is an effective initial approach. In terms of prophylactic treatment, lithium is usually effective, while topiramate, indomethacin, and melatonin have been effective treatments in several reported cases.[2]

Prognosis

Spontaneous remission can occur in some cases of hypnic headache, while others may experience remission with treatment but later relapse. Considering the potential for remission after treatment, periodic trials of discontinuing preventive measures can be justified as a management approach.

Summary

- Diagnosing primary exercise headache, headache associated with sexual activity, primary stabbing headache, nummular headache, and hypnic headaches can pose challenges, typically necessitating neuroimaging to exclude structural lesions.
- Primary exercise headache and primary headache associated with sexual activity may coexist and share similar management strategies, with both conditions having the potential for comorbidity with migraine.
- Multiple explosive headaches occurring during sexual activities should be regarded as headaches attributed to reversible cerebral vasoconstriction syndrome (RCVS) unless proven otherwise.

Primary Headaches

• Primary stabbing headache, characterized by brief, irregular "jabs and jolts," is commonly observed in individuals with migraine and has the shortest duration among all headache disorders.

• When pain is localized to a single round or oval-shaped area on the scalp that remains constant in size and shape, consider the possibility of a nummular headache.

• Hypnic headache, characterized by recurrent and time-dependent episodes during sleep, is the sole headache disorder for which caffeine has been found to have preventive effects.

REFERENCES

1. Pascual J, Gonzalez-Mandly A, Martin R, Oterino A. Headaches precipitated by cough, prolonged exercise or sexual activity: a prospective etiological and clinical study. *J Headache Pain.* 2008;9(5): 259-266.

2. Gonzalez-Quintanilla V, Pascual J. Other primary headaches: an update. *Neurol Clin.* 2019;37(4): 871-891.

3. Headache Classification Committee of the International Headache Society (IHS). *The International Classification of Headache Disorders,* 3rd edition. *Cephalalgia.* 2018;38(1):1-211.

4. Sjaastad O, Bakketeig LS. Exertional headache. I. Vaga study of headache epidemiology. *Cephalalgia.* 2002;22(10):784-790.

5. Pascual J, Iglesias F, Oterino A, Vazquez-Barquero A, Berciano J. Cough, exertional, and sexual headaches: an analysis of 72 benign and symptomatic cases. *Neurology.* 1996;46(6):1520-1524.

6. Frese A, Eikermann A, Frese K, Schwaag S, Husstedt IW, Evers S. Headache associated with sexual activity: demography, clinical features, and comorbidity. *Neurology.* 2003;61(6):796-800.

7. Frese A, Rahmann A, Gregor N, Biehl K, Husstedt IW, Evers S. Headache associated with sexual activity: prognosis and treatment options. *Cephalalgia.* 2007;27(11):1265-1270.

8. Robbins MS, Evans RW. Primary and secondary stabbing headache. *Headache.* 2015;55(4):565-570.

9. Fuh JL, Kuo KH, Wang SJ. Primary stabbing headache in a headache clinic. *Cephalalgia.* 2007;27(9): 1005-1009.

10. Pareja JA, Pareja J, Barriga FJ, et al. Nummular headache: a prospective series of 14 new cases. *Headache.* 2004;44(6):611-614.

11. Schwartz DP, Robbins MS, Grosberg BM. Nummular headache update. *Curr Pain Headache Rep.* 2013;17(6):340.

12. Holle D, Naegel S, Krebs S, et al. Hypothalamic gray matter volume loss in hypnic headache. *Ann Neurol.* 2011;69(3):533-539.

Secondary Headaches

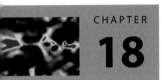

CHAPTER

18

Post-traumatic Headache

Roberto De Icco, Hakan Ashina, Federico Bighiani, and Todd J. Schwedt

Post-traumatic headache (PTH) is a common and incapacitating secondary headache disorder. It arises as a result of traumatic brain injury (TBI), whiplash injury, or craniotomy, as defined by the *International Classification of Headache Disorders,* 3rd edition (ICHD-3).[1] From a clinical perspective, PTH is commonly characterized by recurrent episodes of headache or continuous and unremitting headache that resemble migraine or tension-type headache.[2,3] Patients frequently report symptoms indicative of postconcussive syndrome (PCS), including anxiety, depression, insomnia, and mild cognitive impairment.[2,3]

Epidemiology

Traumatic brain injury (TBI) is a prevalent neurological condition, with an estimated global incidence ranging from 27 to 69 million cases.[4] PTH has been observed to be a more common consequence of mild TBI (mTBI) compared to moderate-to-severe TBI.[3,4] It is noteworthy that up to 90% of patients experience new or exacerbated headaches following mTBI.[4] PTH represents a complication of head trauma, whiplash injury, or craniotomy (see also Chapter 19), and accounts for approximately 4% of all secondary headaches.[4] The lifetime prevalence of PTH is 4.7% in men and 2.4% in women, with a 1-year prevalence of persistent PTH around 0.2% among people with chronic headache between the ages 30 and 44 years.[4]

Pathophysiology

The pathophysiology of PTH remains largely unknown, although various hypotheses regarding its possible causative mechanisms have been proposed.[4,5] One prominent hypothesis focuses on the trigeminovascular system (TVS), which is believed to be the anatomical and physiological substrate underlying PTH pathogenesis.[4] Within the TVS, the expression of calcitonin gene-related peptide (CGRP) and its receptors occurs at multiple levels, and the release of CGRP takes place upon TVS activation.[4] Studies have suggested an upregulation of CGRP molecular signaling in PTH, supported by observations of positive effects on cephalic pain responses in preclinical models treated with drugs targeting the CGRP pathway.[4-6] Furthermore, infusion of CGRP in PTH patients has induced headaches with migraine-like features in a significant majority of subjects.[4]

Another proposed mechanism involves the generation of waves of cortical spreading depression (CSD) as a result of inflammatory mediators and microglial activation following TBI.[4,5] It is hypothesized that CSD may trigger activation and sensitization of the trigeminal system.[4,5] Evidence of CSD events following TBI comes from preclinical models as well as electrocorticography recordings during neurosurgery in patients with traumatic hemorrhage and/or TBI.[4] Several studies have investigated the role of impaired pain processing and modulation in relation to PTH.[6] Advanced neuroimaging techniques, such as MRI, have revealed structural and functional modifications in cortical and subcortical structures of patients with persistent PTH compared to healthy individuals.[4-6] These modifications include alterations in cortical thickness and white matter integrity in brain areas associated with pain processing and sensory integration.[4-6] Additionally, patients with PTH exhibit abnormal activation of somatosensory and pain-related brain areas in response to pain stimuli.[4-6] The severity of PTH has been found to correlate with decreased functional connectivity in pain modulatory areas and increased activity in somatosensory cortices.[4-6]

It is important to consider the presence of methodological differences and conflicting results across studies when interpreting these changes. However, these findings collectively suggest an impairment of the pain matrix and the descending pain inhibitory control system.[4-6] This is supported by evidence of dysfunctional metabolism of endogenous pain modulation in persistent PTH following mild TBI.[4-6] Furthermore, a reduced pain inhibitory capacity observed 1 week after mild TBI has been shown to predict the presence of persistent PTH at 4 months postinjury.[4] PTH may be associated with TBI-induced damage to brain areas involved in the pain control system, such as the spinothalamocortical tract and the brainstem.[4]

Clinical Presentation and Diagnosis

PTH is primarily based on clinical criteria, as outlined in the ICHD-3 (Table 18-1).[1] PTH can be attributed to trauma or injury to the head and/or neck, including mild TBI, moderate-to-severe TBI, whiplash injury, or craniotomy.[1] It is also required that patients report the onset of headache within 7 days of the injury or upon regaining the ability or sense to report pain.[1] Clinicians can also assign a diagnosis of PTH to patients who have preexisting headache disorder, which worsens significantly in frequency and/or severity after the injury.[1] Notably, the ICHD-3 does not specify particular requirements for the headache features of PTH, as it is described simply as "any headache." However, clinicians are encouraged to document information regarding the headache features to facilitate more informed clinical decision-making.[7]

A key aspect of PTH diagnosis involves considering its persistence or remission over time. In "acute PTH," the headache resolves within 3 months of onset or if 3 months have not yet passed since onset.[1] On the other hand, "persistent PTH" refers to cases where the headache persists for more than 3 months.[1] A thorough clinical evaluation, including comprehensive neurological and physical examinations, as well as the exclusion of other possible causes for the headache, is always necessary when evaluating a patient with PTH.[1] If a patient has red flags in the medical history and/or physical examination, clinicians should initiate further testing, for example, blood samples, neuroimaging, and lumbar puncture.[1]

The clinical presentation of PTH is heterogeneous.[2,3] Following mTBI, PTH typically begins within the first couple of days following the injury.[8] For instance, in a study involving 277 PTH patients recruited from an emergency room, 94% reported headache onset on the day of their mTBI or the following day.[8] PTH persists in 23% to 58% of patients, and in these cases, it may persist for up to 12 months in approximately half of the individuals.[4]

PTH is often described based on its similarity to well-known primary headaches.[2,3] Upon careful assessment of clinical features, over 90% of patients with PTH attributed to mTBI exhibit a "migraine-like" phenotype, while the remaining patients are primarily characterized by a "tension-type headache-like" pattern.[7] Other rare PTH phenotypes have also been reported. PTH tends to be bilateral in location with moderate-to-severe intensity.[7] Photophobia, phonophobia, and nausea are

Table 18-1. ICHD-3 Diagnostic Criteria of Headache Attributed to Traumatic Injury to the Head

(A) PTH is initially classified as ACUTE or PERSISTENT	
ACUTE headache attributed to traumatic injury to the head	PERSISTENT headache attributed to traumatic injury to the head
a) Any headache fulfilling criteria C and D	a) Any headache fulfilling criteria C and D
b) Traumatic injury to the head has occurred	b) Traumatic injury to the head has occurred
c) Headache is reported to have developed within seven days after one of the following:	c) Headache is reported to have developed within seven days after one of the following:
1. the injury to the head	1. the injury to the head
2. regaining consciousness following the injury to the head	2. regaining of consciousness following the injury to the head
3. discontinuation of medication(s) impairing ability to sense or report headache following the injury to the head	3. discontinuation of medication(s) impairing ability to sense or report headache following the injury to the head
d) Either of the following:	d) Headache persists for >3 months after its onset
1. Headache has resolved within 3 months after its onset	e) Not better accounted for by another ICHD-3 diagnosis
2. Headache has not yet resolved but 3 months have not yet passed since its onset	
e) Not better accounted for by another ICHD-3 diagnosis	
(B) ACUTE and PERSISTENT PTH are further stratified according to the severity of TBI	
MILD TBI	MODERATE or SEVERE TBI
Injury to the head fulfilling both of the following:	Injury to the head associated with at least one of the following:
1. associated with none of the following:	– loss of consciousness for >30 minutes
– loss of consciousness for >30 minutes	– Glasgow Coma Scale (GCS) score <13
– Glasgow Coma Scale (GCS) score <13	– post-traumatic amnesia lasting >24 hours
– post-traumatic amnesia lasting >24 hours	– alteration in level of awareness for >24 hours
– altered level of awareness for >24 hours	– imaging evidence of a traumatic head injury such as skull fracture, intracranial hemorrhage, and/or brain contusion
– imaging evidence of a traumatic head injury such as skull fracture, intracranial hemorrhage, and/or brain contusion	
2. associated with one or more of the following symptoms and/or signs:	
– transient confusion, disorientation or impaired consciousness	
– loss of memory for events immediately before or after the head injury	
– two or more of the following symptoms suggestive of mild traumatic brain injury:	
– nausea	
– vomiting	
– visual disturbances	
– dizziness and/or vertigo	
– gait and/or postural imbalance	
– impaired memory and/or concentration	

Secondary Headaches

ICHD-3: International Classification of Headache Disorders, 3rd Edition, PTH: post-traumatic headache, TBI: traumatic brain injury.

Note: In this table, the diagnostic criteria for headache attributed to trauma or injury to the head (ICHD-3 code 5.1 & 5.2) are described.

common in PTH patients with a migraine-like phenotype.[7] The pain is frequently localized in the temple or forehead, and up to 60% of PTH cases report neck pain.[7]

Finally, it is important to consider that PTH may represent only one aspect of a complex syndrome that can occur following a traumatic brain injury, commonly known as postconcussive syndrome (PCS).[2,3] PCS may include dizziness, vestibular symptoms, cognitive dysfunction, attentional deficit, reduced concentration, nausea, fatigue, mood alteration, sleep disturbances, post-traumatic stress disorder, anxiety, and depression.[2,3] Based on semistructured interviews conducted with PTH patients and healthy controls, it was found that 85% of PTH patients reported poor quality of sleep (compared to 42% of healthy controls), 52% had at least a probable risk of anxiety.[7]

Treatment

The clinical management of PTH is largely based on expert consensus, as there is very limited data from randomized controlled trials.[2,9] The current recommendation is a phenotype-guided approach, in which patients are treated according to the primary headache phenotype that is most compatible with their clinical picture (e.g., migraine, tension-type headache).[2,9]

For optimal clinical management, all PTH patients should be advised to maintain a written or electronic daily headache diary.[2,9] A prospective and timely recording of headache's clinical characteristics (namely monthly headache days, pain intensity, days and doses of acute drug intake) and associated features will improve treatment monitoring and markedly reduce recall bias.[2] Addressing coexisting sleep, cognitive, autonomic, and psychological symptoms, for example, is often essential for optimizing the patient's health.

Due to the scarcity of data from randomized controlled trials specifically designed to demonstrate effectiveness of acute and preventive treatments in PTH, an empirical expert opinion-based therapeutic approach has been suggested (Table 18-2).[2]

The first important consideration relates to monthly headache frequency. PTH patients with low-frequency headache (namely less than 4 headache days/month) can be managed with acute symptomatic medications, starting with simple analgesics, such as nonsteroidal anti-inflammatory drugs (NSAIDs) or paracetamol/acetaminophen.[2] Triptans or gepants may also represent an alternative for acute PTH treatment, specifically in PTH patients with a "migraine-like" phenotype who do not respond well to NSAIDs.[2] Antiemetics should be prescribed when nausea and vomiting are troublesome symptoms. Conversely, acute medications with a high potential for causing dependence, sensitization, and/or medication overuse headache, such as opioids and barbiturates, should be avoided when treating PTH.[2]

When monthly headache frequency is higher, or when patients suffer from severe and disabling attacks, preventive treatment is generally recommended. Preclinical experiments and expert opinion suggest that starting a preventive treatment early after PTH onset may exert a positive effect on the natural course of acute PTH, by preventing its evolution to a persistent pattern.[2] Using the same criteria that are routinely used for migraine, it seems reasonable to propose a preventive treatment to PTH patients who have 6 or more headache days or 4 or more headache days associated with disability.[2]

This approach is partially reinforced by the observation that PTH shares several pathophysiological similarities with primary headache disorders, although the clinical relevance of this insight is yet to be elucidated.[2,9]

When treating PTH, we suggest avoiding medications that might unintentionally exacerbate other symptoms associated with the TBI, such as exacerbating cognitive dysfunction with topiramate or autonomic dysfunction with amitriptyline.[2,9] A small randomized, placebo-controlled, cross-over study of 40 people with PTH suggested possible benefits with onabotulinumtoxinA.[2] Although results are promising, several limitations (e.g., small sample size, dropout rate, poor compliance in diary completion, and a possible carry-over placebo effect) suggest the need for more definitive studies.[2] CGRP monoclonal antibodies were recently tested and can have a role in the treatment of PTH. An open-label study suggested a positive effect of erenumab, a monoclonal antibody targeting the CGRP receptor, in patients affected by persistent PTH after an mTBI, which occurred on average 5 years

Table 18-2. Proposed Algorithm for Pharmacological Treatment of Post-traumatic Headache[2]

	PTH with tension-type headache-like phenotype	PTH with migraine-like phenotype
ACUTE TREATMENT		
First line	– NSAIDs – Paracetamol/acetaminophen	– NSAIDs – Paracetamol/acetaminophen
Second line	– NSAIDs–paracetamol–caffeine combination drugs	– NSAIDs–paracetamol–caffeine combination drugs – Triptans – Gepants
To be avoided	– Ergot alkaloids – Opioids – Barbiturates	– Ergot alkaloids – Opioids – Barbiturates
PREVENTIVE TREATMENT		
First line	– Amitriptyline	– Propranolol – Amitriptyline – Candesartan – Atenolol
Second line	– Serotonin-norepinephrine reuptake inhibitors (e.g., venlafaxine) – Mirtazapine	– mAbs against CGRP or its receptor – Rimegepant and atogepant – OnabotulinumtoxinA – Serotonin-Norepinephrine Reuptake Inhibitors (e.g., venlafaxine)
To be considered on a case-by-case basis and according to PTH comorbidities	– Anticonvulsants (topiramate, gabapentin, pregabalin) – Extracranial nerve blocks – Physical therapy – Behavioural therapy	

CGRP: calcitonin gene-related peptide, mAbs: monoclonal antibodies, NSAIDs: non-steroidal anti-Inflammatory drugs, PTH: post-traumatic headache.

Note: A stepped-care treatment approach is recommended, therapy should begin with the least intensive treatment and then work upward in case of no or inadequate response, or intolerance due to adverse events. Preventive treatment is recommended if there are at least 8 headache days per month and the patient is negatively affected despite optimize acute medication therapy.

Source: Modified from Ashina H, Eigenbrodt AK, Seifert T, et al. Post-traumatic headache attributed to traumatic brain injury: classification, clinical characteristics, and treatment. *Lancet Neurol.* 2021;20(6):460-469.

before enrolment.[2] In this study, around 30% of patients were responders (i.e., experienced a least 50% reduction in the number of monthly moderate-to-severe headache days) after 3 months of treatment.[2]

Another cardinal point in the clinical management of PTH is the detection and treatment of additional TBI sequelae such as dizziness, nausea, photophobia, vertigo, fatigue, cognitive symptoms, mood alteration, sleep disturbances, post-traumatic stress disorder, anxiety, and depression, which are common in the so-called postconcussion syndrome.[2,9] Comorbidities may also guide the choice of PTH preventive treatment; for example, amitriptyline may represent a first choice in patients with comorbid anxiety, depression, or sleep disturbances. These associated conditions may be markedly disabling and may require specific treatment. Patients with postconcussion syndrome may benefit from a multidisciplinary and/or nonpharmacological approach, such as physical therapy, behavioral therapies, and psychological support.[2]

The last point of discussion is the possible association of PTH with the diagnosis of medication overuse headache (MOH).[2,5] Although PTH is not a primary headache, it cannot be excluded that medication overuse may exert a negative effect on the clinical course and lead to MOH.[2] In this view, we encourage once more the prospective recording of monthly acute drug intake in a headache diary, to educate patients on avoiding medication overuse, and to advise acute medication reductions with preventive medication when MOH is suspected.

Prognosis

In a short-term prospective study, it was observed that 22% of patients who presented with headache following traumatic brain injury (TBI) continued to experience frequent headaches after 1 month. Similarly, in another prospective study with a 1-year follow-up, only 22% of patients diagnosed with PTH had persistent PTH at 3 months. Among this minority, only 24% still reported PTH symptoms at 1 year. These findings suggest that the majority of patients with PTH experience improvement over time, as supported by a prospective study with a 5-year follow-up.[10] Individuals with PTH experience increased disability and a lower quality of life, particularly those who exhibit migraine-like features.[10] The presence of PTH significantly impacts the social lives and work activities of affected individuals, with nearly 35% of patients not returning to work within 3 months after the injury.[4]

Summary

- PTH is characterized by headaches that occur as a result of traumatic brain injury, whiplash injury, or craniotomy.

- The diagnosis of PTH is primarily based on clinical criteria outlined in the 3rd edition of *International Classification of Headache Disorders*.

- The predominant clinical features of PTH are most commonly consistent with a migraine-like phenotype, followed by a tension-type phenotype.

- PTH is often accompanied by symptoms such as sleep disturbances, cognitive dysfunction, anxiety, depression, and post-traumatic stress disorder, collectively known as postconcussion syndrome.

- The pathophysiology of PTH involves trigeminovascular system activation, structural and functional changes in various brain areas, and dysfunction of the pain-descending control system.

- Currently, a phenotype-guided treatment algorithm is considered the most reasonable and feasible approach for managing of PTH.

REFERENCES

1. Langer LK, Bayley MT, Lawrence DW, et al. Revisiting the ICHD-3 criteria for headache attributed to mild traumatic injury to the head: Insights from the Toronto Concussion Study Analysis of Acute Headaches Following Concussion. *Cephalalgia.* 2022;42(11-12):1172-1183.

2. Ashina H, Eigenbrodt AK, Seifert T, et al. Post-traumatic headache attributed to traumatic brain injury: classification, clinical characteristics, and treatment. *Lancet Neurol.* 2021;20(6):460-469.

3. Seifert TD, Evans RW. Posttraumatic headache: a review. *Curr Pain Headache Rep.* 2010;14(4):292-298.

4. Ashina H, Porreca F, Anderson T, et al. Post-traumatic headache: epidemiology and pathophysiological insights. *Nat Rev Neurol.* 2019;15(10).

5. Schwedt TJ. Post-traumatic headache due to mild traumatic brain injury: current knowledge and future directions. *Cephalalgia.* 2021;41(4):464-471.

6. Maleki N, Finkel A, Cai G, et al. Post-traumatic headache and mild traumatic brain injury: brain networks and connectivity. *Curr Pain Headache Rep*. 2021;25(3):20.

7. Ashina H, Iljazi A, Al-Khazali HM, et al. Persistent post-traumatic headache attributed to mild traumatic brain injury: deep phenotyping and treatment patterns. *Cephalalgia*. 2020;40(6):554-564.

8. Nampiaparampil DE. Prevalence of chronic pain after traumatic brain injury: a systematic review. *JAMA*. 2008;300(6):711-719.

9. Larsen EL, Ashina H, Iljazi A, et al. Acute and preventive pharmacological treatment of post-traumatic headache: a systematic review. *J Headache Pain*. 2019;20(1):98.

10. Flynn S, Moore B, Van Der Merwe AJ, et al. Headaches in traumatic brain injury: improvement over time, associations with quality of life, and impact of migraine-type headaches. *J Head Trauma Rehabil*. 2023;38(2).

Secondary Headaches

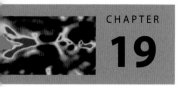

Headache After Craniotomy

Pedro Augusto Sampaio Rocha-Filho and Julio R. Vieira

Neurosurgical procedures including craniotomy are frequently performed for the treatment of various neurological diseases such as brain tumors, refractory epilepsy, and brain aneurysms. With the improvement of surgical, anesthetic, and life support techniques and the consequent decrease in operative mortality, the complications of brain surgery which can lead to a decrease in quality of life began to gain attention. Among these complications, one of the most frequent is postcraniotomy headache (PCH).[1] This type of headache was initially studied in the 1980s and it was recognized by the International Headache Society in 2004. This headache can be debilitating and have a negative impact on patients' lives. It is associated with longer medical follow-up. Those with PCH have a higher frequency of retirement after surgery than those without this headache. Its recognition and management are important to improve quality of life, and to reduce the demand for health services and their economic and social impact.[1]

Epidemiology

In retrospective studies, the prevalence of PCH in patients undergoing neurosurgery has been reported to have a wide range of none to 100%.[1] This great variability most likely occurs due to the lack of standardization on study design and differences in surgical techniques. Most studies reported a prevalence of PCH >30%. The incidence of PCH in prospective studies was 60% within 48 hours postsurgery[2] and 32% after 6 months.[3] Interestingly, others reported PCH incidence of 60% when utilizing the ICHD-3 criteria;[4] however, when utilizing the ICHD-2 classification, which has a more restrictive definition of PCH than the ICHD-3, PCH incidence was lower at 40% to 55% with 11% incidence of acute PCH and 24% to 29% for chronic PCH.[5,6]

Craniectomy, a surgery in which bone is not replaced at its site at the end of the procedure, is associated with a greater risk of developing PCH than craniotomy and cranioplasty.[1] Neurosurgery duration >4 hours was associated with greater risk of developing PCH; however, age, sex, and presurgical history of headache had conflicting results.[1] Patients undergoing intracranial aneurysm neurosurgical repair had a 2.6-fold greater odds of developing PCH than those undergoing endovascular repair.[6]

Cutaneous allodynia at the surgical scar was very prevalent at 82%, although it was only bothersome to 19% of patients with a mean duration of tenderness at the surgical site of 12 months.[7] Over time, PCH prevalence, frequency, and intensity tend to decrease. However, persistent PCH is a debilitating condition that can affect an individual's daily activities (29-60%), sports activities (25%), work (19-38%), social activities (8%), and have a negative impact on mood (15%) and can result in debilitating and incapacitating pain in 22% of patients.[1]

Pathophysiology

PCH is a syndrome, and injuries to intracranial and/or extracranial structures can contribute to its occurrence. The most important pathophysiological component of PCH is the surgical trauma itself (injury to muscles, fascia, periosteum, nerves, meninges, and vessels). Surgical trauma generates inflammation and ischemia that may lead to peripheral sensitization, and, consequently, pain.[1] However, the circulation of bone debris produced during surgery can lead to aseptic meningitis in some cases. Adhesions of the dura mater to the musculature can occur in some patients who have undergone craniectomy, which can also contribute to the pain. Also, hyperalgesia with central sensitization resulting from acute pain may be an important factor for headache persistence.[1]

Clinical Presentation and Diagnosis

Neurosurgery complications that may cause headaches such as surgical wound infection, meningitis, intracranial hypotension secondary to cerebrospinal fluid leak, and subdural and extradural hematoma should be ruled out by obtaining a good history from the patient, adequate clinical and neurological examination, and, if necessary, additional complementary tests.[1] According to the third edition of *International Classification of Headache Disorders (ICHD-3)*, to classify a headache as PCH, a craniotomy must have been performed for a reason other than head trauma and the headache must have started within 7 days following the craniotomy, after the regaining of consciousness following the craniotomy or the discontinuation of medication impairing ability to sense or report headache.[8] If the headache occurs for up to 3 months after craniotomy, it is classified as an "acute headache attributed to craniotomy." If the headache persists for more than 3 months after craniotomy, it is classified as a "persistent headache attributed to craniotomy."

In fact, most headaches that occur as a result of craniotomy start within the first few days after craniotomy (median of 4 days). However, it is possible that the headache could start after the 7 days that have been considered in the ICHD-3.[4] Most patients with prior history of headaches report that newly developed PCH to be different from their previous headaches. This headache often occurs on the same side and at the same site as the craniotomy. The most commonly observed headache pattern is similar to that of tension-type headache. A neuralgic pattern (neuralgia of either the occipital, trigeminal, or intermediate nerves) after posterior fossa surgeries has also been described. The headache can also have migrainous features, especially in the first few months after craniotomy; however, the migraine pattern tends to disappear over time.[1,3-5]

During temporal and frontotemporal craniotomies, there may be an injury to the temporal muscle (scars, ischemia, and hyperalgesia) and consequently, it can cause temporomandibular dysfunction.[9] Patients with temporal muscle injuries are prone to have pain onset during masticatory activities and jaw protrusion, as well as pain reproduction by jaw movements particularly when the jaw is wide open. Patients with PCH had more masticatory muscle tenderness on palpation than those who didn't develop PCH. The presence of pain during jaw movement, limitation of jaw movements, and the presence of pain on palpation of the masticatory muscles indicate the presence of temporomandibular disorders (TMD). Therefore, on physical exam, it is important to examine the temporomandibular joint and to palpate the masticatory muscles, as well as the surgical scar. In general, the highest headache frequency and severity are observed soon after surgery, although there is a tendency for the frequency to decrease over time.

Treatment

Primary headache disorders that were present before surgery should be well characterized to differentiate between an exacerbation of these prior headaches after craniotomy and PCH. In the first case, the treatment consists of medications for prophylactic treatment of the primary headache disorder.[1]

The presence of TMD can contribute to worsening and perpetuating PCH and when identified it should be promptly treated. Headache reproduction after palpation of the surgical scar suggests the occurrence of neurinomas in the scar, which can also perpetuate PCH. There are reports of improvement after infiltration of the surgical scar with local anesthetics. However, this should be avoided in case of non-complete closure of the skull after craniotomy due to the possibility of diffusion of the local anesthetic to the intracranial compartment. Depressive and anxiety disorders are also prevalent after craniotomy and may contribute to headaches, and, therefore, when present they should be treated accordingly.

For pain control, common analgesics such as acetaminophen/paracetamol, nonsteroidal antiinflammatory drugs, and opioids have been used. The use of opioids is typically discouraged due to the risk of complications with this treatment including addiction. A benefit of the use of subcutaneous sumatriptan in patients with PCH with migrainous features has been described.[10]

To this day, there are no clinical trials that have evaluated the prophylactic treatment of PCH. There are anecdotal reports of benefits with the use of verapamil, divalproex, and botulinum toxin A. In analogy to what is done for the treatment of headache attributed to traumatic injury to the head, the most frequent therapy approach is to try matching the pain pattern of PCH with the pattern of primary headaches, and to use the corresponding prophylactic treatment.

If the headache is refractory to medical therapy and the patient has undergone prior craniectomy, there is a possibility of adherence between the dura mater and the musculature, and reoperation should be considered.

Prognosis

Most patients have a good prognosis given that the prevalence and intensity of PCH usually decrease over time after surgery.[5] However, in some patients, it can persist for more than 6 months after surgery.

Summary

- PCH is a frequent complication of neurosurgery and can negatively impact the quality of life of those who suffer from it.

- The risk of occurrence of PCH is greater in those who had major craniotomies, infratentorial compared to supratentorial craniotomies, and in craniectomies as opposed to craniotomies and cranioplasties.

- PCH usually begins within the first few days after craniotomy, and is often at the same side and location of the procedure.

- Clinically, PCH often presents with tension-type headache characteristics.

- Over time, PCH usually shows improvement.

REFERENCES

1. Rocha-Filho PAS. Post-craniotomy headache: a clinical view with a focus on the persistent form. *Headache.* 2015;55(5):733-738.

2. De Benedittis G, Lorenzetti A, Migliore M, Spagnoli D, Tiberio F, Villani RM. Postoperative pain in neurosurgery: a pilot study in brain surgery. *Neurosurgery.* 1996;38(3):466-470.

3. Schankin CJ, Gall C, Straube A. Headache syndromes after acoustic neuroma surgery and their implications for quality of life. *Cephalalgia.* 2009;29(7):760-771.

4. Rocha-Filho PAS, Gherpelli JLD, De Siqueira JTT, Rabello GD. Post-craniotomy headache: a proposed revision of IHS diagnostic criteria. *Cephalalgia.* 2010;30(5):560-566.

5. Rocha-Filho PAS, Gherpelli JLD, De Siqueira JTT, Rabello GD. Post-craniotomy headache: characteristics, behaviour and effect on quality of life in patients operated for treatment of supratentorial intracranial aneurysms. *Cephalalgia.* 2008;28(1):41-48.

6. Magalhães JE, Azevedo-Filho HRC, Rocha-Filho PAS. The risk of headache attributed to surgical treatment of intracranial aneurysms: a cohort study. *Headache.* 2013;53(10):1613-1623.

7. Mosek AC, Dodick DW, Ebersold MJ, Swanson JW. Headache after resection of acoustic neuroma. *Headache.* 1999;39(2):89-94.

8. Headache Classification Committee of the International Headache Society (IHS). *The International*

Classification of Headache Disorders, 3rd edition. *Cephalalgia.* 2018;38(1):1-211.

9. Rocha-Filho PAS, Fujarra FJC, Gherpelli JLD, Rabello GD, de Siqueira JTT. The long-term effect of craniotomy on temporalis muscle function. *Oral Surg Oral Med Oral Pathol Oral Radiol Endod.* 2007;104(5):17-21.

10. Venkatraghavan L, Li L, Bailey T, Manninen PH, Tymianski M. Sumatriptan improves postoperative quality of recovery and reduces postcraniotomy headache after cranial nerve decompression. *Br J Anaesth.* 2016;117(1):73-79.

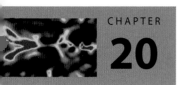

CHAPTER 20

Headache Attributed to Cranial or Cervical Vascular Disorders

Gretchen E. Tietjen

There are multiple types of cranial and cervical vascular disorders, and many are associated with ischemic or hemorrhagic stroke and lasting neurological disabilities. Headache is a common presenting clinical feature of cerebrovascular disorders and early recognition of the underlying condition provides an opportunity to lessen morbidity and mortality.[1] High-intensity headache of abrupt onset, and reaching maximum intensity in less than 1 minute is described as a thunderclap headache (TCH). Although pathognomonic of subarachnoid hemorrhage, TCH may also be associated with expansion of an unruptured cerebral aneurysm, as well as a number of other cerebrovascular conditions, including reversible vasoconstriction syndrome (RCVS), cervical artery dissection (CAD), cerebral venous thrombosis (CVT), pituitary apoplexy, and, on occasion, vasculitis.[1] Nonvascular conditions such as spontaneous intracranial hypotension, Chiari malformation, and colloid cyst in the third ventricle may also present with abrupt, severe headache, as may primary headaches of uncertain etiology, including primary thunderclap headache, primary cough headache, primary exercise headache, and primary headache with sexual activity.[1] Generally, the ICHD-3 criteria for the various types of headache attributed to cranial and cervical vascular disorders requires that (1) a vascular disorder has been established, (2) the headache developed in close temporal relation to other symptoms and/or clinical signs of the vascular disorder diagnosis, (3) the headache significantly improved in parallel with stabilization or improvement of the disorder, and (4) the headache is not better accounted for by another ICHD-3 diagnosis. In many cases, specific characteristics of the headache (e.g., onset, type, location, temporal course) are included in the criteria. In this chapter, headaches attributed to cranial and cervical vascular disorders will be described in terms of clinical presentation, epidemiology, pathophysiology, diagnosis, treatment, and prognosis. This information is summarized in Tables 20-1 and 20-2.

Ischemic Stroke and Transient Ischemic Attack

Headache often occurs in close temporal relationship to signs and symptoms signaling the onset of acute brain ischemia, namely stroke and transient ischemic attacks (TIA). A recent systematic review and meta-analysis of 20 prospective studies enrolling adults with headache associated with ischemic stroke (HAIS) examined the prevalence, features, and clinical outcomes.[2] The prevalence of HAIS ranged from 6% to 44%, with a pooled prevalence of 14%. Headache was documented to occur prior to, during, or after stroke onset, with most headaches occurring on the day of the stroke and at the same time as the neurological deficits. Headache was more common in women and younger adults with stroke. There was an approximately twofold higher prevalence of headache with posterior (vs anterior) circulation infarcts, and with cortical (vs deep) infarcts. Headache was more common in cardioembolic or large vessel origin stroke than in small vessel lacunar infarcts.

Table 20-1. Clinical Presentation, Headache Prevalence, Features and Pathophysiology of Conditions with Headaches Attributed to Cranial and Cerebral Vascular Disorders

Condition	Clinical Presentation	Headache Prevalence	Headache Features	Pathophysiology
Ischemic stroke (IS)	Sudden onset of focal neurological deficits (FND), HTN, +/− HA	14%, pooled (range 6-44%) 85-90% at IS onset, 10-15% with delayed onset HA occurs with posterior (30-75%) > anterior (15-60%) IS; with cortical > subcortical IS; with embolic and LVD > SVD	Usually resembling TTH or M; in BA occlusion: thunderclap onset, neck pain & stiffness *HA resolves in 3 mo*	Arterial occlusion due to cardiac embolism, arterial embolism, or thrombosis (2 degree atherosclerosis, arteritis, dissection, or hypercoagulability)
Transient ischemic attack (TIA)	Sudden onset of transient FND, +/− HA	27%	Usually moderate intensity and w/o defining features; *HA resolves in 24 hours*	Arterial occlusion due to cardiac embolism, arterial embolism, or thrombosis
Intracerebral hemorrhage (ICH), nontraumatic	Sudden onset of FND, HTN, HA (including TCH), N/V, altered consciousness	HA occurs with lobar>deep ICH; with putaminal > caudate, thalamic ICH; common with cerebellar ICH	*TCH +/or maximal on onset day +/or* localized to hemorrhage site, e.g., lobar occipital: ipsilateral orbital & periorbital pain; lobar anterior: periauricular, temporal, frontal pain *HA resolves in 3 mo*	Vascular rupture (e.g., artery, arteriole, AVM, DAVF, cavernous angioma) into parenchyma
Subarachnoid hemorrhage (SAH), nontraumatic	Ruptured aneurysm: TCH, altered consciousness, seizures, FND Unruptured aneurysm: TCH, with retro-orbital location, dilated pupil, oculomotor nerve palsy, if PCOM aneurysm	Headache: 100% with ruptured aneurysm, 20% with unruptured	*Ruptured: Thunderclap HA* *HA resolves in 3 mo* Early bleeding signaling impending rupture termed "sentinel HA" *Unruptured: TCH +/or painful oculomotor nerve palsy; HA worsens with growth, resolves after aneurysm tx*	Vascular rupture (e.g., aneurysm, AVM, DAVF, cavernous angioma) into subarachnoid space

(Continued)

Secondary Headaches

Table 20-1. Clinical Presentation, Headache Prevalence, Features and Pathophysiology of Conditions with Headaches Attributed to Cranial and Cerebral Vascular Disorders (*Continued*)

Condition	Clinical Presentation	Headache Prevalence	Headache Features	Pathophysiology
Arteriovenous malformation (AVM)	Headache, seizures, FND, +/− rupture (ICH, SAH, IVH)	HA: ~50% if unruptured; higher if ruptured; Aura: in up to 58% in women	HA: migraine +/− aura, cluster HA, chronic paroxysmal hemicrania *HA localizes to AVM site* *HA worsens w growth, improves w treatment*	Vascular malformation with 3% annual incidence of rupture (ICH, SAH, IVH). Risk factors for rupture: advanced age, Hispanic ethnicity, deep location, and deep venous drainage
Dural arteriovenous fistula (DAVF)	HA (most common sx), pulsatile tinnitus, FND, seizures; CCF+ symptoms: conjunctival injection, exophthalmos, painful ophthalmoplegia, diplopia	HA: 45%	CCF+: nonmigraine HA CCF−: migraine-like HA *HA localizes to DAVF site* *HA worsens w growth, improves w treatment* *HA w pulsatile tinnitus, +/or ophthalmoplegia, +/− worse in AM hours, w coughing, w bending over*	Vascular malformations fed by dural arteries and draining venous sinuses or meningeal veins. May be caused by CCF (carotid cavernous fistula)
Cavernous angioma	Bleed causes HA (TCH may be 1st symptom), seizures	HA in 4-52% of symptomatic patients	TCH or migraine-like HA *HA localizes to cavernous angioma site* *HA worsens w growth, improves w treatment*	Vascular malformation of brain and spinal cord, with endothelial-lined caverns devoid of smooth muscle; sporadic or autosomal dominant inheritance
Sturge-Weber syndrome (SWS)	HA, epilepsy, stroke-like episodes, learning disorders, behavioral disorders; glaucoma, hearing, and/or vestibular disorders; port-wine stain on face	HA prevalence: 37-71%, about 28% migraine-like	*Migraine-like HA ipsilateral to angioma, worsens w growth* *Aura symptoms contralateral to angioma* Prolonged aura, hemiplegic migraine	Sporadic neurocutaneous disorder 2 degree somatic mosaic mutation in the GNAQ gene, choroidal angioma, dural or leptomeningeal angiomatosis in brain & eye

Table 20-1. Clinical Presentation, Headache Prevalence, Features and Pathophysiology of Conditions with Headaches Attributed to Cranial and Cerebral Vascular Disorders

Condition	Clinical Presentation	Headache Prevalence	Headache Features	Pathophysiology
Primary angiitis of the central nervous system (PACNS)	Subacute-chronic onset of focal deficits, HA Rare: fever, rash, weight loss	60%	Insidious, progressive	HA 2 degree inflammation, IS, SAH. Inflammation is granulomatous, lymphocytic, or necrotizing
Cervical artery dissection (CAD)	Headache, neck pain, Horner's syndrome, +/− stroke symptoms	68-95%; may precede stroke onset; associated w MO > MA	Severe HA, with thunderclap, migraine, or cluster features; *HA precedes signs of retinal +/-or cerebral ischemia* ICA: ipsilateral HA, neck pain, Horner's; VA: occipital HA, neck pain; *resolves in 3 mo*	Separation of arterial-wall layers w stenosis, occlusion, or aneurysm; 2 degree trauma, connective tissue disorder, straining
Cerebral venous thrombosis (CVT)	HA (often 1st, sometimes only, symptom), seizures, FND N/V, papilledema, TVO, abducens nerve palsy 2 degree increased ICP	68-90%	Onset may be thunderclap or subacute; typically, severe, persistent or intermittent, diffuse or unilateral with throbbing and stabbing	Thrombosis of cerebral venous sinus w increased ICP. Varying degrees of venous congestion, which depend not only on the extent of thrombosis in the deep veins but also on the territory of the involved vessels and of venous collaterals
Reversible cerebral vasoconstriction syndrome (RCVS)	Thunderclap HA, +/− FND, seizures, altered MS	Thunderclap HA in >80%; frequent hx of migraine	*Thunderclap HA, +/− triggered by sexual activity, exertion, Valsalva, emotion, bathing, +/− recurrent for ≤1 mo*	Activation of sympathetic NS; diffuse segmental vasoconstriction; no vasculitis
CADASIL	MA: 1st sx in 40-70%; then TIA, IS, seizures, altered mood, and progressive dementia	Migraine in 55-75%, including MA in 40-70%	*MA, with typical, hemiplegic, prolonged, confusional aura*	Monogenic; SVD 2 degree VSMC degeneration, and accumulation of notch 3 receptor protein

(Continued)

Table 20-1. Clinical Presentation, Headache Prevalence, Features and Pathophysiology of Conditions with Headaches Attributed to Cranial and Cerebral Vascular Disorders *(Continued)*

Condition	Clinical Presentation	Headache Prevalence	Headache Features	Pathophysiology
MELAS	HA, stroke-like episodes, encephalopathy, epilepsy, myopathy, DM, short stature, decreased hearing	HA in 70% of persons w mitochondrial diseases. Migraine common in 3243A>G mutation carriers	HA often meets criteria for MO, MA, probable migraine, or TTH; *acute HA precedes or associated w FND +/or seizures*	Insufficient mitochondrial energy production and mitochondrial proliferation-related small vessel angiopathy
Moyamoya disease	HA, IS or HS, seizures, movement disorders	HA in 20-76%	HA usually like migraine (>50% MA) and/or TTH. Occasional cluster HA, hemiplegic migraine, migrainous infarction	Progressive stenosis or occlusion of terminal ICA, ACA, MCA, w small collaterals in "puff of smoke" pattern
Cerebral amyloid angiopathy (CAA)	Migraine aura-like event (often 1st symptom) +/− HA, transient FND, progressive cognitive impairment	Late onset (>50 years old) migraine aura (+/− HA) in ≥50% of CCA carriers, 75% with HA	Aura +/− HA; aura typically precedes symptomatic ICH by several yrs. Auras lasting ≥60 minutes usually signal acute ICH	SVD w amyloid deposition in cortical & leptomeningeal arterial & arteriolar walls; lobar ICH, subcortical microhemorrhages
Pituitary apoplexy	Severe HA (1st sx in 90%), N/V, meningismus, visual sx, impaired mental status, adrenal crisis	Thunderclap HA, retro-orbital; associated with meningismus, N/V	Severe thunderclap HA, often retro-orbital	IS or HS of pituitary, usually in preexisting pituitary adenoma

Note: Script in italics under Headache Features is from *International Classification of Headache Disorders*, third edition.

Abbreviations: ACA, anterior cerebral artery; ACG, anticoagulation; AM, ante meridiem, before midday; AVM, arteriovenous malformation; BA, basilar artery; CAA, cerebral amyloid angiopathy; CADASIL, cerebral autosomal dominant arteriopathy with subcortical infarcts and leukoencephalopathy; CCf, caroid cavernous fistula; CGRP, calcitonin generelated peptide; CSF, cerebrospinal fluid; CT, computed tomography; CTA, CT angiography; CTP, CT perfusion; DAVF, dural arteriovenous fistula; DM, diabetes mellitus; DSA, digital subtraction angiography; FND, focal neurologic deficits; GNAQ, G protein guanine nucleotide binding protein alpha subunit q; HA, headache; HS, hemorrhagic stroke; HTN, hypertension; Hx, history; IA, intra-arterial; ICA, internal carotid artery; ICH, intracerebral hemorrhage; ICP, intracranial pressure; ICH, intracerebral hemorrhage; IVH, intraventricular hemorrhage; IS, ischemic stroke; IV, intravenous; LVD, large vessel disease; M, migraine; MA, migraine with aura; MCA, middle cerebral artery; MELAS, mitochondrial encephalopathy, lactic acidosis, and stroke-like episodes; mo, month; MO, migraine without aura; MRA, magnetic resonance angiography; MRI, MR imaging; MRV, MR venography; MS, mental status; mult, multiple; NS, nervous system; N/V, nausea/vomiting; PCOM, posterior communicating artery; SAH, subarachnoid hemorrhage; SVD, small vessel disease; sx, symptoms; TCH, thunderclap headache; TIA, transient ischemic attack; TTH, tension-type headache; TVO, transient visual obscuration; tx, treatment; VA, vertebral artery; w, with; w/o, without; WM, white matter.

Table 20-2.   Diagnostic Tests, Treatment, and Prognosis of Conditions with Headaches Attributed to Cranial and Cerebral Vascular Disorders

Condition	Diagnostic Tests	Treatment	Prognosis
Ischemic stroke (IS)	Brain CT/CTA/CTP or MRI/MRA	Stroke: IV tPA, IA tPA, thrombectomy HA: acetaminophen	HA for >3 months in up to 23%
Transient ischemic attack (TIA)	Brain CT/CTA/CTP or MRI/MRA	HA: acetaminophen	HA usually resolves in <24 hours
Subarachnoid hemorrhage (SAH)	Brain CT/CTA, MRI/MRA, DSA	HA: acetaminophen, avoid NSAIDs	HA improves with therapeutic intervention of aneurysm, whether ruptured or not
Intracerebral hemorrhage (ICH)	Brain CT/CTA or MRI/MRA	Meds for HA, hypertension, seizures; surgical resection, if indicated	Depends on age, neuro deficits, hemorrhage volume, current use of anticoagulants
Arteriovenous malformation (AVM)	CT/CTA, MRI/MRA, DSA	Meds for HA, seizures; surgical resection, stereotactic radiosurgery, endovascular embolization	Risk of rupture (potentially life-threatening) unless removed
Dural arteriovenous fistula (DAVF)	CTA, MRI/MRA, DSA	Meds for HA, seizures; surgical resection, stereotactic radiosurgery, endovascular embolization	Generally favorable with surgery
Cavernous angioma	Brain MRI	Microsurgical resection or stereotactic radiosurgery	Depends on whether single lesion or multiple lesions
Sturge-Weber syndrome (SWS)	MRI/MRA; ophthalmology exam for glaucoma	Headaches may respond to flunarizine or triptans	May be asymptomatic or cause seizures, developmental delays, cognitive impairment, paresis
Primary angiitis of the central nervous system (PACNS)	CSF (abnormal >95%); MRI (abnormal >90%) with multiple deep>cortical infarcts, WML; Angiography: multiple stenoses, occlusions, irregular lumen; vessel biopsy	Immunosuppressive therapy: corticosteroids +/– cyclophosphamide	HA is usually responsive to treatment

(Continued)

Table 20-2. Diagnostic Tests, Treatment, and Prognosis of Conditions with Headaches Attributed to Cranial and Cerebral Vascular Disorders (*Continued*)

Condition	Diagnostic Tests	Treatment	Prognosis
Cervical artery dissection (CAD)	Head/neck CTA, MRA, DSA, duplex sonography	Antiplatelet or anticoagulation; APAP, antiemetics, ditans for HA; avoid triptans, ergots	Improvement in HA with healing of dissection
Cerebral venous thrombosis (CVT)	MRI/MRA/MRV, CT/CTA, or DSA with venography. Labs: anticardiolipin antibody, factor V Leiden mutation, protein C and protein S deficiency. Evaluation for malignancy, Behcet's disease	Heparin followed by oral ACG for at least 6 months and treatment of the underlying cause, if identified	HA should significantly improve or resolve with resolution of CVT
Reversible cerebral vasoconstriction syndrome (RCVS)	Angiography: sensitivity DSA > CTA or MRA; MRI normal or cortical infarcts, vasogenic edema; CSF: normal, near normal	Supportive, analgesics for HA; calcium channel blockers reverse vasoconstriction	TCH resolves in 1-3 months, but mild-moderate HA persists in 50%
CADASIL	MRI: 100% with diffuse WMH on T2/FLAIR; lacunar infarcts, microbleeds	Empiric symptomatic management but no tx with proven efficacy; safety of CGRP blockers uncertain	Migraine may wane with disease progression; death at 60-70 years
MELAS	Serum: lactic acid, pyruvic acid; CSF: pyruvic acid; mtDNA mutation analysis; muscle biopsy	Triptans for headache. Supplements: nitric oxide precursors (arginine, citrulline), Coenzyme Q10, Vit K-3, Vit K-1, ascorbate, riboflavin, nicotinamide, Dichloroacetate	Slowly progressive with poor prognosis for recovery
Moyamoya disease	MR/MRA, cerebral angiography	Surgical revascularization; avoid triptans, CGRP blockers	93% 5-year survival for >15 years old

(*Continued*)

Table 20-2. Diagnostic Tests, Treatment, and Prognosis of Conditions with Headaches Attributed to Cranial and Cerebral Vascular Disorders (*Continued*)

Condition	Diagnostic Tests	Treatment	Prognosis
Cerebral amyloid angiopathy (CAA)	Blood-sensitive MRI sequences	Migraine prophylaxis (verapamil, topiramate, lamotrigine)	CAA is progressive; migraine prophylaxis may prevent aura
Pituitary apoplexy	MRI, pituitary hormonal evaluation	Symptomatic treatment; intravenous hydrocortisone bolus and maintenance; decompressive surgery, when needed	Mortality <2%; HA and visual symptoms improve with decompression

Abbreviations: ACG, anticoagulation; APAP, acetaminophen; AVM, arteriovenous malformation; CAA, cerebral amyloid angiopathy; CAD, cervical artery dissection; CADASIL, cerebral autosomal dominant arteriopathy with subcortical infarcts and leukoencephalopathy; CGRP, calcitonin gene-related peptide; CSF, cerebrospinal fluid; CT, computed tomography; CTA, CT angiography; CTP, CT perfusion; DSA, digital subtraction angiography; FLAIR, fluid-attenuated inversion recovery; HA, headache; IA, intra-arterial; ICH, intracerebral hemorrhage; IV, intravenous; MELAS, mitochondrial encephalopathy, lactic acidosis, and stroke-like episodes; MRA, magnetic resonance angiography; MRI, MR imaging; MRV, MR venography; mtDNA, mitochondrial deoxyribonucleic acid; mult, multiple; SAH, subarachnoid hemorrhage; TCH, thunderclap headache; TIA, transient ischemic attack; tPA, tissue plasminogen activator; tx, treatment; Vit, vitamin; WMH, white matter hyperintensities; WML, white matter lesions.

Although migraine-like symptoms are not uncommon, the majority of HAIS had tension-type headache features (i.e., bilateral pain and without nausea, vomiting, photophobia, or phonophobia), albeit more intense.[2] The duration of HAIS varied widely, but persisted for months, or even years, in nearly one-quarter of persons, particularly in those who were younger, depressed, or with preexisting primary headache. The phenomenon of HAIS was not associated with worse stroke outcomes or increased risk of recurrent stroke. The prevalence of headache at the onset of transient ischemic attack (TIA) was about 27%, which was similar to the headache prevalence at the onset of stroke. A case-control study of 312 persons, reported an increased prevalence of headache during the week prior to TIA and at the time of TIA. In addition, the 1-year prevalence of migraine was significantly higher in TIA patients than in controls (21% vs 8%).[3]

Intracerebral Hemorrhage

Abrupt onset of headache, often thunderclap in nature, coupled with nausea/vomiting are hallmarks of nontraumatic intracerebral hemorrhage (ICH). Other early symptoms include elevated blood pressure, focal neurological deficits, and altered consciousness, which may obfuscate the report of headache. Risk of headache, which occurs in about half of ICH patients able to provide histories, increases with lobar (vs deep) bleeds, putaminal (vs caudate or thalamic) bleeds, and bleeds within the cerebellum.[1] Further, hematoma location, meningeal signs, and gender were more predictive of headache than hematoma volume. Headache location may in some instances localize the hemorrhage, for example, occipital lobar bleeds are often associated with ipsilateral orbital and periorbital pain, whereas anterior lobar bleeds lead to periauricular, temporal, or frontal area pain. Diagnostic evaluation includes head CT and MRI brain. Due to the increased risk of further hematoma expansion, current guidelines recommend maintaining systolic blood pressure between 140 to 160 mm Hg and patients should avoid using aspirin or NSAIDs. Seizures may occur and are treated with antiepileptic medication. Patients at risk of ICH-related herniation may require surgical resection of the hematoma, or decompression. Overall, prognosis in ICH is determined by age, neurological impairment, hemorrhage volume, and current use of antithrombotic therapy, but studies suggest that headache at onset of ICH may further signal a higher risk of early mortality.[4]

Subarachnoid Hemorrhage

With a TCH prevalence approaching 100%, individuals with a ruptured saccular aneurysm in or near the circle of Willis typically describe it as the "worst headache of life." With subarachnoid hemorrhage (SAH), nausea and vomiting may accompany headache, but these symptoms are less common than in ICH. Other presenting symptoms of aneurysm rupture include altered consciousness, seizures, and in the event of intraparenchymal or cranial nerve involvement, focal neurological deficits. In cases of an early, slow, low-volume bleed, rather than a full-blown aneurysmal rupture, a person may experience abrupt-onset headache in the absence of other symptoms. This has been termed sentinel headache, so named because it signals impending aneurysmal re-bleed, usually within 72 hours. Given the lack of symptoms other than headache, and the serious consequences if not treated, diagnosis requires a high index of suspicion.[1,2] The prevalence of headache is about 20% in persons with unruptured aneurysms. Aneurysm expansion, even without rupture, may still lead to TCH. Based on data from six prospective studies, the increased risk of rupture can be predicted by the PHASES practical risk score, which relies on population type, advanced age, hypertension, aneurysm size, location, and history of prior SAH from a different aneurysm. Aneurysms are most common at the junction of the posterior communicating artery and distal internal carotid artery, and expansion may cause ipsilateral retro-orbital headache, with dilated pupils and painful oculomotor nerve palsy. If presenting acutely (<6 hours), the sensitivity of aneurysmal rupture with SAH on noncontrast CT is nearly 100% (Chapter 2). Traditionally, a negative CT is followed by lumbar puncture with CSF analysis (Chapter 3). Some have advocated for CTA in place of lumbar puncture, based on results of mathematical probability modeling. In either diagnostic paradigm, if these studies are negative, but clinical concerns persist, digital subtraction angiography may be warranted. Treatment strategies to prevent aneurysm rupture or re-rupture, include endovascular coiling, placement of flow diversion stents, or microsurgical clip placement at the aneurysm neck. Headache frequently improves with therapeutic intervention of aneurysm, including in those with unruptured aneurysms and with pre-treatment headache history, but a prospective study of 93 patients experiencing aneurysmal SAH demonstrated that 41% still described headache on mean follow-up of 3 years.[5]

Arteriovenous Malformation

Arteriovenous malformations (AVM) are less prevalent than cerebral aneurysms. In addition to seizures and focal neurological deficits, headache is a frequent presenting symptom of AVM, occurring in about 50%, if unruptured, and higher in the setting of hemorrhage (ICH, SAH, +/or IVH), which occurs at a yearly incidence of 3%. Migraine-like headache and aura ipsilateral to the AVM is common, particularly in women. Infrequently, headache resembles cluster headache or chronic paroxysmal hemicrania.[6] Headache may be episodic or chronic. Diagnostic testing to detect AVM includes CTA, MRA, or digital subtraction angiography (DSA). Surgical resection, stereotactic radiosurgery, or endovascular embolization is used to decrease the risk of hemorrhage.

Dural Arteriovenous Fistula

Headache is reported to be one of the most common symptoms (45%) of dural arteriovenous fistula (DAVF),[7] vascular malformations fed by dural arteries, and draining venous sinuses or meningeal veins. In one study, headaches reported in persons with DAVF related to carotid cavernous fistula (CCF) did not resemble migraine, whereas headache in persons with DAVF related to other causes did.[7] Other common symptoms of DAVF include tinnitus (in transverse and sigmoid sinuses) and conjunctival injection, exophthalmos, diplopia, and painful ophthalmoplegia (in CCF). In persons with DAVF, headache may also be related to hemorrhage or thrombosis of cerebral venous sinus. Diagnostic testing to detect AVM includes CTA, MRA, or DSA. Surgical resection, stereotactic radio-surgery, or endovascular embolization has a favorable prognosis.

Cavernous Angioma

Cavernous angiomas are endothelial-lined vascular malformations of the brain and spinal cord that are devoid of smooth muscle. These malformations may be asymptomatic, but when they bleed, initial clinical presentation includes seizures, focal neurological deficits, and headaches, either TCH or migraine-like in onset.[8] Singular lesions are usually of sporadic etiology, whereas multiple lesions have been ascribed to autosomal dominant inheritance or radiation therapy. Diagnosis is made with brain MRI. Treatment options include microsurgical resection or stereotactic radiosurgery.

Sturge-Weber Syndrome

Facial port-wine stain, choroidal angioma, and dural or leptomeningeal angiomatosis involving the brain and eye are key features of Sturge-Weber syndrome (SWS), a rare, sporadic, neurocutaneous disorder. Headache occurs in up to two-thirds of persons with SWS. In adults, nearly one-third of patients with SWS described migraine, including features suggesting hemiplegic migraine or migraine with prolonged aura. By contrast, migraine features are usually absent in children. Besides headache, common neurological expressions of SWS include seizures, focal neurological deficits, learning and/or behavior disorders, glaucoma, and hearing and vestibular disorders.[9] Diagnostic testing includes brain MRI and MRA and ophthalmological evaluation for glaucoma. The safety and efficacy of migraine therapies have not been established in SWS but there are reports of headache improvement with triptans or flunarizine.

Secondary Headaches

Angiitis of the Central Nervous System

Angiitis of the central nervous system may be primary (PACNS), that is, confined to the brain, meninges, and spinal cord, or secondary (SACNS) to systemic conditions, including infections, connective tissue diseases, inflammatory conditions, neoplasms, drugs, and radiation.[10] PACNS is a rare, idiopathic, inflammatory condition predominantly affecting small and medium more than large vessels, whereas SACNS may affect vessels of any size. Occurring at a median age of 50 years, PACNS typically presents with headache (about 60%), focal neurological deficits, and altered cognition or consciousness, but systemic features such as fever, night sweats, weight loss may be absent. Headache in PACNS has been attributed to inflammation, ischemic stroke, or SAH, and is usually insidious rather than abrupt in onset. Headache is also common in SACNS, with a larger range of possible etiologies, including inflammation, ischemia, hemorrhage, CVT, increased intracranial pressure.[10] Diagnostic studies in PACNS include cerebral spinal fluid analysis (abnormal in >95%, with lymphocytosis, elevated protein, negative cultures), brain MRI (abnormal in >90%, with leptomeningeal enhancement, multiple ischemic infarcts, and deep white matter hyperintensities), angiography (multiple steno-occlusive vascular lesions with beads-on-a-string appearance), and brain biopsy (particularly in small vessels).[10] Headaches usually respond to treatment of PACNS with glucocorticoids +/− cyclophosphamide.[11]

Cervical Artery Dissection

Cervical artery dissection (CAD) involving the carotid or vertebral arteries results from either an intimal tear or from bleeding within the media causing separation of layers of the vessel wall. Neck pain and headache are the most frequent presenting symptoms of CAD (60%), and usually ipsilateral to the dissection, and be accompanied by or precede (by up to 14 days) signs of ischemia in the territories of the affected vessel(s).[12] In internal carotid artery (ICA) dissection, disruption of the sympathetic pathways within the vessel wall may lead to Horner's syndrome with ipsilateral miosis, partial ptosis, anhidrosis, and enophthalmos. Dissection-related headache may present as TCH, migraine, or cluster headache, and may be intermittent or chronic, even daily.[12] In persons with underlying fibromuscular dysplasia, additional symptoms include hypertension, pulsatile tinnitus, and dizziness. Diagnosis is based on CTA or MRA of the head and neck, duplex sonography, or conventional DSA angiography.[13] Antiplatelet and/or anticoagulation therapy have been widely used to treat extracranial ICA and vertebral artery (VA) dissection, but more research is needed to determine the best treatment option. Agents with vasoconstrictive properties such as triptans and ergots are generally avoided.

Cerebral Venous Thrombosis

Cerebral venous thrombosis (CVT) usually occurs in persons (women > men) less than 50 years old, with peak incidence between 20 and 30 years. Headache, the initial and sometimes only symptom, is present in up to 90% of CVT cases and is often without defining features.[14] Onset may be insidious or abrupt (TCH), and pain is typically severe, persistent, and progressive. Although localization is often diffuse, when unilateral with throbbing or stabbing features, it resembles migraine or cluster headache, with worsening when supine or straining. With delay in diagnosis, other neurological symptoms may accompany headache, including seizures, focal neurological deficits (FND), and signs of increased intracranial pressure (nausea, emesis, papilledema, transient visual obscuration, and abducens nerve palsy). Factors that raise the index of suspicion include known hypercoagulable state, such as the use of combined hormonal contraception or prior deep venous thrombosis, and elevated D-dimer. Diagnosis of CVT is based on MRI plus MR angiography/MR venography, CT scan plus CT angiography, or conventional angiography (Chapter 2). Investigations for predisposing prothrombotic states and underlying malignant conditions are recommended. Heparin drip followed by transition to oral anticoagulation for at least 6 months is usually indicated, as is treating the identified underlying cause of CVT. Occasionally, local intravenous thrombolysis, mechanical thrombectomy, and decompressive surgery are necessary. Headache is expected to diminish and/or resolve with improvement of CVT.

Reversible Cerebral Vasoconstriction Syndrome

Thunderclap headache is the initial feature of reversible cerebral vasoconstriction syndrome (RCVS) in >80% of cases and may be recurrent up to 4 to 12 weeks after diagnosis.[13] The condition may be accompanied by seizures, alteration in consciousness, transient FND, ischemic or hemorrhagic stroke. RCVS predominates in women in their fifties and men in their thirties. Conditions causing transient deregulation of cerebral arterial tone (e.g., sympathetic overactivity, oxidative stress, endothelial dysfunction) and accompanying diffuse segmental vasoconstriction include physical exertion, sexual activities, emotional stress, Valsalva maneuvers, bathing, and use of vasoactive substances. RCVS has also been associated with the postpartum period, head and neck trauma, CVT, dissection, surgical procedures, and catecholamine-secreting tumors. The diagnostic finding most typical of RCVS is diffuse segmental vasoconstriction with a beads-on-a-string appearance on CTA, MRA, or DSA, but this is rarely seen at the time of presentation and testing may need to be repeated.[13] Brain MRI may also be normal at the time of presentation, with abnormalities occurring over the course of RCVS, including SAH (typically, over convexity), ICH, borderline ischemic stroke, and reversible brain edema reminiscent of posterior reversible encephalopathy syndrome (PRES). Cerebrospinal fluid is usually normal, or near normal. Headaches in RCVS may respond to simple analgesics, opioids, or to calcium channel blockers used to reverse vasoconstriction. Vasoconstrictive medications such as triptans and ergotamines should be avoided, and corticosteroids have been associated with worse outcomes. Persistent headaches (i.e., those continuing >3 months) of reduced intensity occur in about 50% of patients.[15] RCVS recurs in at least 5% of patients, and risk is higher in those with a history of migraine.

Cerebral Autosomal Dominant Arteriopathy with Subcortical Infarcts and Leukoencephalopathy

The syndrome of cerebral autosomal dominant arteriopathy with subcortical infarcts and leukoencephalopathy (CADASIL) is the most prevalent form of hereditary cerebral ischemia and vascular dementia.[16] Migraine with aura is the predominant (40-70%) initial symptom, but with later age of onset than in general population and often with atypical features, including hemiplegia, confusion, and prolonged duration.[16] Other symptoms of CADASIL include recurrent TIAs, lacunar infarcts, mood disorders, seizures, and progressive dementia.[16] CADASIL is a monogenic (*NOTCH3* gene mutation) small vessel arteriopathy, with the pathognomonic electron microscopic finding of extracellular granular osmiophilic material in vessel media. Besides genotyping and skin biopsy, diagnostic modalities include brain MRI, which is 100% sensitive in symptomatic individuals, showing diffuse white matter hyperintensities (particularly in anterior temporal lobes) on T2/FLAIR +/− lacunar infarcts (subcortical white matter and deep gray structures), and microbleeds.[17] There is no treatment with proven efficacy and management is symptomatic.[16] Anticoagulants are generally contraindicated and safety of calcitonin gene-related peptide (CGRP) ligand and receptor blockers is uncertain.

Mitochondrial Encephalopathy, Lactic Acidosis, and Stroke-Like Episodes

The maternally inherited syndrome of mitochondrial encephalopathy, lactic acidosis, and stroke-like episodes (MELAS) is also often characterized by headache, seizures, focal neurological deficits, hearing impairment, myopathy, diabetes mellitus, and short stature.[17] Headache occurs in 70% of persons with mitochondrial disorders, but headache attributed to MELAS is the only mitochondrial disorder-related headache included in ICHD-3. Headache in MELAS may resemble migraine with and without aura, probable migraine and tension-type headache (TTH).[17] The most common genetic mutation (m.3243A>G) occurs in 80% to 90% of persons diagnosed with MELAS, and has been associated with migraine, but the relationship of the mutation to migraine is uncertain. The pathophysiology of MELAS includes decreased mitochondrial energy production and mitochondrial proliferation-related small vessel angiopathy. Diagnosis is inferred from increased serum lactic acid, serum and CSF pyruvic acid, and characteristic muscle biopsy, with a more definitive diagnosis from mtDNA mutational analysis. Given the guarded prognosis, a variety of supplements are often tried, including nitric oxide precursors (arginine, citrulline), coenzyme Q10, Vitamin K-3, K-1, ascorbate, riboflavin, nicotinamide, and dichloroacetate, despite lack of proven efficacy.

Moyamoya Disease

Moyamoya disease, an angiopathy characterized by bilateral progressive stenosis of terminal ICA, plus the anterior carotid artery (ACA), and/or middle carotid artery (MCA), gets its name from the "puff of smoke" pattern made by the adjacent network of small collaterals. Headache is a frequent (20-76%) presenting symptom, and often resembles migraine (with or without aura) or tension-type headache.[18] Cluster headache, hemiplegic migraine, and migrainous infarction have been described, as have strokes (ischemic or hemorrhagic), seizures, and movement disorders.[18] Diagnosis of moyamoya is made with cerebral MR/MRA and conventional angiography. Treatment involves surgical revascularization and symptomatic treatment of symptoms, generally avoiding the use of triptans and CGRP blockers for headache.[18]

Cerebral Amyloid Angiopathy

Cerebral amyloid angiopathy (CAA), a common sporadic or inherited small-vessel disorder of the aged, is most often associated with progressive cognitive impairment.[19] The pathology of CAA involves amyloid deposition in the walls of small cortical and leptomeningeal arteries and arterioles. These vascular changes predispose to SAH, lobar intracerebral hemorrhage, and subcortical micro-hemorrhages.[19] The initial symptom of CAA is often a transient focal neurological deficit, which in some cases resembles migraine aura with spreading paresthesias and/or positive visual phenomena, with or without headache.[19] The aura-like nature of these events is attributed to cortical siderosis-induced cortical spreading depression (CSD), or when prolonged (≥60 minutes), to acute SAH or ICH. Diagnosis of CAA is made by brain MRI, particularly the blood-sensitive sequences and a recent meta-analysis of symptomatic patients demonstrated that the presence and extent of cortical super-ficial siderosis are the most important risk factors for future ICH. Migraine prophylactic therapies, such as topiramate, lamotrigine, and verapamil, may be effective in preventing symptomatic aura.

Pituitary Apoplexy

Acute ischemic or hemorrhagic infarction of the pituitary (usually into a preexisting macroadenoma) results in a clinical syndrome called pituitary apoplexy, and is usually characterized by severe thunderclap headache, often retro-orbital, and associated with nausea, emesis, and meningismus, and in some cases resembles status migrainosus or the trigeminal autonomic cephalalgias (TACs).[20] Other features of pituitary apoplexy include impaired consciousness, cranial nerve dysfunction (e.g., bitemporal hemianopia, and ophthalmoplegia with diplopia), and additional symptoms due to adrenal crisis (abdominal pain, bradycardia, hypotension, hypothermia, lethargy, and coma).[20] Underlying precipitants of pituitary apoplexy include head trauma, hypertension, pituitary irradiation, pregnancy, and treatment with anticoagulants, estrogen, dopamine receptor agonists, and erectile dysfunction medications. CT and MRI allow for detection of intrasellar pathology. Pituitary hormones should be evaluated on diagnosis and in 4 to 8 weeks. Whether symptomatic or not, acute treatment with intravenous glucocorticoid bolus (100-200 mg hydrocortisone) followed by intermittent (50-100 mg every 6 hours) or continuous (2-4 mg per hour) infusion is recommended. Headache and visual symptoms often improve with conservative management, but also with transsphenoidal resection of the pituitary lesion, when warranted.

Summary

- Headache associated with ischemic stroke often begins at stroke onset, have characteristics of tension-type headaches, and are associated with female sex, young age, and strokes that are in posterior circulation, cortical location, and of cardioembolic or large vessel origin.

- New TCH warrants evaluation for aneurysmal subarachnoid hemorrhage (SAH), but other vascular and nonvascular causes must be considered with primary headache disorders showing TCH symptoms being diagnoses of exclusion.

- Headache associated with ICH and/or SAH may be associated with nausea/emesis, altered consciousness, seizures, and focal neurological deficits.

- Pituitary apoplexy may present with TCH, and have features of status migrainosus, or TACs, as well as visual loss or distortion due to cranial nerve involvement, and symptoms of adrenal crisis.

- Migraine aura-like symptoms may occur with CADASIL, mitochondrial encephalopathy, lactic acidosis, and stroke-like episodes, arteriovenous malformation, moyamoya disease, etc.

- CADASIL is the most prevalent form of hereditary cerebral ischemia and vascular dementia; the predominant initial symptom is migraine with aura, and an MRI brain shows white matter abnormalities by age 30 years.

- TCH in RCVS may recur 4 to 12 weeks after presentation, and its diffuse segmental vasoconstriction with a beads-on-a-string appearance is similar to what is seen in primary angiitis of the central nervous system, but CSF studies and MRI brain may appear normal initially.

- Headache due to cervical artery dissection may be associated with neck trauma and history of migraine without aura, and Horner's syndrome, which is commonly associated with ipsilateral ICA dissection.

- Headache with cerebral venous thrombosis may resemble idiopathic intracranial hypertension with papilledema, and transient visual obscurations.

REFERENCES

1. Rothrock JF, Diener HC. Headache secondary to cerebrovascular disease. *Cephalalgia.* 2021;41(4):479-492.

2. Harriott AM, Karakaya F, Ayata C. Headache after ischemic stroke: a systematic review and meta-analysis. *Neurology.* 2020;94(1):e75-e86.

3. Lebedeva ER, Gurary NM, Olesen J. Headache in transient ischemic attacks. *J Headache Pain.* 2018;19(1):60.

4. Abadie V, Jacquin A, Daubail B, et al. Prevalence and prognostic value of headache on early mortality in acute stroke: the Dijon Stroke Registry. *Cephalalgia.* 2014;34(11):887-894.

5. Huckhagel T, Klinger R, Schmidt NO, Regelsberger J, Westphal M, Czorlich P. The burden of headache following aneurysmal subarachnoid hemorrhage: a prospective single-center cross-sectional analysis. *Acta Neurochir (Wien).* 2020;162(4):893-903.

6. Munoz C, Diez-Tejedor E, Frank A, Barreiro P. Cluster headache syndrome associated with middle cerebral artery arteriovenous malformation. *Cephalalgia.* 1996;16(3):202-205.

7. Corbelli I, De Maria F, Eusebi P, et al. Dural arteriovenous fistulas and headache features: an observational study. *J Headache Pain.* 2020;21(1):6.

8. Malik SN, Young WB. Midbrain cavernous malformation causing migraine-like headache. *Cephalalgia.* 2006;26(8):1016-1019.

9. Cho S, Maharathi B, Ball KL, Loeb JA, Pevsner J. Sturge-Weber syndrome patient registry: delayed diagnosis and poor seizure control. *J Pediatr.* 2019;215:158.e6-e163.e6.

10. Lopez JI, Holdridge A, Chalela J. Headache and vasculitis. *Curr Pain Headache Rep.* 2013; 17(3):320.

Secondary Headaches

11. de Boysson H, Boulouis G, Aouba A, et al. Adult primary angiitis of the central nervous system: isolated small-vessel vasculitis represents distinct disease pattern. *Rheumatology (Oxford)*. 2017;56(3):439-444.

12. Gallerini S, Marsili L, Bartalucci M, Marotti C, Chiti A, Marconi R. Headache secondary to cervical artery dissections: practice pointers. *Neurol Sci*. 2019;40(3):613-615.

13. Schwedt TJ, Matharu MS, Dodick DW. Thunderclap headache. *Lancet Neurol*. 2006;5(7):621-631.

14. Mehta A, Danesh J, Kuruvilla D. Cerebral venous thrombosis headache. *Curr Pain Headache Rep*. 2019;23(7):47.

15. Ling YH, Chen SP. Narrative review: headaches after reversible cerebral vasoconstriction syndrome. *Curr Pain Headache Rep*. 2020;24(12):74.

16. Guey S, Mawet J, Herve D, et al. Prevalence and characteristics of migraine in CADASIL. *Cephalalgia*. 2016;36(11):1038-1047.

17. Kraya T, Deschauer M, Joshi PR, Zierz S, Gaul C. Prevalence of headache in patients with mitochondrial disease: a cross-sectional study. *Headache*. 2018;58(1):45-52.

18. Chiang CC, Shahid AH, Harriott AM, et al. Evaluation and treatment of headache associated with moyamoya disease: a narrative review. *Cephalalgia*. 2022;42(6):542-552.

19. Koemans EA, Voigt S, Rasing I, et al. Migraine with aura as early disease marker in hereditary Dutch-type cerebral amyloid angiopathy. *Stroke*. 2020;51(4):1094-1099.

20. Suri H, Dougherty C. Presentation and management of headache in pituitary apoplexy. *Curr Pain Headache Rep*. 2019;23(9):61.

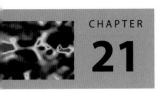

Seizure-Related Headaches

Dana Ionel and Siddharth Kapoor

Epilepsy is a neurological disease characterized by recurrent unprovoked seizures. Similarly, migraine is a neurological disease characterized by recurrent headaches that may also be associated with positive neurological phenomena. Both diseases are characterized by similar clinical episodes that may start with an aura, followed by neurological phenomena and headaches. In certain instances, differentiating between these two conditions can pose a clinical challenge, which has significant implications for management. Seizure-related headaches are more likely after generalized tonic-clonic seizures, or in those who have a secondary generalization of a focal seizure.[1] Interestingly, there is no clear correlation between the duration or frequency of seizures and the incidence of headaches. There is also no established correlation with any epilepsy syndrome.

Epidemiology

There are approximately 3.4 million people in the United States with a diagnosis of epilepsy and 50 million people worldwide.[2,3] There appears to be an increased association of seizure-related headaches with refractory epilepsy, specifically with prevalence increasing with longer duration of epilepsy and a larger number of antiepileptic medications, and the association of these two disorders correlates with worse outcomes in terms of response to treatment. Currently, it is estimated that the frequency of migraine in those with epilepsy ranges from 8.4% to 23%, and the incidence of migraine is 2.4 times higher in those with epilepsy versus those without.[4,5]

Many disability scales designed for assessing disease burden in either epilepsy or migraine often overlook the influence of the other condition. While the Liverpool seizure severity scale is mildly affected by headaches, the concurrent presence of two debilitating diseases with episodic exacerbations can profoundly impact an individual's perceived quality of life.

Headache, Migraine, and Epilepsy: Shared Pathophysiology

The pathophysiology explaining the association between headaches and epilepsy is not known. One theory includes the mechanism of cortical spreading depression that can be seen with both disorders.[6] It has also been postulated that the mechanism may be due to the vasodilation that is typically seen following a seizure. However, this would not explain preictal or ictal headaches, nor would it explain unilateral headaches following generalized seizures.[7] Additionally, more recent data and research are pointing away from the vascular theory of the pathophysiology of migraine, as it is now felt to be a sensory processing disorder affecting the trigeminal pathways.

It is thought that the risk of migraine is at least twice as high in those with epilepsy compared to those without, and evidence has shown that comorbidity between these

Secondary Headaches

two disorders can worsen outcomes, namely, finding that it is less likely to have remission of epilepsy.[8,9] Studies have identified several risk factors or predictors for comorbid epilepsy and migraine, with a history of head trauma being the most common, and focal epilepsy and family history of epilepsy being two other factors.[8] Migraine with aura has been found to be more common in those with epilepsy than migraine without aura, which has led to the question of "migralepsy."[6]

Migraine and Epilepsy: Clinical Presentation and Diagnosis

Frequently a seizure is described as a positive sensorimotor phenomenon evolving over seconds (aura) that may or may not be associated with alteration of awareness (ictal phase) and followed by a postictal state including headache. Depending upon the underlying etiology of the epilepsy, the semiology of a seizure can be very complex. Both focal and generalized seizures can be associated with loss of awareness and followed by headaches. Patients' self-report of loss of awareness is unreliable and poses a challenge to the correct clinical diagnosis. Witness accounts are immensely helpful and consistent aura, when present, can also be of tremendous value. Epigastric rising sensation, when present, can be misinterpreted for nausea, and visual aura can be common to both disorders.

Individuals with migraines may experience episodes accompanied by visual, sensory, motor, and language changes that evolve over a period of more than 5 minutes, as per the criteria of the third edition of the International Classification of Headache Disorders (ICHD-3), and these episodes are often followed by headaches. Table 21-1 provides a comparison of the clinical features of seizures and migraines. Table 21-2 shows the various headache and seizure phenotypes seen in families with similar channelopathies, depending on age and development.

The aura is followed by a headache with prominent migraine features in both conditions. A clear loss of awareness and confusion helps in the diagnosis of seizures but has been reported with migraine and can accompany severe intensity pain. Eventually, one aims to select a diagnosis from the ICHD-3 with precision. This can be achieved through two distinct pathways, as shown in Figure 21-1. The final diagnosis impacts management in myriad ways, including the selection of appropriate medications and the impact on disability secondary to legally mandated restrictions on driving for patient safety. Expert consensus opinion argues against the routine use of EEG in patients with headaches, but a good history should alert the treating physician to appropriate testing in some cases.

Table 21-1. Clinical Feature Comparison: Seizures Versus Migraine

Feature	Seizure	Migraine
Aura duration	Seconds to a minute, rapid onset and progression	>5 minutes to 60 minutes
Aura type		
Auditory	When arising from auditory cortex	Rare, noted in case series
Motor	Excessive movement/dystonia during early part of seizure	Weakness with hemiplegic migraine
Sensory	Positive sensory phenomenon	Numbness
Visual	With seizures originating in visual cortex	Scintillating scotomas
Autonomic	Panayiotopoulos syndrome	Common overlapping symptoms
Olfactory	Common with temporal lobe seizures	

Table 21-2. Different Headache and Seizure Phenotypes Observed in Families with Similar Channelopathies Depending on Age and Development

FHM	Gene	Epilepsy
FHM Type 1	*CACNA1a* gene chromosome19p13	Absence epilepsy, episodic ataxia, spinocerebellar ataxia
FHM Type 2	*ATP1a2* gene chromosome1q23	Benign familial neonatal convulsions and other seizures
FHM Type 3	*SCN1a*	Febrile seizures, generalized epilepsy with febrile seizures, severe myoclonic epilepsy of infancy (Dravet syndrome)
FHM	*PRRT2*	Benign familial infantile seizures, infantile convulsions and choreoathetosis, familial paroxysmal kinesigenic dyskinesia

FHM, familial hemiplegic migraine.

Headaches in Individuals with Epilepsy

Depending upon the timing of the headache, headaches in individuals with epilepsy can be classified into:

- Seizure-related headache
  - Preictal (headache as a warning)
  - Ictal (headache as the sole ictal manifestation)
  - Postictal (ICHD 7.6.2)
- Interictal headache (not occurring within 72 hours of a known seizure)

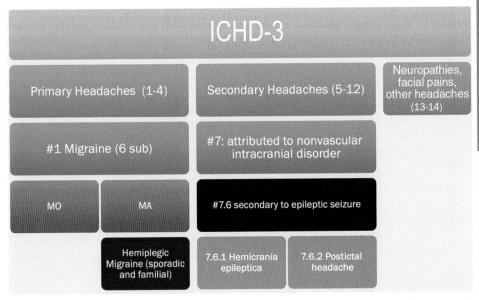

Figure 21-1. Headaches related to seizures/epilepsy listed in the ICHD-3. MO: migraine without aura, MA: migraine with aura.

Preictal Headache

Preictal headaches have been estimated to occur in 5% to 15% of cases of seizure-related headaches.[10] In some studies, headaches preceding seizures were only found in those with focal epilepsy.[7] Interestingly, the rare preictal head pain has been reported to be ipsilateral to the underlying seizure focus in the majority of patients, suggesting potential value in lateralization.

Ictal Headache

Ictal headaches are the rarest of seizure-related headaches and are estimated to occur in 3% to 5% of cases.[10] These may be challenging to characterize and identify because patients may have impaired consciousness due to the seizure itself. The ICHD-3 defines this condition as a headache that arises during a focal seizure. It develops simultaneously with the seizure and is either ipsilateral to the ictal discharge, improves or remits after resolution of the seizure, or both. Some studies indicate that the typical duration of such headaches is between 5 and 10 minutes.[10] Additional symptoms can include confusion, incontinence, brevity, a postictal state, and abnormalities on an EEG.

Another entity that has been described in the literature is the term "migralepsy." The ICHD-3 formally categorizes this as a migraine aura-triggered seizure. The diagnostic criteria specify that a seizure must occur in a patient diagnosed with migraine with aura.

Postictal Headaches

According to current data, the prevalence of postictal headaches, which are the most common seizure-related headaches, ranges between 37% and 51%.[7] The definition by ICHD-3 criteria is a headache following a focal or generalized seizure, which has to have developed within 3 hours of seizure termination, with resolution within 72 hours. These headaches have been found to be most common after generalized seizures, but have also been reported in over 40% of temporal lobe epilepsies and 60% of occipital epilepsies.[7,11] No difference in prevalence has been noted between genders.[1]

Headaches have been described as migraine-like in 30% to 58% of adults, and have been reported by approximately 39% to 50% of adults to cause functional impairment, also being reported in children.[12]

Treatment

Seizure-related headaches, typically with migraine features, can be managed to a large extent with simple analgesics including nonsteroidal anti-inflammatory drugs and medications used for acute migraine. It is possible that calcitonin gene-related peptide (CGRP) small molecule antagonists may also be effective. However, people with epilepsy are typically excluded from clinical trials and hence long-term safety of antimigraine medications is not established. Triptans and ergotamines can cause vasoconstrictions and are contraindicated in hemiplegic migraine. Hence, diagnostic clarity is essential before these agents are utilized for postictal headaches. Ketorolac can also have drug interactions with older antiseizure medications, and caution is advised as use may worsen seizure control. Devices for acute pain control may be utilized, but safety has not been studied in this special population.

Interictal migraine-type headache is also common and poses a particular challenge. Persons with epilepsy have long been excluded from clinical trials for migraine interventions, but the prevalence of this comorbidity is high. Migraine prevention often includes antiseizure medications like valproate and topiramate, but their use is limited in women of childbearing age. Zonisamide can be a useful agent with lower risk based on current pregnancy registry data. While lamotrigine and gabapentin can be helpful in neuropathic type conditions, including trigeminal neuralgia, their efficacy for migraine has limited evidence. Occasionally, medications like lamotrigine and carbamazepine can worsen headaches as a treatment-emergent side effect. Tricyclic antidepressants are relatively contraindicated in epilepsy, but SSRIs/SNRIs may be helpful in managing depression as well migraine (common comorbidity to both migraine and epilepsy). Antihypertensives like propranolol, when tolerated, can be useful. OnabotulinumtoxinA has been used effectively in patients with chronic migraine and epilepsy without any known risk. Newer agents, including CGRP antagonists, though not studied, appear to be safe and effective in reducing headache burden without impacting seizure control. Patients with epilepsy may also have implanted devices like vagal nerve stimulator, deep brain stimulation, and responsive neurostimulator, which may complicate the use of any other devices utilized for headaches. Magnetic interference from external devices can interfere with device programming, and transmagnetic stimulation may be contraindicated for such patients.

Summary

- Epilepsy and migraine have overlapping symptoms, making differentiation challenging but vital for treatment; seizure-linked headaches do not align with seizure patterns or specific syndromes.

- The exact prevalence and incidence of migraine and epilepsy are not known, but it is estimated that the frequency of migraine in those with epilepsy ranges from 8.4% to 23%.

- The pathophysiological relation between headaches and epilepsy is not fully understood, but one theory suggests a shared mechanism of cortical spreading depression in both disorders.

- Differentiating seizures from migraines is complex; seizures typically start with an aura and can alter awareness, while migraine has similar, slower-evolving symptoms per ICHD criteria.

- In individuals with epilepsy, headaches can be classified as seizure-related (preictal, ictal, or postictal) or interictal (those that do not occur within 72 hours of a known seizure).

- In epilepsy patients, headaches are commonly managed with simple analgesics and specific migraine treatments, but their long-term safety is not well studied due to the exclusion of those with epilepsy from clinical trials.

REFERENCES

1. Ekstein D, Schachter SC. Postictal headache. *Epilepsy Behav.* 2010;19(2):151-155.

2. CDC. Epilepsy data and statistics [Internet]. CDC. 2019. Available at https://www.cdc.gov/epilepsy/data/index.html.

3. World Health Organization. Epilepsy [Internet]. World Health Organization. World Health Organization: WHO; 2023. Available at https://www.who.int/news-room/fact-sheets/detail/epilepsy.

4. Bigal ME, Lipton RB, Cohen J, Silberstein SD. Epilepsy and migraine. *Epilepsy Behav.* 2003; 4:13-24.

5. Welch KMA, Lewis D. Migraine and epilepsy. *Neurol Clin.* 1997;15(1):107-114.

6. Leniger T, von den Driesch S, Isbruch K, Diener HC, Hufnagel A. Clinical characteristics of patients with comorbidity of migraine and epilepsy. *Headache J Head Face Pain.* 2003;43(6):672-677.

7. Förderreuther S, Henkel A, Noachtar S, Straube A. Headache associated with epileptic seizures: epidemiology and clinical characteristics. *Headache J Head Face Pain.* 2002;42(7):649-655.

8. Ottman R, Lipton RB. Comorbidity of migraine and epilepsy. *Neurology.* 1994;44(11):2105-2105.

9. Nye BL, Thadani VM. Migraine and epilepsy: review of the literature. *Headache* [Internet]. 2015;55(3):359-380. Available at https://pubmed.ncbi.nlm.nih.gov/25754865/.

Secondary Headaches

10. Saitowitz Z, Flamini R, Berenson F. Ictal epileptic headache: a review of current literature and differentiation from migralepsy and other epilepsies. *Headache J Head Face Pain.* 2014;54(9):1534-1540.

11. Gobel H. 7.6.2 Post-ictal headache [Internet]. ICHD-3. [cited 2023 Aug 27]. Available at https://ichd-3.org/7-headache-attributed-to-non-vascular-intracranial-disorder/7-6-headache-attributed-to-epileptic-seizure/7-6-2-post-ictal-headache/.

12. Velioglu SK, Boz C, Ozmenoglu M. The impact of migraine on epilepsy: a prospective prognosis study. *Cephalalgia.* 2005;25(7):528-535.

CHAPTER 22 Headache and Temporal Arteritis

Umer Najib and Fallon Schloemer

Temporal arteritis (TA), also known as giant cell arteritis, is a condition characterized by inflammation of the blood vessels, particularly in the temples. The typical symptoms of TA include severe headaches, scalp tenderness, jaw pain, and vision problems. However, among these symptoms, headaches are the most common and prominent feature. Headache may be the sole clinical symptom of TA. A new-onset or persistent headache in a patient over 60 years of age should raise concern for TA. It is crucial to diagnose this condition promptly to prevent potential complications such as vision loss and stroke.

Epidemiology

TA is the most common form of systemic vasculitis in patients older than 50 years.[1] It is about three times more common in women with peak incidence between 70 and 80 years of age. The incidence of TA varies globally among different ethnic groups, with Northern Europeans, particularly those of Scandinavian descent, experiencing the highest rates. In comparison, lower rates are observed in Asian, Hispanic, and African American populations. The estimated annual incidence of TA can reach up to 27 cases per 100,000 individuals in certain Northern European populations.[1] Whereas the pooled prevalence of TA is around 52 cases per 100,000 people over age 50. Overall headache is reported by about two-thirds of patients with TA, while it may be the presenting or initial symptom in about one-third of the patients.[2]

Pathophysiology

The pathophysiology of TA involves immune-mediated inflammation of the blood vessels, specifically the medium- and large-sized arteries. The exact cause of this inflammatory response is not fully understood but may involve a combination of genetic susceptibility and environmental triggers. Histopathological examination of affected arteries shows infiltration of immune cells, primarily T-cells and macrophages, into the arterial wall leading to the release of proinflammatory cytokines and other mediators with subsequent vessel wall damage and inflammation. In addition to the intimal thickening resulting from lymphocytic infiltration, biopsy specimens often show large multinucleated giant cells formed by the fusion of activated macrophages (Figure 22-1). These changes eventually lead to impaired blood flow, with ischemia and damage to the surrounding tissues, including organs supplied by the affected arteries.

Clinical Characteristics and Diagnosis

History

According to the American College of Rheumatology clinical criteria, three out of the five following core features are needed for diagnosis of TA: (a) age of onset greater than 50 years,

Secondary Headaches

149

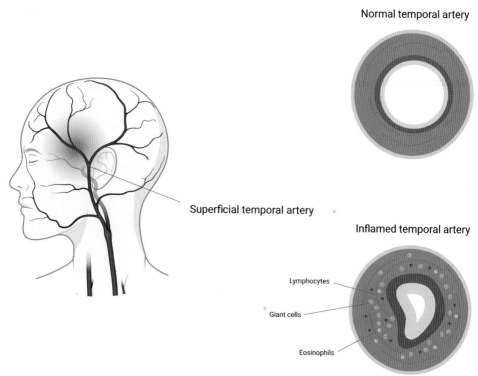

Figure 22-1. Arterial vessel wall changes in Temporal arteritis.

(b) new-onset headache, (c) temporal artery tenderness or decreased temporal artery pulse, (d) elevated erythrocyte sedimentation rate (Westergren) ≥50 mm/h, (e) abnormal temporal artery biopsy (TAB) showing necrotizing arteritis, characterized by a predominance of mononuclear cell infiltrates or a granulomatous process with multinucleated giant cells.[2] Four clinical phenotypes of TA have been described in the literature.[3] There can be substantial overlap between these phenotypes. The most common phenotype is the cranial type, accounting for approximately 80% of cases. It is characterized by cranial arteritis presenting as localized headache in the temporal region, scalp tenderness, tenderness of the temporal arteries, reduced or absent temporal artery pulses, sudden vision loss, and jaw or tongue claudication. While intracranial involvement is not typical in TA, there have been rare reports of transient ischemic attacks and ischemic strokes, typically in the vertebrobasilar distribution. The polymyalgia rheumatica phenotype represents about 40% of cases and is characterized by symptoms such as fatigue, malaise, morning stiffness in the shoulders and neck, and aching of the shoulder and hip girdle. The third phenotype is that of large vessel vasculitis, which manifests with symptoms such as limb claudication, asymmetric peripheral pulses, hypertension, lightheadedness, subclavian steal syndrome, and the potential presence of aortic aneurysms or dissection. Finally, the fourth phenotype is described as a nonspecific systemic inflammatory disease. It is associated with symptoms such as fatigue, malaise, fever, night sweats, and weight loss. It is important to note that these phenotypes serve as a clinical framework and should be considered in conjunction with other diagnostic evaluations to guide appropriate management strategies for patients with TA. The noncranial constellation of findings may precede the classic cranial phenotype, and, therefore, a history of these clinical symptoms should be sought in older patients with new-onset headache.

Headache in TA can manifest as acute or subacute in onset. It is commonly accompanied by scalp tenderness and may exhibit clinical features resembling migraine or trigeminal autonomic cephalalgias. Interestingly, in up to 50% of patients, the headache may localize to regions other than the temporal regions. In addition to the headache, individuals with TA may also experience pain in the jaw or tongue. *The International Classification of Headache Disorders*, 3rd edition, describes the headache in TA in Section 6.4.1, "Headache Attributed to Giant Cell Arteritis" (Box 22-1).[4]

Physical Examination

Although the physical examination findings are typically unremarkable in patients with TA, it is crucial to note that a normal examination does not exclude the diagnosis of TA. To evaluate potential signs of TA, a comprehensive vascular examination should be conducted. Specifically, the temporal arteries should be assessed for tenderness and reduced pulsation through palpation and comparison to the contralateral side. Furthermore, it is important to palpate and auscultate all accessible medium and large arteries, while listening for bruits over the thoracic and abdominal aorta. The scalp and tongue should be inspected for any ischemic changes. During funduscopy, the findings may appear normal, but there is also the possibility of observing a "chalky white" swollen optic disc, which raises concern for anterior ischemic optic neuropathy.

Laboratory Testing

Laboratory data can provide supplementary information and assist in the diagnosis of TA (Chapter 3). Elevated levels of erythrocyte sedimentation rate (ESR) and high-sensitivity C-reactive protein (CRP) are typically observed, but both are nonspecific markers. The majority of patients with TA have an ESR higher than 50 mm/h, with a mean value of 85 mm/h. It is important to consider that the upper normal limit of ESR varies based on age and gender, calculated as (age/2) for men and [(age + 10)/2] for women. However, it should be noted that a normal ESR and CRP do not exclude the diagnosis of TA. In fact, approximately 4% of patients with biopsy-proven TA have normal ESR and CRP levels at the time of diagnosis.[5] A complete blood count can also be informative, as systemic inflammation may lead to normochromic anemia, leukocytosis, thrombocytosis, and elevated hepatic enzymes.

Box 22-1. ICHD-3 Diagnostic Criteria of Headache Attributed to Giant Cell Arteritis (GCA)

Headache caused by and symptomatic of GCA. Headache may be the sole symptom of GCA, a disease most conspicuously associated with headache. The features of the headache are variable.

A. Any new headache fulfilling criterion C

B. GCA has been diagnosed

C. Evidence of causation demonstrated by at least two of the following:
    1. headache has developed in close temporal relation to other symptoms and/or clinical or biological signs of onset of GCA, or has led to the diagnosis of GCA
    2. either or both of the following:
        a) headache has significantly worsened in parallel with worsening of GCA
        b) headache has significantly improved or resolved within 3 days of high-dose steroid treatment
    3. headache is associated with scalp tenderness and/or jaw claudication

D. Not better accounted for by another ICHD-3 diagnosis

Secondary Headaches

Imaging Studies

Imaging techniques such as color Doppler ultrasonography (CDUS), computed tomography with angiography (CTA), magnetic resonance angiography (MRA), and positron emission tomography (PET) can provide valuable information to support the diagnosis of TA. CDUS can be utilized to support the diagnosis of TA by identifying the presence of a halo sign (hypoechoic ring), stenosis, or occlusion of the superficial temporal artery (Chapter 2). When all these findings are present, CDUS can exhibit a sensitivity of up to 87% and a specificity of up to 96%.[6] While the utility of CDUS depends on the expertise of the ultrasonographer, it can still be beneficial in guiding biopsy site selection, particularly as "skip lesions" may be present in affected arteries.

MRA and CTA are particularly useful for evaluating large vessel vasculitis. MRA can reveal edema, wall thickening, or enhancement, while CTA can demonstrate vascular stenosis and dilation. PET can also aid in supporting the diagnosis of TA, as inflamed large arteries typically exhibit increased uptake of fluorodeoxyglucose (FDG). However, it is important to interpret the results of these imaging studies cautiously, as they can be influenced by steroid treatment initiation.

Temporal Artery Biopsy

TAB is considered the gold standard for the diagnosis of TA, with an overall estimated sensitivity of 87%.[7] Although the biopsy itself is a brief and low-risk procedure, it is crucial to ensure technical adequacy. Biopsy should be performed on the artery ipsilateral to the clinical symptoms or any abnormal examination findings, such as tenderness upon palpation. Specific areas with abnormal appearances on CDUS can be targeted for biopsy. Longer biopsy segments are associated with higher diagnostic yield, and a cutoff of 20 mm is typically considered adequate. Positive TAB specimens exhibit intimal thickening resulting from lymphocytic infiltration. While the presence of activated macrophages and multinucleated giant cells is considered classic, they may not always be apparent. False-negative results can occur due to segmental involvement of TA, leading to "skip lesions," or when patients have TA without cranial arteritis. The yield of a second biopsy on the contralateral side is generally low. In cases of high pretest probability, imaging studies and laboratory data can further support the diagnosis. Treatment should never be delayed or withheld while awaiting biopsy results. Studies have indicated that corticosteroid treatment for less than 2 weeks does not reduce the likelihood of obtaining a positive TAB result.

Treatment

High-dose systemic corticosteroids are the recommended treatment for TA. However, in individuals who have comorbidities or contraindications that preclude the use of steroids, alternative options such as steroid-sparing agents can be considered.

Corticosteroids

The initial treatment of TA is often determined by the presence or absence of cranial ischemic manifestations, such as amaurosis fugax, vision loss, or stroke. In cases with these neurological deficits, initial treatment with corticosteroids should be administered intravenously (IV). Two retrospective studies comparing high-dose IV corticosteroids to high-dose oral steroids in patients with giant cell arteritis and cranial manifestations found visual improvements in the IV treatment group.[8,9] An initial intravenous dose of methylprednisolone, ranging from 250 to 1000 mg per day, for 3 to 5 days is typically recommended, followed by oral administration. In cases without cranial ischemic manifestations, high-dose oral glucocorticoids can be initiated as the initial treatment, often starting at a dosage of prednisolone of 1 mg/kg per day (up to a maximum of 60 mg/day). The tapering of steroids should be guided by the patient's response to therapy, with the option of tapering as early as 1 to 2 weeks (to minimize toxicity) or delaying tapering for several weeks to months if clinically necessary.

It is important to note that the literature supporting the efficacy and lower toxicity of moderate-dose glucocorticoids, often in the form of alternate-day dosing, is limited, and therefore, it is not considered a reasonable alternative to high-dose steroids. However, it may be considered in patients at higher risk of complications from steroids. The dosing and duration of therapy may vary among patients, considering their medical comorbidities and the use of steroid-sparing agents. Monitoring the patient's response to therapy is crucial, both clinically and through the measurement of ESR and CRP levels to assess disease activity. The proposed tapering schedule typically starts after 1 month of treatment, with a gradual reduction of prednisolone by 10 mg every 2 weeks until reaching 20 mg. Subsequently, the dose is decreased by 2.5 mg every 2 to 4 weeks until reaching 10 mg, followed by a reduction of 1 mg every 1 to 2 weeks.[10]

Steroid-Sparing Agents

Steroids are not without risk and may need to be avoided in certain patients. Systemic complications of steroids include, but are not limited to, osteoporosis, diabetes, and increased risk of infection. In cases where steroid therapy needs to be minimized or avoided, several steroid-sparing agents can be considered. These agents, such as methotrexate, azathioprine, and hydroxychloroquine, have been studied in clinical trials with small sample sizes.[11] Tocilizumab, a humanized monoclonal antibody targeting interleukin-6 (IL-6), has shown efficacy in reducing disease relapse and decreasing steroid usage. Tocilizumab has received FDA approval for the treatment of GCA.[12] Other treatments that have been considered for TA, although with limited evidence, include antiplatelets such as aspirin and lipid-lowering agents such as statins.

Prognosis

TA is usually a self-limiting disease, but the duration of illness can be variable, lasting months to even years. And some patients can require long-term treatment with glucocorticoids. Relapses can occur, as can therapy-associated complications. Treatment should not be delayed if TA is clinically suspected and should be started even without confirmation through TAB or diagnostic imaging. Any delay in treatment could lead to blindness, which can be irreversible.

Summary

- TA, also called giant cell arteritis, is the most common form of systemic vasculitis in individuals over the age of 50.
- Headache, scalp tenderness, and jaw claudication are hallmark features of TA.
- In individuals over the age of 50 presenting with a new-onset headache, TA should be considered and investigated promptly to avoid misdiagnosis and delayed treatment.
- High-dose corticosteroids remain the primary treatment for TA and should not be delayed while waiting for TAB results.
- Steroid-sparing agents may be considered, although evidence of their efficacy is limited.

REFERENCES

1. Watts RA, Robson J. Introduction, epidemiology and classification of vasculitis. *Best Pract Res Clin Rheumatol.* 2018;32:3-20.
2. Hunder GG, Bloch DA, Michel BA, et al. The American College of Rheumatology 1990 criteria for the classification of giant cell arteritis. *Arthritis Rheum.* 1990;33(8):1122-1128.
3. de Boysson H, Liozon E, Ly KH, et al. The different clinical patterns of giant cell arteritis. *Clin Exp Rheumatol.* 2019;37 Suppl 117(2):57-60.
4. Headache Classification Committee of the International Headache Society (IHS). *The International Classification of Headache Disorders*, 3rd edition. *Cephalalgia.* 2018;38(1):1-211.

5. Smetana GW, Shmerling RH. Does this patient have temporal arteritis? *JAMA*. 2002;287(1):92-101.

6. Karassa FB, Matsagas MI, Schmidt WA, Ioannidis JPA. Meta-analysis: test performance of ultrasonography for giant-cell arteritis. *Ann Intern Med*. 2005;142(5):359-369.

7. Niederkohr RD, Levin LA. A Bayesian analysis of the true sensitivity of a temporal artery biopsy. *Invest Ophthalmol Vis Sci*. 2007;48(2):675-680.

8. Chan CC, Paine M, O'Day J. Steroid management in giant cell arteritis. *Br J Ophthalmol*. 2001;85: 1061-1064.

9. Hayreh SS, Zimmerman B, Kardon RH. Visual improvement with corticosteroid therapy in giant cell arteritis: report of a large study and review of literature. *Acta Ophthalmol Scand*. 2002;80: 355-367.

10. Dasgupta B, Borg FA, Hassan N, et al. BSR and BHPR guidelines for the management of giant cell arteritis. *Rheumatology (Oxford)*. 2010;49:1594-1597.

11. Amol Sagdeo, Ayman Askari, Josh Dixey, Hana Morrissey, Patrick A. Ball. Steroid-sparing agents in giant cell arteritis. *Open Rheumatol J*. 2019; 13:61-71.

12. Stone JH, Tuckwell K, Dimonaco S, et al. Trial of tocilizumab in giant-cell arteritis. *N Engl J Med*. 2017;377(4):317-328.

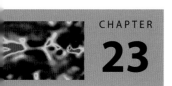

Headache and Idiopathic Intracranial Hypertension

Deborah I. Friedman

The idiopathic intracranial hypertension (IIH), also known as pseudotumor cerebri syndrome (PTCS), encompasses both primary and secondary etiologies.[1,2] The syndrome is characterized by symptoms such as headache, transient visual obscurations, pulsatile tinnitus, and subjective visual loss. Evaluation typically reveals papilledema without hydrocephalus or space-occupying lesions, along with elevated cerebrospinal fluid (CSF) pressure and normal CSF contents. Timely diagnosis and treatment are crucial to prevent permanent visual loss or blindness. Although IIH predominantly affects overweight women of childbearing age, it is essential to note that not all obese women with headaches fall into this category. Adhering to diagnostic criteria is paramount in correctly identifying the condition while avoiding unnecessary overdiagnosis. This chapter presents a systematic approach to diagnosis and management, highlighting potential pitfalls that may lead to unwarranted procedures and treatments.

Epidemiology

The incidence of IIH is estimated to be 5 per 100,000 individuals in the general population, but it rises to 25 per 100,000 in obese women between the ages of 22 and 44.[3] The prevalence in 2017 was 76/100,000 with a sixfold increase since 2003.[4] The female predilection and its association with obesity typically manifest after puberty, while prepubertal boys and girls are equally affected and often maintain a normal weight. IIH is relatively uncommon in men, and its onset after the age of 45 is unusual. It is worth noting that there has been an observed increase in the incidence of IIH over the past 10 to 15 years, with a 108% rise reported between 2002 and 2016 decades.[3] This increase may be attributed to improved detection methods or the concurrent rise in obesity rates witnessed over the past few decades.[3]

Pathophysiology

The pathophysiology of IIH remains uncertain, and various theories have been proposed.[5] One theory suggests an increase in CSF production by the choroid plexus, while another suggests a decrease in CSF absorption by the arachnoid granulations, nasal and dural lymphatics, and glymphatic system. The presence of cerebral venous sinus stenosis in over 90% of IIH cases supports the arachnoid granulation theory. In rodents, nonhuman primates, and humans, CNS lymphatics in the nasal cavity and lymphatic vessels drain approximately 50% of the CSF. Lymphatic vessels in the dura may also play a role. Additionally, paravenous drainage through the glymphatics, which facilitate the exchange of fluid between the brain parenchyma and subarachnoid space, may contribute to the pathophysiology of IIH, although the extent of their involvement is uncertain.[5]

Obesity and recent weight gain are well-established associations with IIH. The predominance of obesity in affected adolescent and adult females raises questions about the contribution of hormonal and metabolic factors. Glucocorticoids, including cortisol, are regulated by the enzyme 11β-hydroxysteroid dehydrogenase type 1 (11β-HSD1). Reduced activation of glucocorticoids by 11β-HSD1 following weight loss has been associated with a decrease in intracranial pressure.[6] Leptin, an adipokine proportional to body fat, influences energy balance and appetite. Studies on CSF leptin levels in IIH have produced conflicting results. Estrogen and progesterone do not appear to play a significant role. However, the high prevalence of polycystic ovary syndrome (PCOS) in patients with IIH raises the possibility that androgens may be contributory. Women with IIH have shown a distinct pattern of androgen excess with increased CSF testosterone and androstenedione, as well as increased serum testosterone, compared to women with simple obesity and PCOS.[7] The specific contribution of androgens to IIH remains uncertain, although androgen receptors are present on choroid plexus epithelial cells.

Furthermore, several medications have been implicated in the development of IIH. These include tetracycline, retinoids/vitamin A, and lithium. Hormonal contraceptives are not causative unless associated with weight gain, although venous sinus thrombosis must be excluded. No apparent commonality has been observed among these medications, providing limited insights into the pathogenesis of IIH. Conditions that impede venous return from the brain to the heart, such as cerebral venous sinus thrombosis, jugular vein thrombosis, or right heart failure, can produce a similar syndrome.

Diagnosis and Clinical Characteristics

Symptoms

The diagnosis of IIH requires a combination of symptoms and signs and cannot be defined by one specific manifestation. Headache, the most common symptom, occurs in approximately 85% to 90% of patients and is often the initial symptom.[8] The headache is typically different from previous headaches and is often severe (Box 23-1). Interestingly, participants in the Idiopathic Intracranial

---

Box 23-1. Diagnostic Criteria of Headache Attributed to Idiopathic Intracranial Hypertension (IIH) According to the *International Classification of Headache Disorders*, Third Edition (ICHD-3)

New headache, or a significant worsening of a preexisting headache, caused by and accompanied by other symptoms and/or clinical and/or neuroimaging signs of idiopathic intracranial hypertension (IIH), with typical features suggestive of IIH.

A. New headache, or a significant worsening of a preexisting headache, fulfilling criterion C

B. Both of the following:
  1. idiopathic intracranial hypertension (IIH) has been diagnosed
  2. cerebrospinal fluid (CSF) pressure exceeds 250 mm CSF (or 280 mm CSF in obese children)

C. Either or both of the following:
  1. headache has developed or significantly worsened in temporal relation to the IIH, or led to its discovery
  2. headache is accompanied by either or both of the following:
    a) pulsatile tinnitus
    b) papilledema

D. Not better accounted for by another ICHD-3 diagnosis

Hypertension Treatment Trial (IIHTT) had a higher prevalence of previous migraine (42%) com-pared to the general population (12% overall, 18% of adult women).[8] The headache phenotype in IIH most commonly resembles migraine without aura or tension-type headache. It may manifest as unilateral or bilateral pain in any location of the head and is frequently associated with neck pain.

Transient visual obscurations (TVOs) are the second most common symptom of IIH. These epi-sodes involve complete or partial visual loss in one or both eyes, often triggered by changes in posture such as arising or bending forward, and typically last for seconds to a few minutes. TVOs are indica-tive of papilledema, although they can also occur in the presence of optic disc drusen, which can mimic papilledema.

Pulsatile tinnitus, experienced as unilateral or bilateral ringing in the ears that coincides with the heartbeat, is often reported by patients with IIH. In some cases, the tinnitus can be intense enough to disrupt sleep, interfere with hearing, or be audible to others. However, pulsatile tinnitus is not exclu-sive to IIH, and its underlying cause is often difficult to identify.

The visual system is commonly affected in IIH. Increased intracranial pressure can result in uni-lateral or bilateral abducens palsy, which serves as a false localizing sign. Some patients with IIH also experience binocular, horizontal diplopia (double vision). Visual loss can affect the central or periph-eral visual fields due to optic disc edema. Decreased visual acuity at presentation is a poor prognostic indicator and requires prompt intervention. Perimetry, a visual field testing method, is essential for diagnosing and monitoring the course of IIH. However, deficits detected on confrontation visual field testing indicate that significant visual field loss has already occurred. Other visual field defects observed in IIH include enlargement of the blind spot, arcuate scotomas, and concentric constric-tion. It is important to differentiate functional visual loss from organic causes to avoid unnecessary interventions.

Many women with IIH also exhibit signs of systemic fluid retention or idiopathic (orthostatic) edema.

Signs

In severe cases of IIH, signs of optic neuropathy may be present, such as decreased visual acuity, a cen-tral scotoma, and abnormal color perception. The pupils may appear normal or demonstrate sluggish reactivity. A relative afferent pupillary defect, which indicates asymmetrical involvement of the two eyes, may be observed. When optic disc edema is severe enough to extend into the macula, blurred and distorted vision (metamorphopsia) can occur. During ocular motility examination, findings may include esophoria (inward deviation of the eyes), esotropia (crossed eyes), or palsy of the lateral rectus muscle. Other patterns of diplopia (double vision) and ophthalmoparesis (weakness or paralysis of eye movements) are rare in IIH.

The hallmark of IIH is the presence of papilledema (Figure 23-1).[5] Detecting subtle papilledema can be challenging with a direct ophthalmoscope, as it can be easily confused with pseudopapill-edema caused by optic disc drusen or tilted optic discs. Therefore, collaboration with an ophthal-mologist or neuro-ophthalmologist is advisable. In addition to indistinct disc margins, other helpful findings on ophthalmoscopy include a dark peripapillary halo (C-shaped in grade 2 papilledema, complete 360-degree halo in grade 3 papilledema), obscuration of a major vessel crossing the disc margin (grade 3), obscuration of a major vessel over the disc (grade 4), or loss of all major vessels crossing the disc margin or over the disc (grade 5). These features aid in grading the severity of pap-illedema. Some cases of IIH lack papilledema. Reasons for the absence of papilledema are (1) resolu-tion of previous papilledema, (2) evaluation very early in the disease course, and (3) preexisting optic nerve damage or atrophy. IIH without papilledema is uncommon, accounting for 5% of IIH patients in a neuro-ophthalmic practice. A definite diagnosis of IIH cannot be made without papilledema (or previously documented papilledema). Imaging findings support a "suggested" diagnosis at best. Incorrect diagnosis of IIH leads to unnecessary diagnostic and therapeutic procedures that may cause harm.[1]

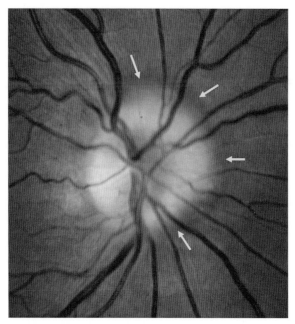

Figure 23-1. Frisén grade 2 papilledema of the right optic disc. There is elevation of the disc margin superiorly, nasally, and inferiorly with a dark C-shaped peripapillary halo (arrows).

Neuroimaging

Magnetic resonance imaging (MRI) of the brain is the standard imaging study for evaluating IIH.[9] It serves to exclude other structural causes of increased CSF pressure and may reveal specific signs associated with IIH. These signs include an enlarged sella turcica with pituitary flattening, expansion of the perioptic subarachnoid spaces, flattening of the posterior sclerae at the junction of the optic nerve and the globe (best visualized on T2-weighted axial images), enlargement of Meckel's caves, meningoencephaloceles, cerebellar tonsillar descent, and protrusion of the optic nerve papilla into the vitreous cavity. It is important to note that some MRI signs, such as pituitary flattening, enlarged Meckel's caves, and perioptic subarachnoid space expansion, can also be observed in individuals without IIH. Therefore, the diagnosis of IIH cannot be solely based on MRI findings.

Magnetic resonance venography (MRV) is useful in excluding venous sinus thrombosis and often reveals venous sinus stenosis, which is a common finding in IIH. In cases where the brain MRI does not adequately visualize the course of the optic nerves, an MRI of the orbits can provide additional information. If MRI is not feasible or contraindicated, computed tomography (CT) of the head with contrast may be considered as an alternative. Although sagittal reconstruction images from current-generation CT scanners have lower resolution compared to MRI, they can still be valuable for assessing changes at the skull base and posterior fossa.

Lumbar Puncture

A diagnostic lumbar puncture (LP) with measurement of the opening pressure is essential for establishing a definitive diagnosis of IIH (Chapter 3). For the most accurate opening pressure reading, the LP procedure is performed with the patient positioned in the lateral decubitus position. Misinterpretation of the LP results, incorrect patient positioning, and use of sedation are common sources of diagnostic error.[1] Although improvement of symptoms after CSF removal can occur, it is not universally observed and should not be relied upon as a diagnostic criterion. Removing enough CSF to reduce the pressure to the mid-normal range (approximately 15 cm CSF) helps prevent a spinal headache that can lead to transient worsening of vision.

Sleep Apnea Assessment

Intracranial pressure can increase during episodes of apnea, which is associated with the retention of carbon dioxide (CO_2). Therefore, it is important to screen patients, particularly males, for obstructive sleep apnea (OSA) in the evaluation of intracranial hypertension.

Treatment

The management of IIH is comprehensive and involves multiple approaches (Box 23-2).[2] If a secondary cause is identified, the first step is to discontinue the medication if possible or address the underlying medical condition responsible for PTCS. However, additional treatment is usually necessary to effectively manage the condition. The primary objective of therapy is to preserve or restore vision. Additionally, separate treatment specifically targeting headaches is often required.

Lowering of CSF Pressure

Pharmacological Treatment

Acetazolamide is the only medication supported by class I evidence for effectively treating IIH. Findings from IIHTT[8] demonstrated statistically significant benefits of acetazolamide compared to placebo in various aspects. These include improvements in visual field loss, papilledema grade, weight loss, general and visual quality of life, as well as LP opening pressure in patients with mild visual field loss. However, there was no significant difference in headache disability improvement between acetazolamide and placebo. The standard initial dosage of acetazolamide is 500 mg taken twice daily, with the option to gradually increase the dose up to 2 g twice daily if necessary. Topiramate (25 mg daily, increasing gradually to 200 mg daily as needed) may be added to acetazolamide for headache control or used as a single agent in cases with mild disc edema, minimal or no visual field loss, and predominant headache. In cases where patients experience intolerable side effects from acetazolamide, alternative medications such as methazolamide (50-200 mg daily) and furosemide (40-160 mg daily) can be considered. It is important to note that a sulfonamide antibiotic allergy does not automatically exclude the use of these alternatives. Thiazide diuretics may also be employed, and limited studies

Secondary Headaches

Box 23-2. Treatment of Idiopathic Intracranial Hypertension

1. Discontinue the causative agent or treat the underlying cause, as applicable
2. Treatments to lower the CSF pressure
   A. Pharmacological
   B. Repeated lumbar punctures
   C. Surgical and interventional
3. Headache treatment
4. Weight loss
   A. Pharmacological
   B. Surgical
5. Treatment of obstructive sleep apnea, as appropriate

suggest the potential use of octreotide. For patients who exhibit an allergy to the sulfonamide group present in the aforementioned medications, alternative diuretic options include spironolactone, triamterene, and ethacrynic acid. It is crucial to closely monitor individuals taking combinations of diuretics, as it may lead to profound hypokalemia. Although corticosteroids can temporarily lower CSF pressure and may be used in urgent cases of impending visual loss, their continued use is counterproductive due to undesired side effects and associated medical risks. Glucagon-like peptide-1 (GLP-1) receptor agonists, which produce rapid weight loss during active treatment, are being investigated for IIH treatment.

Repeated Lumbar Punctures

Repeated LPs may be warranted under specific circumstances.[2] These include cases of rapidly progressive visual loss when a lumbar drain is not feasible, intermittent exacerbations of symptoms, and the need for treatment during pregnancy. However, monitoring CSF pressure as an indicator of treatment efficacy or status is not necessary. The decision to perform an LP should be based on the patient's overall condition and individual clinical factors.

Surgical and Interventional Treatment

Indications for surgical and interventional procedures in the management of IIH include visual acuity loss at presentation, severe visual field loss at presentation, rapidly progressive visual loss, and failure of medical therapy.[5] However, the available evidence supporting these treatments is surprisingly limited.[10] Optic nerve sheath fenestration is a surgical procedure performed by an experienced oculoplastic surgeon. This procedure is indicated in patients with visual acuity or significant visual field loss accompanied by papilledema. The surgery may be performed on one or both eyes, and treating the more severely affected eye may also yield benefits for the fellow eye. Additionally, it is worth noting that headache symptoms sometimes improve after optic nerve sheath fenestration.

Shunting procedures, such as ventriculoperitoneal and lumboperitoneal shunting, directly reduce CSF pressure and are initially effective in most cases. However, shunt failures are relatively common, necessitating repeat operations and potentially leading to shunt dependence. Although headaches may initially improve following shunting, they often recur over time. Consequently, shunts are not recommended as a primary treatment for headaches associated with IIH or PTCS. Venous sinus stenting is an intervention that aims to decrease CSF pressure by reducing cerebral venous sinus pressure and enhancing CSF absorption. Patients are carefully evaluated using venous sinus manometry to assess the pressure gradient across the stenotic area of the vessel, typically the transverse sinus. Higher pressure gradients are indicative of more favorable outcomes. Prior to and for 6 months after stenting, patients receive antiplatelet treatment. It is important to note that re-stenosis can occur adjacent to the stent.

Headache Treatment

No randomized trials have specifically examined medications for the treatment of headaches associated with IIH. The choice of acute and preventive treatments depends on the specific characteristics of the headache experienced by the patient.[2] Topiramate (25 mg daily, gradually increasing to 200 mg daily as needed) and zonisamide (25 mg daily, gradually increasing to 600 mg daily maximum) are two medications that offer potential benefits for IIH-related headaches. In addition to their primary pharmacological actions, they also exhibit carbonic anhydrase inhibition and may contribute to weight loss. Erenumab, as demonstrated in an open-label study, has shown improvement in PTCS-related headaches.[11] It is important to avoid the use of opioids, butalbital, and medications known to be associated with weight gain or peripheral edema (e.g., valproate, corticosteroids, verapamil, pregabalin) in the treatment of IIH-related headaches. Even after successfully controlling CSF pressure, headaches often persist, likely due to central sensitization. In such cases, medications aimed at lowering CSF pressure are generally ineffective, and alternative headache treatments should be considered. It is always essential to consult with a neuro-ophthalmologist for individualized treatment recommendations and guidance.

Weight Loss Treatment

Weight loss is a crucial long-term treatment approach for managing IIH.[5] Achieving a 6% to 10% reduction in body weight, which is a realistic and attainable goal, is associated with improved papilledema and visual field parameters. Medical weight loss strategies involve dietary modifications (low-calorie, low-sodium diet) along with moderate exercise. An endocrinologist may provide additional medication options to facilitate weight loss. It is important to be aware that subsequent weight gain increases the risk of recurrent intracranial hypertension. Bariatric surgery has shown benefits in patients with a BMI >35 kg/m^2, especially when there are other coexisting comorbidities.

Prognosis

The prognosis of patients with IIH is generally favorable, with the majority of patients experiencing a monophasic course.[12] However, it is important to note that some degree of visual field loss persists in approximately 25% of patients, while severe visual loss, legal blindness, or complete blindness occurs in fewer than 10% of cases. Chronic and debilitating headaches are common in patients with IIH and can be challenging to manage effectively. These persistent headaches often require ongoing treatment and may significantly impact the quality of life for affected individuals. Additionally, patients with IIH are prone to developing anxiety and depression, which may necessitate appropriate treatment and support. Recurrences of IIH are possible, highlighting the need for continued monitoring and management of the condition even after initial improvement. In the IIHTT,[8] several poor prognostic factors were identified. These include male sex, high-grade papilledema, presence of optic disc hemorrhages, decreased visual acuity, and assignment to the placebo treatment group. Other factors that may adversely affect the prognosis include uncontrolled systemic hypertension, profound anemia (requiring possible blood transfusion), and renal failure. Overall, understanding the potential challenges and risk factors associated with PTCS allows healthcare providers to provide appropriate monitoring, treatment, and support to improve patient outcomes and minimize long-term complications.

Summary

- The IIH or PTCS is characterized by symptoms such as headache, TVOs, pulsatile tinnitus, and subjective visual loss; the incidence and prevalence of IIH are 5/100,000 and 26/100,000, respectively.
- Timely diagnosis and treatment of IIH are crucial to prevent permanent visual loss or blindness.
- The diagnosis of IIH relies on a combination of symptoms and signs, with collaboration from ophthalmologists to detect papilledema, while MRI and MRV aid in excluding other causes and identifying specific signs, and LP with measurement of opening pressure is essential for diagnosis.
- The management of IIH involves a team approach and multifaceted treatments, including medication (acetazolamide), repeated LPs and surgical/endovascular interventions when indicated (optic nerve sheath fenestration, venous sinus stenting), and individualized headache and weight loss treatments.
- The prognosis of IIH is generally favorable, but some patients may experience persistent visual loss, chronic headaches and other symptoms, and potential recurrences, highlighting the need for effective management to improve outcomes.

REFERENCES

1. Fisayo A, Bruce BB, Newman NJ, Biousse V. Over-diagnosis of idiopathic intracranial hypertension. *Neurology.* 2016;86:341-350.

2. Friedman DI. Contemporary management of the pseudotumor cerebri syndrome. *Expert Rev Neurother.* 2019;19:881-893.

3. Mollan SP, Aguiar M, Evison F, Frew E, Sinclair AJ. The expanding burden of idiopathic intracranial hypertension. *Eye (Lond).* 2019;33:478-485.

4. Miah L, Strafford H, Fonferko-Shadrach B, et al. Incidence, prevalence and healthcare outcomes in idiopathic intracranial hypertension: a population study. *Neurology.* 2021;96:e1251-1261.

5. Wang MTM, Bhatti MT, Danesh-Meyer HV. Idiopathic intracranial hypertension: pathophysiology, diagnosis and management. *J Clin Neurosci.* 2022;95:172-179.

6. Grech O, Mollan SP, Wakerley BR, Alimajstorovic Z, Lavery GG, Sinclair AJ. Emerging themes in idiopathic intracranial hypertension. *J Neurol.* 2020;267:3776-3784.

7. O'Reilly MW, Kempegowda P, Walsh M, et al. AKR1C3-mediated adipose androgen generation drives lipotoxicity in women with polycystic ovary syndrome. *J Clin Endocrinol Metab.* 2017;102:3327-3339.

8. Friedman DI, Quiros PA, Subramanian PS, et al. Headache in idiopathic intracranial hypertension: findings from the idiopathic intracranial hypertension treatment trial. *Headache.* 2017;57:1195-1205.

9. Chen BS, Meyer BI, Saindane AM, Bruce BB, Newman NJ, Biousse V. Prevalence of incidentally detected signs of intracranial hypertension on magnetic resonance imaging and their association with papilledema. *JAMA Neurology.* 2021;78:718-725.

10. Kalyvas AV, Hughes M, Koutsarnakis C, et al. Efficacy, complications and cost of surgical interventions for idiopathic intracranial hypertension: a systematic review of the literature. *Acta Neurochir (Wien).* 2017;159:33-49.

11. Yiangou A, Mitchell JL, Fisher C, et al. Erenumab for headaches in idiopathic intracranial hypertension: a prospective open-label evaluation. *Headache.* 2021;61:157-169.

12. Xu W, Prime Z, Papchenko T, Danesh-Meyer HV. Long term outcomes of idiopathic intracranial hypertension: observational study and literature review. *Clin Neurol Neurosurg.* 2021;205:106463.

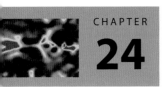

Headache Caused by Low Cerebrospinal Fluid Pressure

Thomas Berk

Headache due to low spinal fluid pressure, also known as intracranial hypotension, is an often overlooked secondary cause of headaches.[1] This condition can manifest in patients with or without a prior history of headaches and may be responsible for "refractory" migraines or other types of headache disorders. The diagnosis and treatment of these headaches can be particularly challenging. However, failure to recognize this condition can result in continued poor health and daily headaches for the patient. Unfortunately, patients with low spinal fluid pressure are often misunderstood by their families and even their doctors when the condition remains undiagnosed. In such cases, the role of the clinician often becomes primarily educational and administrative. Clinicians play a crucial role in teaching the patient and their family about the nature of this condition and what to expect. Additionally, they guide them to other specialists who can perform various diagnostic or therapeutic procedures to further assess and manage the condition.

Epidemiology

Intracranial hypotension has long been underestimated in the general population. The first epidemiological study estimated the incidence of one subtype of intracranial hypotension, spontaneous intracranial hypotension (SIH), at 1 per 50,000, more recent community-based studies report it at 3.7 per 100,000.[2] Cerebrospinal fluid (CSF) leak after dural puncture has been reported to occur between 6% and 36% of any intrathecal procedure.[3,4] A higher incidence is found in women, both after a procedure and spontaneously. Needle size is linked to a greater incidence of low spinal fluid pressure, as is higher BMI. No epidemiological studies have identified a particular socioeconomic group or race with a higher likelihood of intracranial hypotension; the highest risk appears to be in the fourth and fifth decades of life.[5]

People who experience intracranial hypotension have an extremely poor quality of life, often not being able to remain upright for more than a brief period of time. Misdiagnosis is very common; it is thought that a significant percentage of patients in tertiary headache centers thought to have refractory chronic migraine may actually be experiencing intracranial hypotension which can explain a negative response to migraine-specific treatments. This high frequency of misdiagnosis makes determining the incidence of this disorder particularly challenging.

Pathophysiology

The normal physiology of the CSF is complicated but essential to normal brain function.[6] CSF is renewed about four times every 24 hours, and a reduction of the CSF turnover rate can lead to the accumulation of proteins in the brain and CSF that are associated with neurodegenerative diseases. The mean CSF volume is 150 mL, primarily secreted by the choroid plexus and absorbed by the arachnoid villi via the venous and lymphatic system.

CSF pressure is typically maintained between 10 and 20 mm Hg, although a number of factors can affect CSF pressure, and variants of high- and low-pressure conditions have been reported at many different measurements of spinal fluid pressure.

The most prevalent causes of CSF leaks are iatrogenic in nature, often arising as complications from epidural anesthesia or lumbar puncture procedures. Another leading cause is trauma to the mid or low back, which should be taken into consideration, particularly in cases of refractory positional headaches following motor vehicle accidents. While less common, SIH has been well documented. Rarely, intracranial hypertension can indirectly lead to low CSF pressure. This may occur when increased pressure within the spinal fluid causes leakage in the cranial region.

The decrease in spinal fluid pressure leads to a sag, or pulling down, of the structures of the brain that sit closest to the posterior fossa. This activates nociceptive A-delta and C-fibers of the dura. This activation is starting to propagate the production of inflammatory neurotransmitters, leading to significant pain when upright. There may be an increase in vasodilation secondary to sag of the blood vessels around these structures, and this is thought to lead to a more throbbing quality of pain. Increased fluid intake may influence increased production of spinal fluid, caffeine is thought to decrease spinal fluid reabsorption, and, as we will see below, these can improve symptoms to a lesser extent.

Diagnosis and Clinical Presentation

The classic presentation of intracranial hypotension is characterized by a positional headache that worsens shortly after assuming an upright position from a reclining or supine position.[1] Typically, the headache pain is localized to the occipital region and is accompanied by neck pain, often described as a "pulling" sensation upon assuming an upright posture. While a positional headache raises suspicion for intracranial hypotension, making a formal diagnosis can be challenging. *The International Classification of Headache Disorders* (ICHD-3) provides diagnostic criteria for headaches attributed to low CSF pressure, which include three subtypes: postdural puncture headache, CSF fistula headache, and headache attributed to SIH (Box 24-1).[9] Confirmation of low spinal fluid pressure is most reliably achieved through a lumbar puncture, which measures the opening pressure (Chapter 3). However, it is important to note that the opening pressure can exhibit significant variation. It is possible to encounter cases where a CSF leak is associated with an elevated opening pressure or even cases of intracranial hypertension with a low opening pressure.

Box 24-1. Diagnostic Criteria of Headache Attributed to Low Cerebrospinal Fluid (CSF) Pressure According to *The International Classification of Headache Disorders*, Third Edition (ICHD-3)

Orthostatic headache caused by low cerebrospinal fluid (CSF) pressure (either spontaneous or secondary), or CSF leakage, usually accompanied by neck pain, tinnitus, changes in hearing, photophobia, and/or nausea. It remits after normalization of CSF pressure or successful sealing of the CSF leak.

A. Any headache fulfilling criterion C

B. Either or both of the following:
   1. Low cerebrospinal fluid (CSF) pressure (<60 mm CSF)
   2. Evidence of CSF leakage on imaging

C. Headache has developed in temporal relation to the low CSF pressure or CSF leakage, or led to its discovery

D. Not better accounted for by another ICHD-3 diagnosis

It is important to consider the possibility of a cranial leak in CSF patients present with unexplained fluid discharge from their nose or ears, particularly if they have a history of sinus or ear surgeries. A definitive diagnosis can be made by testing the fluid for beta-2 transferrin, which confirms the presence of CSF. Depending on the clinical context, additional confirmatory tests may be employed (Figure 24-1) (see also Chapter 2). Magnetic resonance imaging (MRI) of the spine is a valuable tool for identifying the source of a potential spinal leak, especially when contemplating a targeted epidural blood patch procedure. Myelogram can be considered to rule out a CSF fistula. Cisternogram, although not commonly utilized, is reserved for confirming a cranial leak.

When intracranial hypotension is suspected, international guidelines recommend an initial diagnostic step of performing a brain MRI with contrast. The BERN (Brain Engorgement Responsive to Noradrenaline) score is a predictive measure used to assess the likelihood of intracranial hypotension based on imaging findings.[7] Patients are classified into groups at low, intermediate, or high

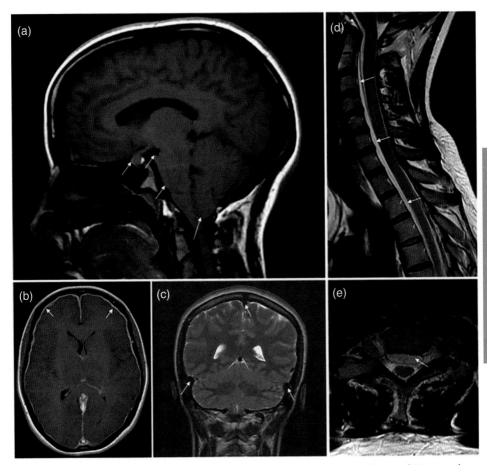

Figure 24-1. Typical MRI findings of spontaneous intracranial hypotension (SIH). (a) Sagittal T1 image showing enlargement of the pituitary, decreased mamillopontine distance, sagging of the brainstem, and cerebellar tonsillar descent. (b) Axial T1 postcontrast image showing diffuse smooth dural thickening and pachymeningeal contrast enhancement. (c) Coronal T2 image showing distension of the dural venous sinuses. (d) Sagittal T2 image showing extensive ventral spinal longitudinal epidural collection (SLEC) extending from the upper cervical to thoracic regions. (e) Axial T2 image showing ventral SLEC.

Box 24-2. The BERN (Brain Engorgement Responsive to Noradrenaline) Scoring Scale

Major criteria	
Engorgement of venous sinuses	2
Pachymeningeal enhancement	2
Suprasellar cistern ≤4 mm	2
Minor criteria	
Subdural fluid collection	1
Prepontine cistern ≤5 mm	1
Mamillopontine distance ≤6.5 mm	1
Sum	9
Low risk ≤2 points	
Intermediate risk 3-4 points	
High risk ≥5 points	

probability of having a spinal CSF leak, with total scores of 2 points or fewer, 3 to 4 points, and 5 points or more, respectively, on a scale of 9 points. The scoring scale is presented in Box 24-2.

Treatment

Consensus guidelines recommend a conservative approach to managing intracranial hypotension during the initial 7 to 14 days after symptom onset.[3,4] This entails several key components, including bed rest, adequate hydration, the consumption of caffeinated beverages, the use of abdominal binders, and the avoidance of Valsalva maneuvers. If symptoms do not improve during this conservative period, a nontargeted epidural blood patch (EBP) should be offered.

For patients with a clinical and/or imaging diagnosis of SIH, a nontargeted EBP is recommended after a maximum of 2 weeks of conservative management. If there is no response or only a transient response to the initial EBP, a second EBP may be considered before proceeding to myelography after 2 to 4 weeks. During a nontargeted EBP, approximately 40 mL of autologous blood is injected.

Targeted EBP should be recommended if the patient continues to remain symptomatic after the initial nontargeted procedures, and there is a causative lesion identified on myelography. Often the myelogram and targeted EBP are performed together. Targeted EBP can also be performed with fibrin. In cases where the patient continues to experience symptoms following initial nontargeted procedures and a causative lesion is identified through myelography, it is advisable to recommend targeted EBP as a treatment option. Often, myelography and targeted EBP are performed concurrently. Alternatively, targeted EBP can also be performed using fibrin. One potential complication of EBP is rebound intracranial hypertension, which can manifest hours to weeks after the procedure.[8] Patients often describe a headache pattern that is nearly the opposite of their previous experience. Headache pain is typically localized in the frontal regions and behind the eyes and worsens when lying down. In severe cases, papilledema (optic disc swelling) may be observed, and intervention with CSF-lowering agents such as acetazolamide and topiramate may be necessary.

In some instances, surgical or endovascular interventions may be necessary.[4] If imaging reveals the presence of a CSF-venous fistula, endovascular treatment is typically considered as the first-line approach. Surgical repair of SIH may be recommended if a lesion is identified on myelography, and the patient remains unresponsive to targeted EBP.

Prognosis

The prognosis following a diagnosis of low CSF pressure varies significantly depending on the underlying cause of the hypotension.[4] In the case of postdural puncture headache, it is generally believed that approximately 80% of these headaches will resolve spontaneously with conservative management. The resolution can occur even more rapidly after undergoing EBP treatment. For cases involving CSF-venous fistula, the prognosis is also favorable following endovascular intervention. On the other hand, SIH can exhibit varied prognoses, and early intervention appears to yield the most beneficial long-term outcomes. Around 60% of SIH cases show a positive response to an initial high-volume, nontargeted EBP. However, if EBP proves ineffective after multiple attempts, surgical intervention can be the most helpful alternative, although some patients may continue to experience symptoms despite this intervention. Unfortunately, the longer a patient remains symptomatic, the higher the likelihood of experiencing disability.

Summary

- Headache due to low CSF pressure is often misdiagnosed and leads to severe disability and poor quality of life.
- Sagging and pulling down of the central brain structures around the posterior fossa leads to the activation of nociceptive fibers in dura and vasodilation.
- The diagnosis can be difficult to make; use the BERN score to predict the likelihood of intracranial hypotension.
- This diagnosis should be considered when headaches are refractory, primarily occipital, and positional in nature.
- It is essential to make this diagnosis appropriately, as treatments that target other headache conditions will not improve the symptoms of intracranial hypotension.
- Consensus guidelines advise conservative management for intracranial hypotension, followed by nontargeted and targeted EBP if symptoms persist, and surgical or endovascular interventions if needed.
- The prognosis of this condition is varied and depends often on the responses to intervention.

REFERENCES

1. Schievink WI. Spontaneous spinal cerebrospinal fluid leaks and intracranial hypotension. *JAMA*. 2006;295(19):2286-2296.
2. Mokri B. Spontaneous low pressure, low CSF volume headaches: spontaneous CSF leaks. *Headache*. 2013;53(7):1034-1053.
3. Cheema S, Anderson J, Angus-Leppan H, et al. Multidisciplinary consensus guideline for the diagnosis and management of spontaneous intracranial hypotension. *J Neurol Neurosurg Psychiatry*. 2023;jnnp-2023-331166.
4. Patel R, Ivan Urits, Vwaire Orhurhu, et al. A comprehensive update on the treatment and management of postdural puncture headache. *Curr Pain Headache Rep*. 2020;24(6).
5. Schievink WI, Maya MM, Moser FG, Simon P, Nuño M. Incidence of spontaneous intracranial hypotension in a community: Beverly Hills, California, 2006-2020. *Cephalalgia*. 2022;42(4-5):312-316.
6. Filis AK, Aghayev K, Vrionis FD. Cerebrospinal fluid and hydrocephalus: physiology, diagnosis, and treatment. *Cancer Control*. 2017;24:6-8.
7. Dobrocky T, Grunder L, Breiding PS, et al. Assessing spinal cerebrospinal fluid leaks in spontaneous intracranial hypotension with a scoring system based on brain magnetic resonance imaging findings. *JAMA Neurol*. 2019;76(5):580-587.
8. Kranz PG, Amrhein TJ, Gray L. Rebound intracranial hypertension: a complication of epidural blood patching for intracranial hypotension. *AJNR Am J Neuroradiol*. 2014;35:1237-1240.
9. Headache Classification Committee of the International Headache Society (IHS). *The International Classification of Headache Disorders*, 3rd edition. *Cephalalgia*. 2018;38(1):1-211.

Secondary Headaches

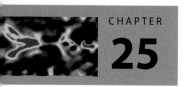

CHAPTER

25

Headache and Chiari Malformation

Ashley Alex and Melissa Rayhill

Chiari malformations, particularly Chiari malformation type I (CMI), are the most common craniocervical junction abnormalities observed in adults.[1] While Chiari malformations II-IV typically present in infancy with severe neurologic manifestations, CMI can remain asymptomatic or present in adulthood with headache and/or focal neurologic deficits. CMI is a congenital deformity stemming from inadequate development of the posterior cranial fossa during fetal development.

Epidemiology

The incidence of Chiari malformation type I (CMI) is estimated to be around 1 in 1000 births.[2] This is likely an underestimate as many individuals remain asymptomatic and do not present until adulthood, but diagnosis is increasing with the increased availability of magnetic resonance imaging (MRI).[3] Chiari I malformation occurs in approximately 0.5% to 3.5% of patients undergoing MRI.[4] There is a slight female predominance, with a ratio of 1.3 females to 1 male,[1] and the presence of a syrinx is observed in approximately 34% to 40% of individuals with CMI.[5]

Pathophysiology

Impaired cerebrospinal fluid (CSF) flow between the cranial and spinal compartments, caused by tonsillar herniation and foramen magnum crowding, leads to a pressure dissociation with increased intracranial pressure, heightened venous volume and pressure during Valsalva maneuvers, and subsequent head pain due to obstruction, traction, and compression of the C1-C2 nerve roots.[5-7] Moreover, vessel dilation prompts the release of endothelial factors from nerve fibers, resulting in neurogenic inflammation, while the altered flow dynamics can lead to the accumulation of CSF within the spinal cord, resulting in syringomyelia.[2,3,7,8]

Diagnosis and Clinical Presentation

Chiari malformation type I (CMI) is often incidentally detected in individuals presenting with nonspecific symptoms or unrelated head and neck pain, with approximately 31% of those meeting radiologic criteria being asymptomatic.[9] Headache is the predominant symptom in up to 50% of symptomatic cases, with the characteristic headache attributed to CMI resembling primary cough headache but lasting longer; it presents as brief episodes (<5 min) of lancinating pain in the occipital/suboccipital region triggered by cough or other Valsalva maneuvers (Box 25-1).[6,10] The 3rd edition of the *International Classification of Headache Disorders* (ICHD-3) provides specific criteria to aid in recognition and diagnosis, as outlined in Box 25-1.[10] While this represents the classic headache pattern associated with CMI, individuals may describe other headache phenotypes such as migraine or tension-type headache.[11] The specific characteristics of the headache are significant as they may influence the success of surgical intervention.

Box 25-1. ICHD-3 Diagnostic Criteria for Headache Attributed to Chiari Malformation Type I

Headache caused by Chiari type I malformation, usually occipital or suboccipital, of short duration (less than 5 min) and provoked by cough or other Valsalva-like maneuvers. It remits after the successful treatment of the Chiari malformation.

A. Headache fulfilling criterion C

B. Chiari malformation type I (CMI) has been demonstrated

C. Evidence of causation demonstrated by at least two of the following:
   1. either or both of the following:
      a) headache has developed in temporal relation to the CMI or led to its discovery
      b) headache has resolved within 3 months after successful treatment of the CMI

   2. headache has one or more of the following three characteristics:
      a) precipitated by cough or other Valsalva-like maneuver
      b) occipital or suboccipital location
      c) lasting <5 min

   3. headache is associated with other symptoms and/or clinical signs of brainstem, cerebellar, lower cranial nerve, and/or cervical spinal cord dysfunction

D. Not better accounted for by another ICHD-3 diagnosis

Apart from headaches, individuals with CMI can exhibit a range of additional symptoms. Direct compression of the brainstem can lead to lower cranial nerve palsies, resulting in visual abnormalities, vertigo, nystagmus, ataxia, dysphagia, and sleep disturbances (Table 25-1).[6] The occipital head pain can also radiate down and cause significant neck and scapulothoracic pain, especially if there is involvement of the cervical spine. CMI cases associated with a syrinx and cervical cord compression may also cause weakness, atrophy, sensory deficits, pain, urinary/bowel incontinence, or autonomic dysfunction.[3] Cerebrospinal fluid (CSF) disturbances can manifest as pseudotumor-like episodes or hydrocephalus.[6]

Radiologically on MRI, CMI is defined by a 5-mm caudal descent of the cerebellar tonsils or 3-mm caudal descent of the cerebellar tonsils plus crowding of the subarachnoid space at the craniocervical junction as evidenced by: compression of the CSF spaces posterior and lateral to the cerebellum, reduced height of the supraocciput, increased slope of the tentorium, or kinking of the medulla oblongata.[10] The descending tissue typically appears peg-like or pointed (Figure 25-1).

Secondary Headaches

Table 25-1. Clinical Manifestations of Chiari I Malformation

Meningeal Irritation	Headache
Brainstem compression (Cranial neuropathies)	Hoarseness, vocal cord paralysis, dysarthria, palatal weakness, nystagmus, oscillopsia, sleep-related breathing disorder, hiccups, syncope
Hydrocephalus	Headache, vomiting, lethargy, irritability
Cervical cord compression	Neck pain, myelopathy, weakness, spasticity, hyperreflexia, Babinski response
Syringomyelia (cervical cord)	Scoliosis, gait disturbance, radicular pain, dysesthesia, upper motor neuron signs (legs), lower motor neuron signs (arms)

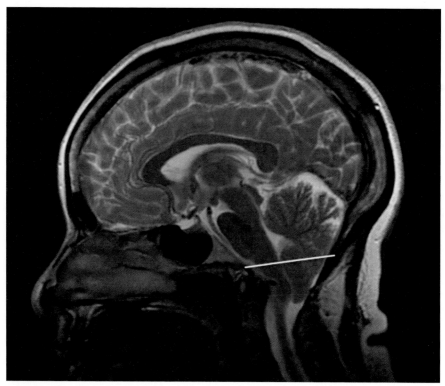

Figure 25-1. Chiari malformation type I. Sagittal T2-weighted image of the brain demonstrating an extension of the cerebellar tonsils ~15 mm below the basion-opisthion line (white line), medullary kinking, and peg-like tonsillar appearance.

Measurement of caudal descent is done as the perpendicular distance below the basion-opisthion line.[11] These abnormalities are best visualized on midsagittal brain MRI, particularly high-resolution T2-weighted images that provide detailed visualization of CSF spaces at the craniocervical junction.[5] If MRI is not available, computed tomography or radiographs can be used to assess associated bony abnormalities. Additionally, cine phase-contrast analysis can quantitatively assess flow abnormalities and demonstrate the pulsatile downward motion of the tonsils causing obstruction.[5,7] MRI of the cervical spine is also valuable for identifying syringomyelia and cervical compression.[5] Table 25-1 describes clinical correlates to these radiological findings. Differentiating acquired causes from CMI is important, as CSF pressure disorders, such as idiopathic intracranial hypertension and intracranial hypotension with CSF leak, can exhibit a similar presentation of Valsalva-induced headaches and share similar radiological findings.

Treatment

For individuals with asymptomatic or mild symptoms, conservative management is the preferred approach. Surgical intervention may be beneficial for improving symptoms of ataxia and cough headache, but it is less likely to alleviate nausea and nonspecific symptoms.[1] In cases of atypical headaches, treatment should focus on addressing the comorbid headache disorder (e.g., tension-type, migraine) rather than relying solely on surgical decompression. Indomethacin can be considered as a treatment option for cough headaches, as it may possibly inhibit neurogenic inflammation and reduce intracranial pressure by constricting precapillary resistance vessels.[8]

The surgical management of CMI requires a multidisciplinary approach involving neuroradiology and neurosurgery teams. As there are no randomized, controlled studies comparing surgical versus conservative management, the decision to proceed with surgery should be carefully considered, taking into account the individual's symptoms, impact on quality of life, and the potential risks of surgical complications.[1] Surgery is typically recommended for individuals exhibiting signs and symptoms of brainstem or cerebellar compression, progressive syringomyelia, or poorly controlled cough headache associated with CMI.[6] The traditional surgical approach involves posterior fossa decompression through suboccipital craniectomy and C1 laminectomy, with or without expansile duraplasty or cerebellar tonsillar resection.[2] Potential complications of surgery include meningitis, pseudomeningocele, wound infection, stroke, hydrocephalus, and CSF fistula.[1]

Prognosis

CMI is not necessarily a progressive condition, and symptoms may remain stable or improve over time. In those undergoing surgery, results have typically been favorable with approximately 62.5% reporting improvement of cough-related headache symptoms at the 1-year mark.[8] However, decompression surgery failed to improve headaches in individuals with nonobstructive flow. While occipital headaches showed no recurrence after surgery, 57% of those with frontal headaches reported recurrence.[7]

Summary

- CMI is the most prevalent abnormality affecting the craniocervical junction in adults.
- CMI can be an incidental finding on brain imaging in individuals with primary headache disorders.
- Pathophysiology of CMI involves impaired CSF flow due to tonsillar herniation and foramen magnum crowding, resulting in increased intracranial pressure, headache from nerve compression and obstruction, and possible formation of syringomyelia.
- Headaches associated with CMI commonly manifest as cough headache, or headache provoked by Valsalva maneuver, but can also present with other atypical headache phenotypes.
- Conservative management is the preferred approach for individuals with asymptomatic or mild symptoms.
- Surgical management should be considered on a patient-to-patient basis and tends to have better success rates in those with typical cough headache with obstructed CSF flow.

REFERENCES

1. Langridge B, Phillips E, Choi D. Chiari malformation type 1: a systematic review of natural history and conservative management. *World Neurosurg.* 2017;104:213-219.

2. Liu, PP, Nelson CI, Arnon, GD, et al. Surgery for Chiari Type I Malformation. In *Monitoring the Nervous System for Anesthesiologists and Other Health Care Professionals*, A Koht, TB Sloan, JR Toleikis (eds). Springer International Publishing, 2017, 435-444.

3. Harris SB, Ellenbogen RG. *Chiari Syndrome, in Emergency Approaches to Neurosurgical Conditions,* A Agrawal and G Britz (eds). Springer International Publishing, 2014, 79-88.

4. Sadler B, Kuensting T, Strahle J, et al. Prevalence and impact of underlying diagnosis and comorbidities on Chiari 1 malformation. *Pediatr Neurol.* 2020;106:32-37.

5. Bezuidenhout AF, Chang Y-M, Heilman CB, Bhadelia RA. Headache in Chiari malformation. *Neuroimaging Clin N Am.* 2019;29(2):243-253.

6. Beretta E, Vetrano IG, Curone M, et al. Chiari malformation-related headache: outcome after surgical treatment. *Neurol Sci.* 2017;38(S1):95-98.

7. Robbins MS, Grosberg BM, Lipton RB. Secondary headache disorders encountered in clinical practice. In: *Headache.* Chichester, England: Wiley-Blackwell; 2013:45-46.

Secondary Headaches

8. Bates JE, Augustine EF. Pearls & Oy-Sters: Cough headache secondary to Chiari malformation type I. *Neurology.* 2014;83(16).

9. Elster AD, Chen MY. Chiari I malformations: clinical and radiologic reappraisal. *Radiology.* 1992;183(2):347-353.

10. Headache Classification Committee of the International Headache Society (IHS). *The International Classification of Headache Disorders*, 3rd edition. *Cephalalgia.* 2018;38(1):1-211.

11. Thunstedt DC, Schmutzer M, Fabritius MP, et al. Headache characteristics and postoperative course in Chiari I malformation. *Cephalalgia.* 2022;42(9): 879-887.

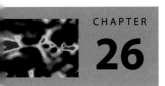

CHAPTER
26

Headache and Noninfectious Inflammatory Diseases

Athena Kostidis and Amara Mian

Headache in noninfectious inflammatory diseases includes a range of conditions such as neurosarcoidosis, aseptic (noninfectious) meningitis, lymphocytic hypophysitis (LH), systemic lupus erythematosus (SLE), and the syndrome of transient headache and neurological deficits with cerebrospinal fluid (CSF) lymphocytosis (HaNDL). Inflammatory diseases affecting the central nervous system (CNS) can also lead to secondary headaches in affected patients.

Neurosarcoidosis

Sarcoidosis is characterized by the development of granulomatous inflammation in various organs. Although the involvement of the CNS is relatively uncommon, it can affect both the CNS and peripheral nervous system. Neurological complications arise in approximately 5% of individuals with sarcoidosis, manifesting either centrally or peripherally.[1] The clinical presentation of neurosarcoidosis can vary significantly depending on the specific region of the nervous system affected. Possible sites of involvement include the cranial nerves, brain, spinal cord, meninges, and peripheral nerves. Headaches associated with neurosarcoidosis are thought to arise from nerve granulomas, resulting in elevated intracranial pressure or granulomatous basal meningitis.[2,3] These headaches can be diffuse and nonpulsating, occur almost daily, lack typical migraine-associated symptoms, and show no response to steroid treatment. The clinical presentation of these headaches may resemble chronic tension-type headache.[2] The *International Classification of Headache Disorders*, 3rd edition (ICHD-3), outlines diagnostic criteria for headaches attributed to neurosarcoidosis, as outlined in Box 26-1.[4]

Aseptic (Noninfectious) Meningitis

Drug-induced aseptic meningitis is a known complication associated with the administration of nonsteroidal anti-inflammatory drugs, intravenous immunoglobulins, and certain antibiotics. The pathophysiology of this condition is believed to involve a hypersensitivity reaction or the release of cytokines. Clinical presentation of aseptic meningitis typically includes symptoms such as headache, meningismus (neck stiffness), and alterations in mental status. CSF analysis commonly reveals elevated protein levels, normal to low glucose levels, and a white cell count ranging from several hundred to several thousand cells, with a predominance of neutrophils.[1] The ICHD-3 provides detailed criteria for diagnosing this condition, which are outlined in Box 26-2.[4] Patients diagnosed with aseptic or viral meningitis commonly exhibit headaches that are characterized by their severity and bilateral nature. These headaches may have an abrupt onset or be described by the patients as the most intense they have ever experienced.[5] It is crucial to consider aseptic meningitis as a potential cause when patients present with a severe headache that worsens suddenly or exhibits an abrupt onset.

Box 26-1. ICHD-3 Diagnostic Criteria for Headache Attributed to Neurosarcoidosis

Headache caused by and associated with other symptoms and signs of neurosarcoidosis

A. Any headache fulfilling criterion C

B. Neurosarcoidosis has been diagnosed

C. Evidence of causation demonstrated by at least two of the following:
   1. Headache has developed in temporal relation to the onset of neurosarcoidosis
   2. Either or both of the following:
      a) Headache has significantly worsened in parallel with the worsening of the neurosarcoidosis
      b) Headache has significantly improved in parallel with the improvement in neurosarcoidosis
   3. Headache is accompanied by one or more cranial nerve palsies

D. Not better accounted for by another ICHD-3 diagnosis

Box 26-2. ICHD-3 Diagnostic Criteria for Headache Attributed to Aseptic (Noninfectious) Meningitis

Headache caused by aseptic meningitis, associated with other symptoms and/or clinical signs of meningeal irritation. It resolves after the resolution of the meningitis.

A. Any headache fulfilling criterion C

B. Aseptic meningitis has been diagnosed by cerebrospinal fluid (CSF) examination

C. Evidence of causation demonstrated by at least two of the following:
   1. Headache has developed in temporal relation to the onset of aseptic meningitis or led to its discovery
   2. Either or both of the following:
      a) Headache has significantly worsened in parallel with worsening of the aseptic meningitis
      b) Headache has significantly improved in parallel with improvement in the aseptic meningitis
   3. Headache is accompanied by other symptoms and/or clinical signs of meningeal inflammation including neck stiffness (meningismus) and/or photophobia

D. Not better accounted for by another ICHD-3 diagnosis

Other NonInfectious Inflammatory Intracranial Disease

The primary disorders in this category include SLE, antiphospholipid antibody syndrome, and Behcet's disease. Approximately 20% of patients with SLE experience migraine-like headaches, which are attributed to active lupus and require diagnostic procedures such as lumbar puncture or brain vascular imaging such as magnetic resonance arteriography or computer tomography angiography.

The term "lupus headache" refers to a severe and persistent headache that may exhibit migrainous characteristics and does not respond to narcotic analgesia.[6] Various types of primary headaches, such as migraine and tension-type headache, are more common in SLE patients compared to the general population. The presence of headaches in SLE is associated with a negative impact on the individual's quality of life. Treatment for true lupus-related headaches typically involves the use of steroids.[7]

Behcet's disease is a chronic multisystem disorder primarily mediated by T cells.[3] It is associated with specific human leukocyte antigen (HLA) types, namely, HLA-B5 and B51, and its underlying pathophysiology is characterized by a vasculitic pattern. Neurological involvement is observed in 22% to 50% of Behcet's disease cases, and headaches are a commonly reported manifestation of this disease.[3] Treating the underlying condition can potentially lead to an improvement in headache symptoms.

Lymphocytic Hypophysitis

LH is characterized by the initial occurrence of acute inflammation and edema in the pituitary gland. This inflammatory process can lead to the development of headaches and, in more severe cases, compression of the optic chiasm. Patients with LH may also experience various endocrine abnormalities, including hypopituitarism, diabetes insipidus, and hyperprolactinemia.[8] LH is considered a rare disorder that predominantly affects women. While it commonly arises during late pregnancy or the postpartum period, it can also manifest in prepubertal or postmenopausal women. The exact cause of LH remains uncertain and subject to ongoing debate, but an autoimmune etiology is likely. A definitive diagnosis of LH requires a biopsy. Clinical presentation typically involves headaches, hypopituitarism, and visual field defects. Headaches, a frequent complaint among LH patients, are believed to be linked to the mass effect of the pituitary lesion. With timely and adequate treatment involving steroids and/ or surgery, the headaches can rapidly resolve, leading to a favorable outcome.[1,8]

Syndrome of Transient Headache and Neurological Deficits with Cerebrospinal Fluid Lymphocytosis (HaNDL)

Transient headache and neurologic deficits with CSF lymphocytosis syndrome (HaNDL) is a headache disorder characterized by moderate to severe headache attacks, neurological symptoms, and an elevation in white blood cells in the CSF. The exact etiology of HaNDL remains unclear, although it has been proposed to be a severe variant of migraine. Some speculate that the condition may have either an inflammatory or infectious origin, but extensive investigations have provided limited support for these hypotheses.[9] Unilateral vasospasm in the intracranial blood vessels has also been suggested as a possible mechanism. HaNDL syndrome predominantly affects females, and the most common neurological symptom is a hemisensory deficit, although hemiparesis and aphasia can also occur. The right-sided deficits are more frequently observed than left-sided deficits. Headaches associated with HaNDL syndrome may be unilateral or bilateral, and they can exhibit migrainous features. Patients typically remain asymptomatic between episodes.[10] The condition typically resolves within 1 to 3 weeks, leading to a favorable prognosis. Therefore, treatment primarily focuses on managing symptoms.

Summary

- Neurosarcoidosis, a rare complication of sarcoidosis, can affect the central and peripheral nervous system, leading to variable clinical presentations including headaches that resemble chronic tension-type headache and do not respond to steroid treatment.
- Drug-induced aseptic meningitis can present as severe headaches, meningismus, and mental status changes.
- Migraine-like headaches are common in SLE, which is also comorbid with primary headaches, especially migraine and tension-type headache.

Secondary Headaches

- Headaches are a common manifestation of Behcet's disease, a chronic multisystem disorder with neurological involvement.

- LH, a rare condition, is characterized by acute inflammation and edema in the pituitary gland, often leading to headaches, endocrine abnormalities, and visual field defects, which can be treated with steroids and/or surgery.

- HaNDL is a headache disorder predominantly affecting females, characterized by moderate to severe headache attacks, neurological symptoms, and elevated white blood cells in the CSF.

REFERENCES

1. McGeeney B. Classification and diagnosis of secondary headaches: altered intracranial pressure, neoplasm, and infection. In: Levin M, ed. *Comprehensive Review of Headache Medicine*. New York: Oxford University Press; 2008:154-157.

2. Curone M, Tullo V, Peccarisi C, et al. Headache as presenting symptom of neurosarcoidosis. *Neurol Sci*. 2013;34:183-185.

3. La Mantia L, Erbetta A. Headache and inflammatory disorders of the central nervous system. *Neurol Sci*. 2004;25(Suppl 3):S148-S153.

4. IHS Classification ICHD-3. Available at: https://ichd-3.org/.

5. Lamonte M, Silberstein SD, Marcelis JF. Headache associated with aseptic meningitis. *Headache*. 1995;35(9):520-526.

6. Elolemy G, Al Rashidi A, Youssry D, et al. Headache in patients with systemic lupus erythematosus: characteristics, brain MRI patterns, and impact. *Egypt Rheumatol Rehabil*. 2021;48:31.

7. Johns Hopkins Lupus Center: How lupus affects the nervous system. Available at: https://www.hopkinslupus.org/lupus-info/lupus-affects-body/lupus-nervous-system/.

8. Yang MG, Cai HQ, Wang SS, Liu L, Wang CM. Full recovery from chronic headache and hypopituitarism caused by lymphocytic hypophysitis: a case report. *World J Clin Cases*. 2022;10(3):1041-1049.

9. Säflund M, Sjöstrand C, Sveinsson O. HaNDL – viktig men gåtfull differentialdiagnos med svår migränliknande huvudvärk – Förknippat med neurologiska symtom och lymfocytär pleocytos [The syndrome of transient headache and neurologic deficits with cerebrospinal fluid lymphocytosis (HaNDL)]. *Lakartidningen*. 2018;115: EWPH. Swedish.

10. Armstrong-Javors A, Krishnamoorthy K. HaNDL syndrome: case report and literature review. *J Child Neurol*. 2019;34(3):161-167.

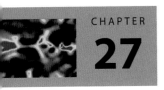

Headache Attributed to a Substance or Its Withdrawal

Abigail L. Chua

Headache associated with a substance or its withdrawal, classified as a secondary headache disorder in the International Classification of Headache Disorders, 3rd edition (ICHD-3), occurs after exposure to or withdrawal from a substance known to trigger headaches.[1] To meet diagnostic criteria, these headaches must exhibit at least two of the following features: (1) the headache has occurred in close temporal relation to the exposure or withdrawal of the substance, (2) the headache has improved or resolved when the substance is discontinued or completely withdrawn, and (3) the headache has characteristics typical of headaches caused by exposure to or withdrawal from that particular substance. It is important to note that there are numerous drugs and substances that can induce headaches. For medication overuse headaches, see Chapter 28.

Headache Attributed to Use of or Exposure to a Substance

See Table 27-1 for an overview of headaches attributed to the use of or exposure to a substance. Headaches can be induced by various substances, including histamine and calcitonin gene-related peptide (CGRP). This section focuses only on clinically relevant substances and the headaches associated with them.

Nitric Oxide Donors

Nitric oxide (NO) is a gaseous signaling molecule that plays a significant role in various biological processes throughout the body. The involvement of NO in the pathogenesis of headaches has been established in migraine, tension-type headache (TTH), and cluster headache (CH).[2] Administration of NO donors such as sodium nitroprusside and glyceryl trinitrate causes immediate headaches in individuals with or without a primary headache disorder, while individuals with migraine, TTH, or CH may experience delayed headaches. These induced headaches were previously referred to as "nitroglycerine headache," "dynamite headache," and "hot dog headache." Typically, these attacks manifest as throbbing pain in the frontotemporal region, ranging from mild to moderate in intensity, and can worsen with routine physical activities. Immediate headaches caused by NO donors occur within an hour of drug absorption and subside approximately 1 hour after the release of NO ceases. On the other hand, the delayed headache subtype arises 2 to 12 hours following exposure and resolves 72 hours after usage. Discontinuing use of the offending NO donor is often the primary step in managing these headaches. Once the exposure is stopped, the headache symptoms may gradually improve and eventually resolve. Acute and preventive treatment will vary depending on the specific characteristics and features of the headache.

Table 27-1. Headache Attributed to the Use of or Exposure to a Substance

Substance	Drug Examples	Immediate Headache	Delayed Headache	Headache Onset (from Time of Exposure)	Headache Cessation	Headache Features	Clinical Pearls
NO donor	NTG, GTN	Yes		Within 1 hour	Within 1 hour after the NO release ends	At least one of the following: - Bilateral - Mild to moderate - Pulsating - Aggravated by physical activity	Tolerance develops within 1 week of chronic NTG use
			Yes	Within 2-12 hours, and after NO is cleared from the system (in 1-2 hours in those with CH)	Within 72 hours after exposure	Clinically resembles the phenotype of primary headache	Occurs in those with a primary headache disorder (migraine, TTH, CH)
PDE inhibitor	Sildenafil, dipyridamole			Within 5 hours	Within 72 hours	At least one of the following: - Bilateral - Mild to moderate - Pulsating - Aggravated by physical activity	Typically, TTH phenotype but can resemble migraine without aura in those with migraine
CO				Within 12 hours	Within 72 hours after CO eliminated	Depends on level of COHb: - 10-20%: mild headache - 20-30%: moderate pulsating headache, irritability - 30-40%: severe headache, nausea, vomiting, blurred vision	COHb levels above 40% cause loss of consciousness

Substance	Drug Examples	Immediate Headache	Delayed Headache	Headache Onset (from Time of Exposure)	Headache Cessation	Headache Features	Clinical Pearls
Alcohol		Yes		Within 3 hours	Within 72 hours after exposure	At least one of the following: - Bilateral - Pulsating - Aggravated by physical activity	The amount and type of alcohol needed to trigger a headache is variable
			Yes	Within 5-12 hours	Within 72 hours after headache onset	At least one of the following: - Bilateral - Pulsating - Aggravated by physical activity	More common than the immediate onset
Cocaine				Within 1 hour	Within 72 hours	At least one of the following: - Bilateral - Mild to moderate - Pulsating - Aggravated by physical activity	Occurs with any route of exposure
Exogenous acute pressor agent	Norepinephrine, epinephrine, phenylephrine, vasopressin			Within 1 hour	Within 72 hours after administration	Typically bilateral and throbbing in nature	Headache occurs during, and caused by, acute elevation in blood pressure
Occasional use of nonheadache medication	Nicotine, atropine, hydralazine, imipramine			Minutes to hours depending on the drug	Within 72 hours	Not well defined—usually dull, continuous, diffuse, moderate to severe intensity	Features of headache likely vary based on causative agent

(Continued)

Table 27-1. Headache Attributed to the Use of or Exposure to a Substance *(Continued)*

Substance	Drug Examples	Immediate Headache	Delayed Headache	Headache Onset (from Time of Exposure)	Headache Cessation	Headache Features	Clinical Pearls
Chronic use of nonheadache medication	Exogenous hormones, tetracyclines			Variable depending on the drug	Variable—may not resolve	Not well defined—likely resembles migraine or preexisting primary headache	Headache is present for at least 15 days per month
Other (for homeopathic use): Herbs Animal Products Organic and inorganic compounds	Valerian root, camphor			Within 12 hours	Within 72 hours	Not well defined—usually dull, continuous, diffuse, moderate to severe intensity	Features of headache likely vary based on causative agent

CH, cluster headache; CO, carbon monoxide; COHb, carboxyhemoglobin; GTN, glyceryl trinitrate; NO, nitric oxide; NTG, nitroglycerin; PDE, phosphodiesterase; TTH, tension-type headache.

Phosphodiesterase Inhibitors

Phosphodiesterases (PDEs) are enzymes that play a crucial role in regulating cellular signal transduction. They achieve this by degrading cyclic adenosine monophosphate (cAMP) and cyclic guanosine monophosphate (cGMP), which are secondary messengers involved in a wide range of cellular processes throughout the body. In the nervous system, PDEs are involved in critical functions such as memory formation, pain perception, mood regulation, neurogenesis, and synaptic plasticity.[3] PDE inhibitors, including medications like sildenafil and dipyridamole, work by blocking the activity of PDE enzymes. As a result, the levels of cAMP and cGMP increase, leading to enhanced signaling within cells. However, it has been observed that PDE inhibitors can cause headaches in both healthy individuals and those with migraine and CH.[4] Headache induced by PDE inhibitors typically resembles TTH. However, in individuals with preexisting migraine or CH, the headache attack may manifest in a manner similar to their primary headache disorder. The onset of the headache usually occurs within 5 hours after drug exposure, and typically resolves within a span of 72 hours. The treatment approach for this headache is similar to the management of NO donor-induced headaches.

Carbon Monoxide

Commonly referred to as "warehouse worker's headache" in the past, this type of secondary headache typically emerges within 12 hours of carbon monoxide (CO) exposure. CO is an odorless and tasteless gas that exhibits a strong affinity for binding to hemoglobin and heme-containing proteins. As a result, it leads to a widespread decrease in oxygen delivery, as well as the formation of free radicals and inflammation within the body. The effects of acute CO poisoning can range from mild symptoms like headaches, fatigue, decreased concentration, and nausea/vomiting to more severe consequences such as loss of consciousness, myocardial infarction, brain injury, and even death.[5] Survivors of CO poisoning often report long-term impairments, including memory deficits, chronic fatigue, depression, vestibular dysfunction, and motor impairment, even up to 6 years following the initial exposure. Diagnosing milder or chronic cases of CO poisoning can be challenging due to the presence of nonspecific symptoms, occurrence throughout both winter and warmer months, and low levels of carboxyhemoglobin (COHb) resulting from insidious exposure.[6] Headaches induced by CO exposure typically manifest as bilateral pain that changes severity depending on the level of toxicity. The headache usually resolves within 72 hours once the body has eliminated the CO. The standard treatment for CO poisoning involves administering 100% normobaric or hyperbaric oxygen, which helps to facilitate the removal of CO from the body and restore normal oxygenation.

Alcohol

Alcohols, most notably beer and wine, are often cited as common migraine triggers.[7] The consumption of alcohol can lead to the onset of headaches, either immediately within 3 hours of exposure or more commonly as a delayed "hangover" headache occurring 5 to 12 hours later.[1] These headaches typically subside within 72 hours after onset. Although the exact mechanism by which alcohol induces headaches is not fully understood, several factors are believed to contribute, including dehydration, sleep disturbances, the release of CGRP, and effects on adenosine, histamine, amines, sulphites, serotonin, tyramine, and flavonoids.[7] Alcohol-induced headaches generally exhibit bilateral pulsating pain that can worsen with physical activity. Management of alcohol-induced headaches includes hydration, electrolyte replenishment, and symptomatic treatment with analgesics.

Cocaine

Cocaine is a widely used naturally occurring stimulant that is regarded as illegal for personal use in all states in the United States except one (small amounts of cocaine are decriminalized in Oregon).[8] Acute use results in a wide range of symptoms such as tremors, seizures, hyperthermia, hypertension, strokes, and headaches. Chronic exposure to cocaine is linked to neurodegeneration, depression, and damage to blood vessels.[9] Headaches, a common consequence of cocaine use, can manifest after a single dose and affect up to 90% of chronic users. They are primarily caused by acute vasoconstriction and the depletion of norepinephrine, dopamine, and serotonin. Attacks can occur immediately after use or during a period of abstinence in chronic users. Headaches can be bifrontal or occipital and are associated with photophobia, nausea, and sometimes vomiting. Resolution usually occurs within 72 hours after exposure. Various treatment options have been proposed for cocaine-induced headaches, including doxepin, amlodipine, corticosteroids, and endonasal surgery.[9]

Pressor Agents

Pressor agents, such as norepinephrine, epinephrine, phenylephrine, and vasopressin, are vasoconstrictors that have numerous clinical applications. Intravenous vasopressors are administered in cases of shock, cardiac arrest, or anaphylaxis, while other formulations are utilized for nasal decongestion, pupil dilation, and asthma treatment. The systemic use of these agents can trigger headaches within 1 hour of drug administration, primarily attributed to an acute rise in blood pressure, typically exceeding a systolic pressure of 180 mm Hg and a diastolic pressure of 120 mm Hg or higher.[10] Headaches due to elevated blood pressure are typically bilateral, throbbing in nature, and generally resolve within 72 hours of onset.

Nicotine

Nicotine is a naturally occurring alkaloid known for its addictive stimulant and antinociceptive properties.[11] It is present in tobacco products and utilized in replacement therapies for smoking cessation. Acute exposure to nicotine can result in symptoms such as dizziness, confusion, tachycardia, hypertension, and headache.[11] Headaches can manifest within minutes to hours following the administration of one or more doses of the drug. These headaches are typically characterized by diffuse, nonpulsatile pain of moderate to severe intensity. Resolution of the headache occurs within 72 hours after discontinuation of nicotine exposure.

Other Medications and Substances

Various medications, including exogenous hormones and antibiotics such as tetracyclines, can trigger headaches. A relationship between sex hormones and primary headaches has been observed in migraine,[12] CH,[12] hemicrania continua,[13] and paroxysmal hemicrania.[14] The use of exogenous hormones for contraception, hormone replacement therapy, and gender-affirming treatment can exacerbate existing primary headaches or provoke new-onset attacks (Chapters 36 and 51). These headaches can occur with estrogen-only, estrogen-progesterone combinations, and testosterone treatment. However, the risk may be higher in individuals with a significant personal or family history of headaches prior to initiating treatment.[12] Doxycycline and minocycline are tetracyclines commonly used to treat various conditions such as infections, acne, and rheumatoid arthritis. Both are known to cause headaches due to their ability to cross the blood–brain barrier.[15] Tetracyclines are also associated with symptoms of altered mental status, dizziness, changes in vision, and also the development of pseudotumor cerebri.[15] Headaches attributed to these medications share features of migraine and can improve once the offending drug is discontinued, although the headache may not always be reversible.[1]

Organic and Inorganic Compounds

Headaches can also be induced by herbs, animal products, and various organic and inorganic compounds.[1] Valerian root and camphor are notable examples. Valerian root is a perennial plant commonly used as an herbal remedy for sleep and mood disorders.[16] Its sedative effects are thought to be mediated through gamma-aminobutyric acid receptors.[16] Although rare, toxicity can occur, especially when combined with other sedating medications or GABAergic agents. Adverse reactions to valerian root may include fatigue, headache, abdominal cramps, hepatotoxicity, vivid dreams, marked somnolence, and encephalopathy.[16] Camphor, a waxy aromatic ketone, can be absorbed through the skin, eyes, respiratory tract, and gastrointestinal system.[17] It also crosses the placenta and thus should be avoided during pregnancy. Over-the-counter treatments containing camphor are used to alleviate joint pain, itching, congestion, and cough. However, exposure to camphor can be toxic, resulting in symptoms ranging from headache to vomiting, delirium, seizures, and even coma.[17] Headaches falling into this subtype are generally described as dull, holocranial (affecting the entire head), and moderate to severe in intensity and typically develop within 12 hours of exposure. The headache usually resolves within 72 hours after the exposure has ended.

Headache Attributed to Substance Withdrawal

See Table 27-2 for an overview of headaches attributed to substance withdrawal.

Caffeine-Withdrawal Headache

Caffeine, a naturally occurring stimulant, is rapidly absorbed within 30 to 120 minutes after oral consumption.[18] Its effectiveness as an abortive treatment for migraine stems from its ability to antagonize adenosine receptors. Additionally, caffeine enhances the analgesic effects of other medications, making it a common addition to therapies containing acetaminophen, ibuprofen, and aspirin.[18] Guidelines recommend limiting daily caffeine intake to no more than 400 mg for males and 300 mg for nonpregnant females (with exceptions for certain occupations such as the military) or up to 5.7 mg/kg/day for nonpregnant adults.[19] It is important to note that popular over-the-counter treatments marketed for TTHs, hangover headaches, and migraine contain caffeine doses ranging from 65 to 150 mg per dose. Therefore, individuals using these medications should consider these caffeine amounts when calculating their daily intake. For individuals who consume at least 200 mg of caffeine per day for 2 weeks, abrupt cessation can lead to caffeine-withdrawal headache that typically starts within 24 hours of the last caffeine intake.[1] This headache may exhibit migraine-like features and will typically resolve completely after 1 week of caffeine avoidance or within 1 hour of consuming at least 100 mg of caffeine.

Opioid-Withdrawal Headache

Opioids, such as morphine, oxycontin, and codeine, are widely used for pain management. Chronic use of these medications can result in systemic effects such as drug dependence, constipation, sleep-disordered breathing, hyperalgesia, dizziness (which increases the risk for fractures due to falls), depression, and androgen deficiency.[20] Frequent use of opioids can also be associated with development of medication overuse headache (see Chapter 28). Opioid-withdrawal headaches manifest within 24 hours of sudden cessation in individuals with a history of daily exposure for a duration of 3 months or longer.[1] The headache typically resolves spontaneously within 7 days after the last opioid use. However, pharmacological interventions may be necessary for those experiencing more pronounced withdrawal symptoms, including fever, vomiting, myalgia, diarrhea, tachycardia, hypertension, hyperthermia, disorientation, and agitation.[20]

Estrogen-Withdrawal Headache

A treatment regimen involving combined oral contraceptive pills typically follows a 21/7 dosing schedule, which consists of 21 days of active hormonal treatment followed by 7 days of placebo.[21] During this hormone-free interval (HFI), there is a notable increase in pelvic pain, breast tenderness, bloating, and analgesic use.[21] Headaches experienced during the HFI are more severe, frequent,

Table 27-2 Headache Attributed to Substance Withdrawal

Substance	Drug Examples	Headache Onset (from Last Use)	Headache Cessation	Headache Features	Clinical Pearls
Caffeine	Coffee, tea, energy drinks, chocolate	Within 24 hours	7 days after total withdrawal 1 hour after 100 mg of caffeine	Not clearly defined, likely shares features with TTH or migraine	Occurs with daily caffeine consumption of at least 200 mg for 2 weeks or more
Opioid	Morphine, oxycontin, codeine	Within 24 hours	Within 1 week	Not clearly defined, likely shares features with TTH or migraine	Headache spontaneously resolves but pharmacologic treatment may be needed for other withdrawal symptoms
Estrogen	Combined oral contraceptives, hormone replacement	Within 5 days	Within 72 hours	Not clearly defined, likely shares features with TTH or migraine	Headaches more severe and longer in duration during hormone-free interval
Chronic use of other substances	Corticosteroids, TCAs, SSRIs, NSAIDs	Within 1 week, depending on the half-life of the drug	Weeks to months	Not clearly defined, likely shares features with TTH or migraine	Long taper over several weeks or months may prevent withdrawal headache

NSAIDs, nonsteroidal anti-inflammatory drugs; SSRIs, selective serotonin reuptake inhibitors; TTH, tension-type headache; TCAs, tricyclic antidepressants.

and prolonged, usually occurring within 5 days of estrogen withdrawal.[1,21] These headaches exhibit phenotypic characteristics resembling migraine or TTHs and tend to resolve within 3 days of onset. Managing estrogen-withdrawal headaches may involve initiating "mini-prophylaxis" with long-acting triptans starting on the last day of active pills or shortening the HFI by using a 24/4 or 26/2 dosing schedule.[22] See also Chapter 36.

Headache Attributed to Withdrawal from Chronic Use of Other Substances

Withdrawal headaches have been documented with various medications, including tricyclic antidepressants (TCAs) and selective serotonin reuptake inhibitors (SSRIs).[1] In fact, all major classes of antidepressants can lead to a condition referred to as antidepressant discontinuation syndrome (ADS), also known as withdrawal.[23] ADS affects around 20% of individuals who experience a delay or cessation of antidepressant treatment and is believed to occur after at least 6 weeks of medication usage.[23] Symptoms of ADS encompass headache, flu-like illness, myalgias, disturbed sleep, nausea, vertigo, dysesthesia, anxiety, and agitation. The onset of ADS typically occurs within 3 days of discontinuation but can commence as early as hours after the last dose, depending on the drug's half-life.[23] Withdrawal symptoms typically resolve spontaneously within 2 weeks. The specific characteristics of withdrawal headaches are not precisely defined but are likely similar to either TTHs or migraine. Other substances thought to induce withdrawal headaches include corticosteroids and nonsteroidal anti-inflammatory drugs.

Summary

- Recognizing substance-related headaches can be challenging due to the numerous potential offending agents and the high prevalence of primary headaches that can occur alongside them.

- Substances known to induce headaches include NO donors, PDE inhibitors, carbon monoxide, alcohol, cocaine, pressor agents, nicotine, tetracyclines, valerian root, and camphor.

- Substances known to induce withdrawal headaches include caffeine, opioids, estrogen, and antidepressants.

- Headaches resulting from substances can have features of migraine, TTH, or trigeminal autonomic cephalalgias.

- Treatment varies with each substance but typically involves symptomatic treatment and management of any life-threatening effects.

REFERENCES

1. Gobel H. 8. *Headache Attributed to a Substance or its Withdrawal [Internet].* ICHD-3. [cited 2022 Jul 9]. Available at: https://ichd-3.org/8-headache-attributed-to-a-substance-or-its-withdrawal/.

2. Olesen J. The role of nitric oxide (NO) in migraine, tension-type headache and cluster headache. *Pharmacol Ther.* 2008;120(2):157-171.

3. Puzzo D, Sapienza S, Arancio O, Palmeri A. Role of phosphodiesterase 5 in synaptic plasticity and memory. *Neuropsychiatr Dis Treat.* 2008;4(2):371-387.

4. Lin G-Y, Lee J-T, Peng G-S, Yang F-C. Sildenafil can induce the onset of a cluster headache bout. *Can Urol Assoc J.* 2014;8(5-6):E378-E380.

5. Rose JJ, Wang L, Xu Q, et al. Carbon monoxide poisoning: pathogenesis, management, and future directions of therapy. *Am J Respir Crit Care Med.* 2017;195(5):596-606.

6. Keleş A, Demircan A, Kurtoğlu G. Carbon monoxide poisoning: how many patients do we miss? *Eur J Emerg Med.* 2008;15(3):154-157.

7. Nicoletti P, Trevisani M, Manconi M, et al. Ethanol causes neurogenic vasodilation by TRPV1 activation and CGRP release in the trigeminovascular system of the guinea pig. *Cephalalgia.* 2008;28(1):9-17.

8. *Drug Decriminalisation Across the World [Internet].* TalkingDrugs. [cited 2022 Jul 10]. Available at: https://www.talkingdrugs.org/drug-decriminalisation.

9. Farooque U, Okorie N, Kataria S, Shah SF, Bollampally VC. Cocaine-induced headache: a review of pathogenesis, presentation, diagnosis, and management. *Cureus.* 2020;12(8):e10128.

10. Arca KN, Halker Singh RB. The hypertensive headache: a review. *Curr Pain Headache Rep.* 2019;23(5):30.

11. Carstens E, Carstens MI. Sensory effects of nicotine and tobacco. *Nicotine Tob Res.* 2022;24: 306-315.

12. Ailani, J. Updates on management of headache in women and transgender women. *Curr Opin Neurol.* 2021;34:339-343.

13. Prakash S, Shah ND. Pure menstrual hemicrania continua: does it exist? A case report. *Cephalalgia.* 2010;30(5):631-633.

14. Maggioni F, Palmieri A, Viaro F, Mainardi F, Zanchin G. Menstrual paroxysmal hemicrania, a possible new entity? *Cephalalgia.* 2007;27(9): 1085-1087.

15. Ferrari A. Headache: one of the most common and troublesome adverse reactions to drugs. *Curr Drug Saf.* 2006;1:43-58.

16. Freitas C, Khanal S, Landsberg D, Kaul V. An alternative cause of encephalopathy: valerian root overdose. *Cureus.* 2021;13(9):e17759.

17. Zuccarini P. Camphor: risks and benefits of a widely used natural product. *J Appl Sci Environ Manage [Internet].* 2010 Jun 8 [cited 2022 Jul 17]; 13(2). Available at: http://www.bioline.org.br/pdf?ja09027.

18. Lipton RB, Diener H-C, Robbins MS, Garas SY, Patel K. Caffeine in the management of patients with headache. *J Headache Pain.* 2017;18(1):107.

19. Knapik JJ, Trone DW, McGraw S, Steelman RA, Austin KG, Lieberman HR. Caffeine use among active duty navy and marine corps personnel. *Nutrients [Internet].* 2016;8(10):620.

20. Baldini A, Von Korff M, Lin EHB. A review of potential adverse effects of long-term opioid therapy: a practitioner's guide. *Prim Care Companion CNS Disord [Internet].* 2012;14(3):PCC.11m01326.

21. Graziottin A. The shorter, the better: a review of the evidence for a shorter contraceptive hormone-free interval. *Eur J Contracept Reprod Health Care.* 2016;21(2):93-105.

22. Silberstein SD, Holland S, Freitag F, et al. Evidence-based guideline update: pharmacologic treatment for episodic migraine prevention in adults: report of the Quality Standards Subcommittee of the American Academy of Neurology and the American Headache Society. *Neurology.* 2012; 78(17):1337-1345.

23. Warner CH, Bobo W, Warner C, Reid S, Rachal J. Antidepressant discontinuation syndrome. *Am Fam Physician.* 2006;74(3):449-456.

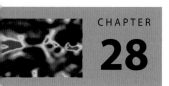

CHAPTER

28 Medication-Overuse Headache

Nicholas Tzikas and Hans-Christoph Diener

Medication-overuse headache (MOH) was first described in 1951 and has been known by various terms such as rebound headache, drug-overuse headache, drug-induced headache (International Classification of Diseases, Tenth Revision or ICD-10), medication-misuse headache, or medication-adaptation headache.[1] It is now classified as a secondary headache disorder according to the *International Classification of Headache Disorders*, including the latest 3rd edition, ICHD-3 (see Preface). MOH is commonly associated with episodic migraine and tension-type headaches, often worsening with increased acute medication intake. It can also exacerbate other primary and secondary headache disorders. Interestingly, MOH does not typically occur in patients without preexisting headaches. MOH is a preventable and treatable condition, although many clinicians are not fully aware of its risks and management strategies. The term MOH has faced criticism, including that it is potentially blaming patients, but its use continues due to the lack of a widely accepted alternative.

Epidemiology

The prevalence of MOH is substantial, with more than half of patients presenting with chronic headache having this condition.[1] Global estimates from the Global Burden of Disease Study in 2015 indicate that approximately 59 million individuals worldwide are affected by MOH. Epidemiological studies have reported varying prevalence rates, ranging from 1% to 2% in the general population but reaching up to 7.2% in certain populations. In specialized headache centers, the prevalence of MOH can be as high as 50% to 80%. Interestingly, there are differences in the prevalence of MOH among ethnic groups within European countries, with higher rates observed among migrants, which could be due to genetic, cultural, or socioeconomic factors such as differences in healthcare access, migration-related stress, and language/communication difficulties.[2] Women and individuals in their 30s to 50s are most commonly affected by MOH. The incidence of MOH was found to be 0.72 per 1000 person-years based on the Nord-Trøndelag Health Survey (HUNT), with no consideration for potential resolution of cases during the study period.[1]

This disabling headache disorder imposes a significant burden on individuals and society, ranking among the top 20 diseases causing years of life lost due to disability. Medication overuse is associated with higher pain intensity and rates of cutaneous allodynia in individuals with migraine, with a higher likelihood observed in users of triptans, opioids, and barbiturates. Longitudinal studies indicate that increasing daily doses of opioids and barbiturates in people with migraine increases the risk of chronic headache onset. Several risk factors have been identified for the development of MOH, including regular use of tranquilizers, analgesics, and sleep-inducing medications, as well as comorbidities such as chronic musculoskeletal and gastrointestinal complaints, high levels of anxiety and depression, insomnia, smoking, physical inactivity, younger age, female gender, low education level, and a history of migraine or other/nonmigraine headaches.

Secondary Headaches

Pathophysiology

The pathophysiology of MOH is not fully understood, but several mechanisms have been proposed.[3,4] Genetic factors may play a role, although extensive genome-wide association studies are lacking. Abnormalities in metabolic pathways, serotonergic and dopaminergic transmission, and drug dependence-related genes have been suggested as potential genetic risk factors. Structural, functional, and metabolic brain changes have been observed in regions such as the hippocampus, periaqueductal gray area (PAG), posterior cingulate cortex, thalamus, cerebellum, orbitofrontal cortex (OFC), and the mesocorticolimbic reward system. Alterations in cortical excitability, including increased susceptibility to cortical spreading depression, changes in serotonin (5-HT) modulation, and upregulation of vasoactive and proinflammatory mediators, may contribute to MOH. Acute headache medications have been shown to enhance net descending facilitation in pain modulatory pathways and induce sensitization of peripheral and central pain pathways. Animal studies have demonstrated persistent hypersensitivity, latent sensitization, and generalized cutaneous allodynia in response to chronic exposure to medications such as triptans.

Diagnosis and Clinical Presentation

The diagnosis of MOH requires a comprehensive assessment, including a thorough history and examination to identify potential secondary headache causes. Diagnostic evaluation may involve blood tests, neuroimaging, and cerebrospinal fluid testing in the presence of "red flags" (Chapters 1-3). The ICHD-3 criteria are used to diagnose MOH, which necessitate the presence of a preexisting primary headache, the development of a new headache, or worsening of the preexisting headache due to medication overuse, headaches occurring on ≥15 days per month, and regular overuse of acute or symptomatic headache medications for >3 months (Table 28-1). The diagnosis of MOH is assigned in conjunction with the preexisting primary headache diagnosis. The number of medication days required for a diagnosis varies depending on the type of medication used. It is important to note that determining the causal relationship between medication overuse and headache worsening can be challenging, and headache improvement following medication discontinuation supports the diagnosis of MOH but is not mandatory according to the ICHD criteria. The current diagnostic criteria have limitations, including the lack of consideration for medication dosage and consecutive days of use, as well as the variable thresholds for defining medication overuse.[1]

Those presenting to specialized headache centers tend to have daily or near-daily headaches. Patients with MOH typically present with a chronic or frequent headache oftentimes highlighted by migraine semiology, particularly in cases where migraine is the underlying disorder. In cases of analgesic overuse, patients are more likely to develop a diffuse holocranial dull-pressing headache, often lacking associated migraine symptoms. On the contrary, triptan overuse can lead to a daily migraine-like headache that typically occurs in the morning, subsides rapidly after triptan use, but reappears within a few hours or the next day. Some patients who overuse triptans may report an increase in the frequency of migraine attacks exclusively. The characteristics of the headache can evolve as the number of headache days increases, and individuals with migraine may experience fewer associated symptoms such as nausea, vomiting, photophobia, and phonophobia. At the time of seeking medical attention, patients with MOH have usually been experiencing the headache disorder for approximately 20 years, with overmedication occurring for about 6 years. Raising awareness among patients and clinicians about the nature and consequences of MOH is crucial, as misdiagnosis and unsuccessful treatment attempts with different acute and preventive strategies can perpetuate the cycle of irrational use of headache medications.

Table 28-1. Diagnostic Criteria for Medication-Overuse Headache According to the *International Classification of Headache Disorders*, Third Edition (ICHD-3)

All forms of Medication-Overuse Headache must meet criteria A, B, and C below. Criterion B varies with the type(s) of medication(s) overused.	
Criterion A	Headache occurring on ≥15 days/month in a patient with a preexisting headache disorder
Criterion B	Regular overuse for >3 months of one or more drugs that can be taken for acute and/or symptomatic treatment of headache taken above a specified threshold
Ergotamine-overuse headache	Regular intake of ergotamine on ≥10 days/month for >3 months
Triptan-overuse headache	Regular intake of one or more triptans, in any formulation, on ≥10 days/month for >3 months
Acetaminophen/paracetamol-overuse headache	Regular intake of acetaminophen/paracetamol on ≥15 days/month for >3 months
NSAID-overuse headache	Regular intake of one or more nonsteroidal anti-inflammatory drugs (NSAIDs) (other than acetylsalicylic acid) on ≥15 days/month for >3 months
Acetylsalicylic acid-overuse headache	Regular intake of acetylsalicylic acid on ≥15 days/month for >3 months
Nonopioid analgesic-overuse headache	Regular intake of a nonopioid analgesic other than paracetamol or nonsteroidal anti-inflammatory drugs (including acetylsalicylic acid) on ≥15 days/month for >3 months
Opioid-overuse headache	Regular intake of one or more opioids on ≥10 days/month for >3 months
Combination-analgesic-overuse headache	Regular intake of one or more combination-analgesic medications (nonopioid analgesics with opioids, butalbital, and/or caffeine) on ≥10 days/month for >3 months
Medication-overuse headache attributed to multiple drug classes	Regular intake of any combination of ergotamine, triptans, nonopioid analgesics and/or opioids for a total of ≥10 days/month for >3 months without overuse of any single drug or drug class alone
Medication-overuse headache attributed to unspecified or unverified overuse of multiple drug classes	Regular overuse, on ≥10 days/month for >3 months, of one or more medications other than those described earlier, taken for acute or symptomatic treatment of headache
Criterion C	Not better accounted for by another ICHD-3 diagnosis

Treatment

MOH can be one of the most difficult headache conditions to treat as patients have become dependent on their abortive medication, which at this juncture likely provides transient relief and requires frequent use with escalated dosing. The treatment of MOH includes nonpharmacologic approaches, pharmacological treatment, and discontinuation of the overused medication.[1] Nonpharmacologic interventions, such as education and awareness of MOH, have been shown to reduce medication use and headache frequency.

It is necessary for patients to understand that overusing acute medication (paradoxically) leads to increased headache frequency, which leads to more medication use, a vicious cycle in which the treatment propagates the disease. The overused medicine can be stopped immediately if it is a simple analgesic, triptan, or ergot. However, long-term use of barbiturates, opiates, and benzodiazepines will require a slow tapering of the drug to prevent serious withdrawal symptoms which can also include life-threatening seizures secondary to benzodiazepine and barbiturate withdrawal.[5] When possible, the overused medication is abruptly discontinued, preventive therapy is started/optimized, and alternative acute headache abortive medication is administered in place of the overused medication (as long as it is a different class than the offending agent—triptan substituted for analgesic and vice versa). The concept of reducing acute medications may be uncomfortable, but it has been shown to be an effective treatment for MOH. Medication reduction can be done in outpatient settings, although inpatient treatment may be necessary for certain cases. Switching to an alternative acute medication with limited frequency can help manage ongoing headaches. The "Raskin protocol" is one such regimen that compared intravenous dihydroergotamine (DHE) and metoclopramide every 8 hours versus diazepam in patients with MOH and it demonstrated that DHE was beneficial (89% headache free in 48 hours and 71% at 16 months) during the detoxification phase of MOH; however, it is contraindicated in those with vascular disease.[6] Several recent studies have found that steroids have little to no impact on MOH withdrawal symptoms but are slightly better than placebo.

Preventive treatment may be initiated during acute medication withdrawal, and regular follow-up visits are important to prevent relapse into medication overuse. Preventive treatments including topiramate, onabotulinumtoxinA, and monoclonal antibodies against CGRP or the CGRP receptor have demonstrated efficacy in reducing headache days and medication use in MOH patients.[1,7] Valproic acid has shown effectiveness in treating MOH with a history of migraine after detoxification. OnabotulinumtoxinA has been more effective than placebo in reducing overall headache days, migraine days, and cumulative monthly headache hours. Monoclonal antibodies against CGRP or the CGRP receptor have shown positive results in reducing monthly migraine days and acute headache medication use. The use of beta-blockers, flunarizine (not available in the United States), tricyclic antidepressants, and candesartan for MOH treatment lacks randomized trial evidence but are commonly used in practice. Studies on preventive treatment of migraine with gepants have also demonstrated decreased use of headache abortive medications. While neuromodulatory treatments have not been studied specifically in MOH, they may be considered as an alternative treatment option. Further randomized trials are needed to evaluate the use of neuromodulation, long-acting nonsteroidal anti-inflammatory drugs, and gepants for MOH treatment.

Prognosis

If MOH is effectively treated, it can lead to highly rewarding outcomes for both the patient and the healthcare provider. The prognosis for patients with MOH is generally favorable, with 50% to 70% of patients showing improvement after withdrawal therapy, particularly when combined with preventive medication.[1,8] However, relapse rates of 10% to 40% within 5 years after withdrawal have been reported. The first year following withdrawal is considered critical in predicting long-term success, emphasizing the importance of close monitoring during this period to prevent relapse. Several factors have been identified as predictive factors for relapse, including the combination of migraine and tension-type headache, overuse of opioids, longer duration of regular acute medication intake, a high number of acute treatments, lack of improvement after 2 months of withdrawal, smoking, alcohol use, patient-reported poor sleep quality, and high levels of body pain. Psychiatric comorbidity, high dependence score, and overuse of barbiturates, benzodiazepines, and opioids predicted a poorer outcome of withdrawal therapy.[5]

Summary

- MOH is a common secondary headache disorder which constitutes a great proportion of chronic headaches.

- MOH remains underdiagnosed and undertreated, and can be associated with a substantial burden and decreased quality of life.

- Medication overuse is a modifiable risk factor for the progression or persistence of headaches, and the risk of MOH is highest with opioids, butalbital, and combination analgesics.

- The diagnosis of MOH is primarily clinical, based on the criteria outlined in ICHD-3, and typically involves increased headache frequency in individuals with a preexisting primary headache disorder and frequent use of analgesics.

- MOH does not have distinctive phenotypic characteristics that distinguish it from other chronic daily headache conditions, but it commonly exhibits features of migraine or TTH.

- The treatment plan for MOH involves patient education, discontinuation of the overused acute headache medication, implementation of effective preventive treatment, consideration of bridge therapy if necessary, and regular follow-up to prevent relapse.

REFERENCES

1. Ashina S, Terwindt GM, Steiner TJ, et al. Medication overuse headache. *Nat Rev Dis Primers.* 2023; 9:5.

2. Westergaard ML, Munksgaard SB, Bendtsen L, Jensen RH. Medication-overuse headache: a perspective review. *Ther Adv Drug Saf.* 2016;7:147-158.

3. Vandenbussche N, Laterza D, Lisicki M, et al. Medication-overuse headache: a widely recognized entity amidst ongoing debate. *J Headache Pain.* 2018;19:50.

4. Sun-Edelstein C, Rapoport AM, Rattanawong W, Srikiatkhachorn A. The evolution of medication overuse headache: history, pathophysiology and clinical update. *CNS Drugs.* 2021;35:545-565.

5. Loder E, Biondi D. Oral phenobarbital loading: a safe and effective method of withdrawing patients with headache from butalbital compounds. *Headache.* 2003;43:904-909.

6. Tepper D. Medication overuse headache. *Headache.* 2017;57:845-846.

7. Diener HC, Antonaci F, Braschinsky M, et al. European Academy of Neurology guideline on the management of medication-overuse headache. *Eur J Neurol.* 2020;27:1102-1116.

8. Chiang CC, Schwedt TJ, Wang SJ, Dodick DW. Treatment of medication-overuse headache: a systematic review. *Cephalalgia.* 2016;36:371-386.

Secondary Headaches

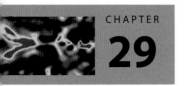

Headache Attributed to Infection

Eileen Yu, Eric Bhaimia, and Zubair A. Ahmed

While the majority of headaches are of primary or migraine origin, it is crucial not to overlook the potentially life-threatening nature of secondary headaches caused by systemic or intracranial infections. The accurate diagnosis of infection-related secondary headaches relies on precise anatomical localization and identification of the specific pathogen involved. A thorough assessment, encompassing a detailed medical history, comprehensive neurological examination, and evaluation of serum, cerebrospinal fluid (CSF), and imaging findings, facilitates the development of an informed treatment plan and prognosis. The following questions can aid clinicians in the diagnosis and management of secondary headaches attributed to infection.

1. Is the infection primarily within the central nervous system (CNS), or is it due to a systemic infection?
2. Is the illness acute, subacute, or chronic?

Bacterial Meningitis

Epidemiology

In the United States, there are 1.38 cases of meningitis per 100,000 people and approximately 500 deaths from bacterial meningitis annually.[1] The leading causes of bacterial meningitis across all age groups are *Streptococcus pneumoniae* and *Neisseria meningitidis*. Nosocomial infections are commonly acquired following neurosurgery, penetrating head trauma, or basilar skull fracture. They consist primarily of gram-positive organisms with the remainder being gram-negative organisms.[2] *Listeria monocytogenes* and gram-negative bacilli (such as *Escherichia coli* and *Klebsiella* spp.) are more commonly associated with older adults (>50 years) and neonates. *Haemophilus influenzae* type b predominantly affects individuals who have not undergone vaccination. Other risk factors for bacterial meningitis include crowded living conditions, close contacts, and immunocompromised states (i.e., HIV/AIDS, complement deficiency, sickle cell anemia, asplenia, hypogammaglobulinemia, pregnancy, and alcoholism).

Pathophysiology

The pathogenesis of bacterial meningitis involves the invasion of the CNS by bacteria through direct (e.g., neurosurgery or head trauma) or indirect routes.[3] In the latter, bacteria colonize the nasopharynx and mucosa before entering the brain. This entry can occur via hematogenous spread to the subarachnoid space or through contiguous pathways such as the middle ear or sinuses. Infection of the CNS leads to inflammatory processes that compromise the blood–brain barrier, leading to increased cortical permeability, cerebral edema, and increased intracranial pressure. The release of bacterial toxins and neuroinflammatory pain mediators further contribute to meningeal irritation and the development of headaches.

Diagnosis and Clinical Presentation

Severe headache is a prominent symptom in 84% of patients with meningitis/encephalitis, making it one of the most common clinical features for diagnosis. Other common symptoms include fever, nausea/vomiting, and sensitivity to light and sound. The presence of altered sensorium, such as behavioral/personality changes or hallucinations, suggests a diagnosis of encephalitis. Focal neurological deficits may also be observed. The lumbar puncture (LP) is the diagnostic method of choice for meningitis (Chapter 3) (Table 29-1). However, in cases where neuroimaging is indicated before LP (e.g., in immunocompromised individuals, those with a history of mass lesions or stroke, papilledema, new-onset seizure, altered mental status, or focal neurologic deficit),[4] prompt initiation of empiric antibiotics must not be delayed.

Treatment

The treatment approach for bacterial meningitis involves prompt administration of antibiotics tailored to the patient's clinical context, along with dexamethasone if *S. pneumoniae* meningitis is suspected.[5] In cases where *Listeria* spp. is suspected, such as in pregnancy, newborns, the elderly, or immunocompromised individuals, ampicillin should be added to the antibiotic regimen. The spirochetes *Treponema pallidum* and *Borrelia burgdorferi* causing syphilis and Lyme disease, respectively, may also present with headache and suspicion may be raised on history. Once the causative pathogens are identified, antibiotic therapy can be adjusted accordingly. The prognosis for bacterial meningitis can vary depending on factors such as age, comorbidities, and the causative organism.

Viral Meningitis and Encephalitis

Epidemiology

Viral meningitis is generally self-limiting and less severe as compared to bacterial meningitis. The annual incidence of viral meningitis is around 2.73 cases per 100,000 people, with a higher prevalence among children and in areas with low vaccination rates.[6] Nonpolio enteroviruses (e.g., coxsackievirus and echovirus) are the most common cause of viral meningitis, followed by herpesviruses (such as HSV1, HSV2, WNV, and VZV). HSV-1 is more commonly associated with encephalitis, while HSV-2 is linked to benign recurrent lymphocytic meningitis, also known as Mollaret meningitis, and is discussed later in this chapter.[3] Other viral causes include lymphocytic choriomeningitis virus (LCMV), paramyxoviruses (e.g., measles and mumps), arboviruses (e.g., West Nile virus and tickborne encephalitis virus), St. Louis encephalitis virus, California encephalitis virus, Western equine encephalitis virus, dengue virus, and influenza virus. Infection with human immunodeficiency virus (HIV) may also present with meningitis and is discussed in a separate section of this chapter. It is important to note that the majority (around 70%) of infectious encephalitides are viral in nature.

Pathophysiology

Viral spread to the CNS can occur through various routes. Most viruses enter the body and replicate peripherally before hematogenous spread to the brain. Several herpesviruses and the rabies virus may travel retrograde along nerve endings to reach the CNS. Furthermore, HSV can establish a dormant state in the dorsal root ganglia. Reactivation of HSV in the ophthalmic branch of the trigeminal ganglia can lead to threatened vision. The exact pathophysiology of the development of headaches in viral meningitis is not fully understood, but inflammation of the meninges is a possible explanation.

Diagnosis and Clinical Presentation

Identifying features of viral encephalitis, particularly HSV, include focal seizures with subsequent secondary generalization. Both HSV and VZV may be accompanied by vesicular lesions or rash. LCMV can present with flu-like illness and rarely orchitis, parotitis, myopericarditis, or arthritis.

Table 29-1. Cerebrospinal Fluid (CSF) Characteristics and Recommended Diagnostics

	CSF Analysis	Labs/Diagnostics	Neuroimaging/MRI
Meningitis/Encephalitis			
Bacterial	Cloudy, purulent appearance	CSF culture, PCR, and antigen testing	Leptomeningeal enhancement
- *Streptococcus pneumoniae*	↑ Opening pressure, PMNs, protein, lactate	*Listeria* cultures can have low sensitivity	
- *Listeria monocytogenes*	↓ Glucose		
Viral	Clear appearance	EBV, HIV, VZV, WNV, CMV	Temporal/frontal involvement (for HSV meningitis/encephalitis)
	↑ Lymphocytes	PCR	
	Variable opening pressure, protein, lactate	Enterovirus, HSV-1 and 2, HHV-6 PCR	
	Normal glucose		
Fungal/parasitic	Variable appearance	Cryptococcus: antigen testing, culture with India ink	Possible hydrocephalus, ring-enhancing lesions
	↑ Opening pressure, lymphocytosis, ↑ protein, ↓ glucose	Histoplasmosis: culture, antigen testing, serology	
		Coccidioides: culture, serology, antigen testing	
		Toxoplasmosis: Wright or Giemsa stain	
		Taeniasis: eosinophilia on CBC, eggs, and/or worms on stool culture	
		Angiostrongylus: eosinophilic meningitis, surgical specimen pathology	
Benign recurrent lymphocytic meningitis	↑ Lymphocytes (initial PMN predominance may be present)	HSV-2 PCR	
	Large, irregularly shaped monocyte-like cells with Papanicolaou stain		
	PCR for HSV DNA detection		
Neurosyphilis	↑ Lymphocytes, protein	VDRL	MRA differentiates between parenchymal vs. arterial pathology
- *Treponema pallidum*	CSF VDRL (screening)	TP-PA or FTA-ABS	
	CSF FTA-ABS (confirmatory)		

	CSF Analysis	Labs/Diagnostics	Neuroimaging/MRI
Localized Brain Infections			
Fungal infections/TB - Endemic mycoses (histoplasma, blastomyces, *Cryptococcus, Coccidioides*)	↑ Opening pressure, lymphocytes, protein, lactate	Blood or sputum cultures (variable sensitivity), serology, urine Ag	Possible abscess, meningeal enhancement, granuloma formation, ring-enhancing lesions +/− hemorrhage (indicates intracranial mass lesions) *Mycobacterium tuberculosis*: thickened basilar meninges on T1w MRI
Brain abscess - *Staphylococcus, Streptococcus,* anaerobes, GNRs - *Nocardia* (immunocompromised)	↑ WBC, protein Normal glucose Negative cultures	Aspiration or drainage of brain lesion (confirmatory) ↑ CRP and ESR Blood cultures	DWI on MRI shows hyperintense ring-enhancing lesions
Subdural empyema	Commonly negative CSF cultures Possible ↑ lymphocytes, protein	Possible ↑ WBC	Crescent-shaped hypointense area on T1 MRI with gadolinium. Check for signs of mass effect or midline shift
HaNDL	↑ Lymphocytes Common ↑ opening pressure, protein Possible ↑ IgG or oligoclonal bands present	Broad spectrum labs to rule out other etiologies	Nonspecific findings or leptomeningeal enhancement on CT or MRI
Systemic infections			
HIV/AIDS	Negative cultures Viral load	Variable HIV-1/2 Ab differentiation immunoassay HIV-1 quant viral load CD4+ count	Usually negative findings Neuroinflammation, tumor, hemorrhage, and other abnormalities on CT or MRI

Abbreviations: Ag, Antigen; AIDS, Acquired Immunodeficiency Syndrome; CBC, complete blood count; CMV, cytomegalovirus; CRP, C-reactive protein; CSF analysis, cerebrospinal fluid analysis; CT, computed tomography; DNA, deoxyribonucleic acid; DWI, diffusion-weighted imaging; EBV, Epstein-Barr virus; ESR, erythrocyte sedimentation rate; FTA-ABS, fluorescent treponemal antibody-absorption; GNRs, gram-negative rods; HaNDL, headache with neurological deficits and CSF lymphocytosis; HIV, human immunodeficiency virus; HSV, herpes simplex virus; IgG, immunoglobulin G; MRA, magnetic resonance angiography; MRI, magnetic resonance imaging; PCR, polymerase chain reaction; PMNs, polymorphonuclear neutrophils; TB, tuberculosis; TP-PA, *Treponema pallidum* particle agglutination; VDRL, Venereal Disease Research Laboratory; VZV, varicella-zoster virus; WNV, West Nile virus.

Diagnosis of viral encephalitis is typically confirmed through CSF analysis (Table 29-1). MRI brain findings often reveal asymmetric involvement of the limbic system, insula, medial temporal lobes, and inferolateral frontal lobes.

Treatment

Treatment of viral meningitis and encephalitis is generally supportive. Given the overlap in presentation with bacterial meningitis, empiric antibiotics should be administered until bacterial causes are ruled out. In the case of HSV encephalitis, intravenous acyclovir has been shown to decrease morbidity and mortality.[7] Depending on the etiology, viral meningitis usually resolves without treatment within 7 to 10 days. Rarely, patients may experience neurologic sequelae such as sensorineural hearing loss, cognitive deficits, or epilepsy.

Tuberculous Meningitis

In the United States, tuberculous meningitis accounts for approximately 1% of all tuberculosis cases and is characterized by *Mycobacterium tuberculosis* crossing the blood–brain barrier where a resultant subependymal tubercle may rupture, leading to a severe and potentially life-threatening form of basilar meningitis. The pathogenesis of headache during tuberculous meningitis may involve mechanisms such as meningeal irritation, tuberculoma formation, and the development of obstructive hydrocephalus, similar to those observed in other bacterial meningitis cases.

Tuberculous meningitis can have a subacute clinical progression over a period of weeks to months. While patients often present with the classic meningitis triad, the fever in tuberculous meningitis tends to develop more gradually and may be intermittent. Other signs and symptoms associated with tuberculous meningitis include cranial nerve palsies (predominantly CN VI, as well as CN III, VII, VIII), focal neurological deficits, and seizures. CSF analysis typically shows a mixed pleocytosis with a lymphocytic predominance, low glucose, and elevated protein levels. Confirmation of the diagnosis is achieved through CSF staining for acid-fast bacilli and cultures, while CSF polymerase chain reaction (PCR) may be employed in reference laboratories when there is a high clinical suspicion (Table 29-1). Positive tuberculin skin testing or interferon-gamma release assay may support the diagnosis. Neuroimaging findings may show hydrocephalus, ring-enhancing lesions on T1 MRI brain with gadolinium, and thickening of the basilar meninges.

Treatment for tuberculous meningitis typically includes rifampin, isoniazid, pyrazinamide, and ethambutol (RIPE therapy) for 2 months, followed by isoniazid and rifampin for up to 10 months. In cases where patients display neurologic deficits or progressive neurologic deterioration, corticosteroids are recommended as an adjunctive therapy. It is important to note that tuberculous meningitis is often fatal if left untreated, with a mortality rate ranging from 55% to 75%. The risk of mortality increases with age and in individuals with compromised immune systems. Complications associated with tuberculous meningitis include obstructive hydrocephalus and vasculitis.

Cryptococcal Meningitis

Cryptococcal meningitis is a common opportunistic infection in AIDS and immunocompromised patients, with *Cryptococcus neoformans* being the most common causative fungus. The infection is typically acquired through inhalation of fungal spores present in soil, trees, and bird droppings, followed by dissemination to the CNS via the bloodstream. Similar to tuberculous meningitis, cryptococcal meningitis often affects the basilar regions of the brain, with a gradual onset over months to years, and is frequently associated with hydrocephalus and cranial nerve abnormalities. CSF analysis reveals lymphocytic pleocytosis, elevated protein levels, and low glucose (see Table 29-1). Treatment consists of amphotericin B and flucytosine induction, followed by fluconazole consolidation and maintenance therapy for 12 months. Overall, cryptococcal meningitis carries a poor prognosis and may be associated with neurological sequelae. Adherence to the treatment regimen and timely management are crucial in preventing relapse and improving outcomes.

Recurrent Benign Lymphocytic Meningitis

Benign recurrent lymphocytic meningitis (RBLM) is a rare aseptic meningitis with a variable presentation and acuity, with the onset of symptoms occurring anywhere from hours to weeks after inoculation.[8] A limited number of case series have reported a female-predominant patient population with an average age of approximately 37 years. While many herpes viruses have been implicated, RBLM is most commonly associated with HSV-2. The diagnosis of RBLM is defined by recurrent (three or more) episodes of meningismus that occur over weeks to years. These episodes are self-resolving and typically last hours to days. Other symptoms include altered mental status, seizures, hallucinations, cranial nerve deficits, and diplopia.

The presence of large, irregularly shaped monocyte-like cells on the Papanicolaou stain of CSF is a hallmark of the syndrome, although these cells may only be detectable within the first 24 hours of disease onset. PCR identification of HSV-2 can provide supportive evidence for the diagnosis. Given the self-resolving nature of RBLM, treatment is controversial and may be reserved for those with concerning neurologic signs or evidence of encephalitis. The use of antiviral prophylaxis to prevent recurrence may be considered on an individual basis, as there is conflicting data regarding its efficacy.[2] Some patients have been documented to develop intractable migraines, which require further treatment and prophylaxis.

Neurosyphilis

While the majority of common bacterial etiologies of CNS infections present acutely, neurosyphilis (infection of the CNS due to *T. pallidum*) may present as both acute and chronic meningitis. Based on symptomatology and clinical findings, syphilis may be divided into several categories, with neurosyphilis occurring during any stage of infection. While most patients experience CNS invasion with infection, only about 10% of individuals develop symptomatic infection. Persons living with HIV (PLWH) and other forms of immunosuppression increase the risk of neurologic complications. Neurosyphilis can manifest in acute forms, such as meningitis and meningovascular disease, or chronic forms with parenchymal involvement, such as tabes dorsalis and general paresis.

As the meninges are affected earlier in the disease progression, headache is a common feature of acute presentations. In addition to meningismus, other potential findings may include vertigo, tinnitus, and signs associated with thrombosis and infarction. Involvement of the spinal cord can lead to spasticity, muscular atrophy, and sensory deficits.

Neurosyphilis should be considered in any patient presenting with neurological symptoms, and confirmatory serologic testing is important for diagnosis. CSF fluorescent treponemal antibody-absorbed test (FTA-ABS), a highly sensitive test, may be performed when there is high clinical suspicion for neurosyphilis as the alternative CSF Venereal Disease Laboratory Research (VDRL) test has low sensitivity, but higher specificity. MRI and cerebral angiography can help differentiate between parenchymal disease and arteritis.

Treatment involves intravenous penicillin administered every 4 hours for 10 to 14 days. Patients with acute meningeal syphilis usually experience a full recovery. Meningovascular syphilis and later forms of neurosyphilis generally improve but may be accompanied by lasting complications.

Localized Fungal Infections

In addition to meningitis, fungal infections of the CNS can give rise to various manifestations, including abscesses, vasculitis, and parenchymal syndromes, all of which can present with headache. These infections predominantly affect immunocompromised individuals, such as those with HIV/AIDS, hematologic malignancies, and advanced age. Notably, diabetic patients are particularly suscep-tible to infections by *Mucorales* spp., *Cryptococcus, Candida, Aspergillus,* dimorphic endemic fungi (*Histoplasma, Blastomyces, Coccidioides*), and dematiaceous molds (*Exophiala* spp. and *Cladophialophora* spp.), which are among the causative agents of CNS fungal infections. Fungal spores are typically inhaled and initially invade the respiratory mucosa. Subsequently, dissemination to the CNS occurs through the bloodstream or via direct entry through the sinuses, middle ear, or orbits. These infec-tions can lead to various serious complications, including cavernous sinus syndrome, cerebral infarc-tion, hemorrhage, and stroke. Common clinical presentations include headache (particularly in the presence of a brain abscess), neurological deficits, fever, papilledema, and seizures. Neuroimaging studies may reveal the presence of abscesses, meningeal enhancement, or granuloma formation. Intracranial mass lesions, with or without hemorrhage (such as cryptococcoma and aspergilloma), typically appear as ring-enhancing lesions on MRI. Culture-negative CSF is frequently observed, although specialized tests such as India ink stain for *Cryptococcus* or mannan antigen and antibody tests for *Candida* may aid in the identification of certain species (Table 29-1). Treatment primar-ily involves antifungal therapy, possibly complemented by surgical removal of localized lesions. The mortality rate for CNS fungal infections is high, ranging from 40% to 80%. Immunocompromised patients are at a significantly higher risk of developing severe or fatal complications.

Headaches Attributed to Systemic Infections

Headache is a common symptom in systemic infections unrelated to the CNS. In certain etiologies such as Rickettsioses, Lyme disease (*Borrelia burgdorferi*), Psittacosis (*Chlamydophila psittaci*), Brucellosis (*Brucella* spp.), Leptospirosis (*Leptospira* spp.), and Q fever (*Coxiella burnetii*), up to 90% of patients experience headache. Other systemic infections associated with headache include influenza, Legionnaire's disease (*Legionella* spp.), atypical pneumonia (e.g., *Mycoplasma pneumoniae*), and ehrlichiosis (*Ehrlichia chaffeensis*). The exact pathophysiology of headaches in the context of systemic infection remains unclear. It is likely attributed to a combination of factors, including fever, the inflammatory cascade induced by lipopolysaccharides, and the release of other pain mediators.

Differentiating headaches caused by systemic infections from intracranial infections is impor-tant. In systemic infections, headaches are typically diffuse and nonspecific. Patients may also exhibit flu-like symptoms, fever, malaise, and laboratory findings indicative of systemic infection. Notably, the absence of neck stiffness, focal symptoms, and signs suggestive of encephalitis helps distinguish systemic infection-related headaches. An LP should be performed to exclude intracranial infections. Treatment for systemic infection-related headaches is primarily symptomatic and involves managing the underlying infection. Analgesics and antipyretics are commonly used.

Headaches Related to HIV Infection/AIDS

Headaches in PLWH can be associated with both intracranial and systemic HIV infection. It is esti-mated that 12.5% to 55% of PLWHs experience headaches.[9] Various factors can contribute to head-aches in PLWH, including primary headache disorders independent of HIV infection. Headache is also a common manifestation of acute retroviral syndrome. Multiple studies have shown a correla-tion between neurological symptoms and HIV-1 viral load in CSF, with aseptic meningitis occurring regardless of CD4 cell count. In advanced HIV/AIDS, patients are more susceptible to opportunistic infections that can invade the CNS and cause headaches.

Headaches related to HIV infection often present as bilateral and dull, resembling tension-type headaches, although the specific phenotype can vary. It is crucial to maintain a high level of suspicion for opportunistic infections when managing headaches in PLWH. CSF analysis and neuroimaging should be conducted to identify potential causative opportunistic infections, and treatment should be tailored accordingly. Organisms such as *Cryptococcus, Candida, Coccidioidomycosis,* CMV, John Cunningham virus, and *Toxoplasma gondii* are among those that may be implicated. If no infection is detected, symptomatic treatment can be initiated as needed, or treatment should follow recommendations for managing primary headaches.

Summary

- A wide range of systemic infections can manifest with headaches; when appropriate, LP should be performed to differentiate between headaches of intracranial and systemic infectious origin.
- Bacterial and viral etiologies account for the vast majority of meningitis, while most cases of encephalitis are of viral etiology.
- Understanding the risk factors and acuity of presentation for causative organisms can facilitate the selection of suitable diagnostic tests and prompt initiation of management.
- Tuberculous and fungal meningitis present subacutely and are more common in immunocompromised individuals.
- Recurrent benign lymphocytic meningitis is most commonly associated with HSV-2; consensus regarding treatment and prophylaxis is controversial, and episodes are typically self-resolving.
- Headaches may arise in PLWH as a primary headache disorder, a symptom of HIV infection, or the manifestation of an opportunistic infection.

REFERENCES

1. Thigpen MC, Whitney CG, Messonnier NE, et al. Bacterial meningitis in the United States, 1998-2007. *N Engl J Med.* 2011;364(21):2016-2025.

2. Srihawan C, Lopez Castelblanco R, Salazar L, et al. Clinical characteristics and predictors of adverse outcome in adult and pediatric patients with healthcare-associated ventriculitis and meningitis. *Open Forum Infect Dis.* 2016;3(2):ofw077.

3. Bhimraj A, Bloch KC, Hasbun R. *Diagnostic Approach to a Patient with Suspected CNS Infection.* Switzerland: Humana Cham; 2021:3-11.

4. Hasbun R. Clinical features and diagnosis of acute bacterial meningitis in adults. In: Tunkel AR, Mitty J, eds. *UpToDate [Internet].* 2023. Available at: https://www.uptodate.com/contents/clinical-features-and-diagnosis-of-acute-bacterial-meningitis-in adults?search=meningitis&sectionRank=1&usage_type=default&anchor=H3&source=machineLearning&selectedTitle=1~150&display_rank=1#H11.

5. Gans JD, Beek DVD. Dexamethasone in adults with bacterial meningitis. *N Engl J Med.* 2002;347:1549-1556.

6. McGill F, Griffiths MJ, Bonnett LJ, et al. Incidence, aetiology, and sequelae of viral meningitis in UK adults: a multicentre prospective observational cohort study. *Lancet Infect Dis.* 2018;18(9):992-1003.

7. Raschilas F, Wolff M, Delatour F, et al. Outcome of and prognostic factors for herpes simplex encephalitis in adult patients: results of a multicenter study. *Clin Infect Dis.* 2002;35(3):254-260.

8. Rosenberg J, Galen BT. Recurrent meningitis. *Curr Pain Headache Rep.* 2017;21(7):33.

9. Weber JR, Sakai F. Headache attributed to infection. In Olesen J, Goadsby PJ, Ramadan NM, Tfelt-Hansen P, Welch KMA, eds. *The Headaches.* Lippincott Williams and Wilkins; 2005.

Secondary Headaches

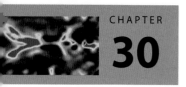

CHAPTER

30

Headache and COVID-19 Infection

Amanda Macone and Hayrunnisa Bolay

Coronavirus disease 2019 (COVID-19) is caused by novel and severe acute respiratory syndrome coronavirus 2 (SARS-CoV-2).[1] The World Health Organization officially declared the global outbreak as a pandemic on March 11, 2020. Headache has emerged as a commonly reported symptom associated with COVID-19, and it is now recognized as the most common neurological symptom of the infection.[2] The presentation of headaches in COVID-19 can vary, with some individuals experiencing short-lived headaches that resolve alongside other viral symptoms, while others may suffer from persistent headaches lasting for months, either as isolated daily persistent headaches or as part of a constellation of symptoms referred to as long-COVID or postacute COVID syndrome.

Epidemiology

The prevalence of headaches during acute COVID-19 infection has been reported in various studies, with rates ranging from 12% to 74%.[3] These variations in the frequency of headaches can be attributed, at least in part, to differences in study design, the severity of illness among the population being studied, and potentially underlying genetic variations within the population. Although there are variations between studies, it appears that headaches associated with acute COVID-19 infection are more commonly observed in females and younger patients. Additionally, while many COVID-19 patients with headaches do not have a history of prior headaches, those with existing primary headache disorders seem to be at a higher risk of experiencing headaches during the infection. Some individuals may continue to experience persistent headaches following their recovery from COVID-19, while others may develop delayed persistent headaches even after their COVID-19 symptoms have resolved. The prevalence of persistent headaches following COVID-19 infection also varies, occurring in up to 38% of patients at 4 to 6 weeks after the illness. These persistent headaches can occur on their own or in conjunction with other persistent symptoms lasting more than 4 weeks after the acute illness, which is commonly referred to as long COVID in the literature. Studies indicate that approximately 75% of individuals will experience at least one persistent symptom after recovering from COVID-19.[4] In the postacute phase, headaches are more frequently observed in females and are highly associated with fatigue and cognitive impairment.

Pathophysiology

Headaches during viral infections indicate the activation of the trigeminovascular system, either directly or indirectly, by the pathogen. In the case of SARS-CoV-2, the virus binds to angiotensin-converting enzyme 2 (ACE2) receptors on host cells, disrupting normal angiotensin II-mediated events and triggering nociceptive, vasoactive, and inflammatory signals. Direct invasion of the trigeminal nerve by the virus seems unlikely based on current evidence. Instead, inflammatory mediators released by infected cells in the nasal and oral cavities likely sensitize trigeminal nociceptors, leading to headaches and possible anosmia. The dysregulated immune response in COVID-19, including cytokine storm, plays a significant role. Studies suggest a stronger innate immune response in COVID-19 patients with headaches, with elevated levels of NOD-, LRR and pyrin domain-containing protein 3 (NLRP3), high mobility group box 1 (HMGB1), and Interleukin-6 implicated in trigeminal nociceptor activation. However, the use of inflammatory cytokine levels as headache severity markers has yielded inconsistent results. Circulating calcitonin gene-related peptide levels appear similar in COVID-19 patients with and without headaches, indicating a minor role for CGRP in COVID-19-associated headaches. Thus, the evidence indicates that headaches during the acute phase of COVID-19 are likely a result of trigeminal activation by dysregulated inflammatory signals, whether locally or systemically.[5] Similarly, post-COVID headaches may be related to a persistent immune response and the release of nociceptive and inflammatory mediators that sensitize the trigeminovascular system, resulting in headaches that phenotypically resemble migraine attacks.

Diagnosis and Clinical Presentation

Headaches commonly manifest within 72 hours of symptom onset in COVID-19, and they can be the initial or sole symptom in 25% of patients.[2,6] The description of headache characteristics is often heterogenous and can change during the course of the illness. However, certain characteristics are more frequently associated with acute COVID-19 infection. Headaches are often described as holocranial, with a predominant bifrontal or temporal distribution. The pain intensity is frequently moderate to severe (90%), typically rating around 7 out of 10 on the visual analog scale, and it is disabling with a poor response to analgesics (approximately 50%). The pain is commonly described as a persistent pressing sensation but can also be pulsating (<57%), throbbing, or aching. Patients often report worsened pain with physical activity, head movement, Valsalva maneuver, or coughing throughout the course of the illness.[2,6] A majority of patients experience a tension-like pressing quality (<80%), but migrainous features such as photophobia (30-63%), phonophobia (27-41%), nausea, and vomiting can also be present. The coexistence of headache with anosmia and/or ageusia strongly suggests COVID-19. Headache associated with COVID-19 affects both sexes, with a female-to-male ratio lower than that of migraine.

Some studies suggest that patients with a preexisting diagnosis of migraine may have earlier onset, longer-lasting, and more intense headaches in association with COVID-19. However, the headache characteristics during acute COVID-19 infection often differ from their typical headache pattern. Many patients with primary headache disorders also find their pain resistant to traditional over-the-counter analgesics, such as ibuprofen or paracetamol. Associations between headaches and other features such as fever, presence of inflammatory markers, and anosmia/ageusia have shown variations in the literature. Overall, individuals experiencing headaches tend to have a better overall outcome, with less severe illness, lower risk of ICU admission, and lower mortality compared to those without headaches upon initial presentation. However, these reports may be biased as severely ill COVID-19 patients in the ICU, who may struggle with other symptoms like dyspnea, may be unable to report headaches. One study[5] found that COVID-19 patients hospitalized without ICU need and experiencing headaches exhibited a stronger circulating innate immune response, including the presence of pronociceptive molecules like HMGB1 and NLRP3. Elevated circulating inflammatory and nociceptive molecules such as NLRP3, HMGB1, and IL-6 could contribute to headaches and have implications for clinical outcomes.

While most individuals with headaches during acute COVID-19 infection have normal neurological examinations, secondary headache disorders can occur and should be considered based on the clinical picture. Secondary etiologies may include encephalitis, meningitis, and acute cerebrovascular events such as cerebral venous thrombosis (CVT). Patients with secondary headaches often present with a more severe COVID-19 illness and additional features such as focal neurological deficits, alterations in mental status or consciousness, or seizures. Depending on the presentation,

Secondary Headaches

further diagnostic workup may involve brain imaging studies (CT, MRI, MRV), lumbar puncture, and electroencephalogram (Chapter 2).

Treatment

Acetaminophen (paracetamol) is the most commonly used drug for treating headaches in the acute phase. Initial concerns about the use of nonsteroidal anti-inflammatory drugs (NSAIDs) have been clarified since the early stages of the pandemic. However, approximately half of individuals with COVID-19-related headaches do not respond to analgesics. In a study of 34 patients unresponsive to 1000 mg of paracetamol, relief was achieved in 85% of cases through greater occipital nerve blocks.[7] Corticosteroids or indomethacin have also been successful in improving headaches in some patients. Treating headaches in the postacute phase can be challenging, with about 30% of patients experiencing difficulty in finding effective treatment. When determining a treatment strategy and considering preventive medications, it is crucial to take into account the specific headache phenotype (migraine-like, tension-like, etc.), any underlying primary headache disorder, and the potential for medication overuse.

Prognosis

The average duration of headache in hospitalized COVID-19 patients is approximately 1 to 2 weeks, although exact figures for outpatients are not known. After 3 months, up to 20% of COVID-19 patients may still experience headaches. While prevalence tends to decrease over time, some studies report that 8.4% to 16.8% of patients continue to have headaches at 6 months postillness. These headaches can be of the migraine or tension-like type. The occurrence of headaches does not appear to differ between hospitalized and nonhospitalized patients, nor is it more common in individuals with preexisting primary headache disorders. However, persistent headaches are more common in individuals who had headaches during their acute illness and those who experienced severe headache intensity at that time.[4]

Headaches can occur independently or in combination with other symptoms in the context of long COVID. Patients who had headaches during their acute illness are more likely to experience a higher number of long-COVID symptoms. Fatigue, dyspnea, cough, headache, and generalized weakness are among the most commonly reported symptoms.[4]

Long-COVID symptoms are more frequently observed in females, individuals who had more than five symptoms during their acute illness, those who experienced earlier dyspnea, and those with underlying psychiatric disorders. The severity of the initial COVID-19 infection and age do not appear to be significant contributing factors, although findings have varied across studies. It is currently difficult to predict the duration of postacute COVID symptoms. Persistent symptoms, including headaches, have been reported for months to years following other viral illnesses, including previous coronaviruses such as middle east respiratory syndrome (MERS) and severe acute respiratory syndrome (SARS).

Summary

- Headache is an early and important symptom of acute SARS-CoV-2 infection.
- Headache associated with COVID-19 has a heterogeneous presentation, including features commonly seen in secondary headache disorders, tension-type headache, and /or migraine.
- Headache associated with COVID-19 can occur in those both with or without an underlying primary headache disorder and can be persistent following resolution of acute illness.
- While most individuals with headaches during acute COVID-19 infection have normal neurological examinations, secondary headache disorders can occur and should be considered based on the clinical presentation.

- Post-COVID headache can present with various phenotypes and may be accompanied by additional symptoms such as fatigue and brain fog, particularly in cases of long COVID, and can be difficult to treat.

- Treatment of headaches due to COVID-19 can be challenging, as many patients do not respond to standard pain relief medications, necessitating targeted therapies focused on specific headache phenotypes.

REFERENCES

1. Heymann DL, Shindo N; WHO Scientific and Technical Advisory Group for Infectious Hazards. COVID-19: what is next for public health? *Lancet.* 2020;395:542-545.
2. Membrilla JA, de Lorenzo Í, Sastre M, Díaz de Terán J. Headache as a cardinal symptom of coronavirus disease 2019: a cross-sectional study. *Headache.* 2020;60:2176-2191.
3. Gonzalez-Martinez A, Fanjul V, Ramos C, et al. Headache during SARS-CoV-2 infection as an early symptom associated with a more benign course of disease: a case-control study. *Eur J Neurol.* 2021;28:3426-3436.
4. Fernández-de-Las-Peñas C, Gómez-Mayordomo V, Cuadrado ML, et al. The presence of headache at onset in SARS-CoV-2 infection is associated with long-term post-COVID headache and fatigue: a case-control study. *Cephalalgia.* 2021;41:1332-1341.
5. Bolay H, Karadas Ö, Oztürk B, et al. HMGB1, NLRP3, IL-6 and ACE2 levels are elevated in COVID-19 with headache: a window to the infection-related headache mechanism. *J Headache Pain.* 2021;22:94.
6. Uygun Ö, Ertaş M, Ekizoğlu E, et al. Headache characteristics in COVID-19 pandemic-a survey study. *J Headache Pain.* 2020;21(1):121.
7. Karadaş Ö, Öztürk B, Sonkaya AR, Taşdelen B, Özge A, Bolay H. Latent class cluster analysis identified hidden headache phenotypes in COVID-19: impact of pulmonary infiltration and IL-6. *Neurol Sci.* 2021;42:1665-1673.

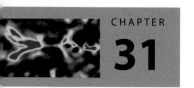

Headache and Neck Disorder

Yury Khelemsky and Henrik Schytz

Neck pain is a frequently encountered complaint in clinical practice. It refers to discomfort or distress experienced in the neck region, which includes various structures such as muscles, ligaments, nerves, and vertebrae. The localization and characteristics of neck pain can vary, ranging from aching, stiffness, and limited range of motion to sharp, shooting sensations.

There are several reasons that can contribute to the development of neck pain. Muscular strain or tension, often caused by poor posture, prolonged sitting, or repetitive movements, is a common culprit. Other factors such as trauma, degenerative changes in the cervical spine, herniated discs, and inflammatory conditions like arthritis can also lead to neck pain. Interestingly, neck pain can coexist with or be a symptom of various types of headaches. Migraine, tension-type headache (TTH), and other forms of headache, including secondary headaches like post-traumatic headaches, are well known to be associated with neck pain. One specific type of headache associated with neck pain is cervicogenic headache, which is defined by the third edition of the *International Classification of Headache Disorders* (ICHD-3), and is caused by a disorder or lesion within the cervical spine or soft tissues of the neck, which is known to be able to cause headache.[1] Understanding the relationship between neck pain and headaches is important for accurate diagnosis and effective management of these conditions.

Epidemiology

Neck pain is a highly prevalent neurological complaint in the general population and is recognized as one of the major causes of disability in the United States.[2] Its prevalence in the general population over 1-year period is estimated to range from 4.8% to 79.5%, with a higher incidence observed among females.[3] The variation in prevalence estimates can be attributed to variations in case definitions and methodologies employed in different studies.

Epidemiological studies show a higher prevalence of coexistent neck pain in individuals with migraine and TTH compared to those without headaches.[4] Neck pain is reported by approximately 76% of individuals with migraine, making it 12 times more common in this group than in those without headaches. The prevalence of neck pain is significantly elevated in individuals with chronic migraine compared to those with episodic migraine. Likewise, about 90% of individuals with TTH experience coexisting neck pain, with odds of neck pain four times higher in individuals with TTH compared to those without headaches. Studies also demonstrate a positive correlation between headache frequency and the presence of neck pain, as both increase with higher headache frequency. Moreover, coexistent neck pain has been associated with transformation of episodic migraine and episodic TTH to chronic forms, and it may contribute to disability and reduced effectiveness of headache treatments.

Anatomy

The association between neck pain and headaches can be explained by the anatomy and function of the trigeminocervical complex (TCC).[5] In this complex, cervical spinal nerves carrying pain inputs from the periphery converge with those from the trigeminal nerve on second-order neurons in the brainstem and cervical spine. One of the main contributors to chronic neck pain and pain that leads to headaches (including cervicogenic headache) through this pathway is dysfunction of the upper cervical facet joints.[6] Pathologies affecting these joints and the associated innervating upper cervical nerves can result in pain that radiates to various areas of the head.

Pathophysiology

Pathologies affecting structures of the cervical spine can give rise to both localized and referred pain in the occipital region. Nociception in neck region structures is mediated by thin myelinated (Aδ) and unmyelinated (C) fibers that can become activated through noxious and innocuous stimuli, including inflammatory pain from joints, neuropathic pain, muscle strain or contraction, inflammation, and ischemia.[7] If nociceptive activity is maintained, this may lead to sensitization of nociceptors and thereby further increase in pain perception. Moreover, through the TCC, pain originating from the facet joints can be referred to different regions of the head. The sensitization of second-order neurons in the TCC and decreased antinociceptive or modulating activity from supraspinal structures may further enhance neck pain and referred headache. It has been suggested that nociceptive input from this area may serve as a trigger for primary headaches. Interestingly, migraine patients have been shown to have increased neck muscle stiffness and tenderness even outside of attacks.[8] Whether a true direct causal relationship exists has not been systematically investigated, and should be explored in future studies. Thus, it is important to recognize that cervical spine pathology can not only manifest as cervicogenic headaches but may also contribute to the exacerbation of multiple primary headaches, secondary headaches, facial pain, and cranial neuralgias. In addition, cervical radiculopathy can cause or trigger headaches through a process of referred pain.

Cervicogenic Headache: Epidemiology, Diagnosis, and Clinical Characteristics

Cervicogenic headache is characterized by a disorder affecting the cervical spine, including its bony, disc, and soft tissue components, often accompanied by neck pain. The ICHD-3 diagnostic criteria of cervicogenic headache are outlined in Box 31-1.[1] This secondary headache disorder has been reported to have a prevalence ranging from 1% to 4% in the general population.[9] The diagnosis of cervicogenic headache has been widely debated for several reasons. Imaging findings in the upper cervical spine are common in patients without headache. Tumors, fractures, infections, and rheumatoid arthritis of the upper cervical spine have not been formally validated as causes of headache. Cervical range of motion has also been shown to be decreased in migraine, and the cervical flexion-rotation test has small to moderate effect on the probability of a patient having cervicogenic headache.[5,10] Diagnostic blockade of cervical structures requires expertise and a specialized set-up, which is often not available at many neurologist practices. Further research is warranted to establish cervicogenic headache as a valid diagnosis and to enhance our understanding of its treatment. Currently, there is a lack of solid clinical trials specifically focused on treating cervicogenic headache.

Treatment/Prognosis

The treatment approach for neck pain should be comprehensive and involve multiple strategies.[5] Physical therapy plays a crucial role, focusing on core strengthening exercises and correcting poor posture, especially considering the contribution of ergonomic factors in work and daily life. However, the evidence for the effect of such interventions is still sparse in both migraine and TTH, as

Box 31-1. ICHD-3 Diagnostic Criteria of Cervicogenic Headache

Headache caused by a disorder of the cervical spine and its component bony, disc, and/or soft tissue elements, usually but not invariably accompanied by neck pain.

A. Any headache fulfilling criterion C

B. Clinical and/or imaging evidence of a disorder or lesion within the cervical spine or soft tissues of the neck known to be able to cause headache

C. Evidence of causation demonstrated by at least two of the following:
   1. Headache has developed in temporal relation to the onset of the cervical disorder or appearance of the lesion
   2. Headache has significantly improved or resolved in parallel with improvement in or resolution of the cervical disorder or lesion
   3. Cervical range of motion is reduced and headache is made significantly worse by provocative maneuvers
   4. Headache is abolished following diagnostic blockade of a cervical structure or its nerve supply

D. Not better accounted for by another ICHD-3 diagnosis

well as cervicogenic headache. It is important to use anti-inflammatory and analgesic medications judiciously to avoid medication overuse and potential medication overuse headache that can exacerbate the pain cycle. In the management of facet-mediated neck pain, early consideration should be given to interventions such as cervical medial branch blocks, radiofrequency ablation, and pulsed radiofrequency ablation, as these can serve both diagnostic and therapeutic purposes without significant systemic effects.[11,12] The management of neuropathic pain or pain associated with radiculopathy often involves the use of pregabalin, gabapentin, and duloxetine, which are commonly recommended for this purpose.[12] These medications have demonstrated efficacy in reducing neuropathic pain and can be beneficial in the overall management of neck pain related to radiculopathy, but the effect on headache has not been clearly demonstrated. Trigger point injections may also be useful in treating accompanying myofascial pain (Chapter 44). Furthermore, it is noteworthy that patients may experience multiple headache disorders simultaneously, underscoring the importance of a multidisciplinary approach involving a team of healthcare professionals to address the diverse components of headache disorders, ultimately leading to improved treatment outcomes.

Overall, the prognosis for treating neck pain associated with local alterations appears to be favorable, especially in the short term. However, there is a clear need for further high-quality studies to provide more robust evidence in this area.

Summary

- Pathology affecting the cervical facets can lead to chronic neck pain and headaches associated with the neck.
- Neck pain is a common symptom in various headache types, including migraine, TTH, and secondary headaches.
- When managing headaches, it is important to address any accompanying neck pain.

- A multidisciplinary team approach including neurologists and pain physicians may be of benefit to patients with difficult-to-treat headache and associated neck pain.
- There is a limited evidence available regarding the treatment of neck pain and headache in primary headache disorders.

REFERENCES

1. Headache Classification Committee of the International Headache Society (IHS). *The International Classification of Headache Disorders*, 3rd edition. *Cephalalgia*. 2018;38:1-211.

2. Collaborators GN. Global, regional, and national burden of neurological disorders, 1990-2016: a systematic analysis for the Global Burden of Disease Study 2016. *Lancet Neurol*. 2019;18:459-480.

3. Hoy DG, Protani M, De R, Buchbinder R. The epidemiology of neck pain. *Best Pract Res Clin Rheumatol*. 2010;24:783-792.

4. Al-Khazali HM, Younis S, Al-Sayegh Z, Ashina S, Ashina M, Schytz HW. Prevalence of neck pain in migraine: a systematic review and meta-analysis. *Cephalalgia*. 2022;42:663-673.

5. Al-Khazali HM, Krøll LS, Ashina H, et al. Neck pain and headache: pathophysiology, treatments and future directions. *Musculoskelet Sci Pract*. 2023:102804.

6. Manchikanti L, Boswell MV, Singh V, Pampati V, Damron KS, Beyer CD. Prevalence of facet joint pain in chronic spinal pain of cervical, thoracic, and lumbar regions. *BMC Musculoskelet Disord*. 2004;5:15.

7. Ashina S, Mitsikostas DD, Lee MJ, et al. Tension-type headache. *Nat Rev Dis Primers*. 2021;7:24.

8. Hvedstrup J, Kolding LT, Younis S, Ashina M, Schytz HW. Ictal neck pain investigated in the interictal state: a search for the origin of pain. *Cephalalgia*. 2019;40:614-624.

9. Bogduk N, Govind J. Cervicogenic headache: an assessment of the evidence on clinical diagnosis, invasive tests, and treatment. *Lancet Neurol*. 2009;8:959-968.

10. Demont A, Lafrance S, Benaissa L, Mawet J. Cervicogenic headache, an easy diagnosis? A systematic review and meta-analysis of diagnostic studies. *Musculoskelet Sci Pract*. 2022;62:102640.

11. Hurley RW, Adams MCB, Barad M, et al. Consensus practice guidelines on interventions for cervical spine (facet) joint pain from a multispecialty international working group. *Reg Anesth Pain Med*. 2022;47:3-59.

12. Peene L, Cohen SP, Brouwer B, et al. 2. Cervical radicular pain. *Pain Pract*. 2023.

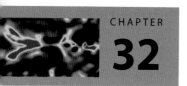

Headache and Sinuses

*Frederick A. Godley, III and Jennifer Robblee**

Current explanations regarding the interrelationship between migraine disease and symptoms associated with the paranasal sinuses and nose are insufficient. Within the headache community, infection and inflammation within the paranasal sinuses are recognized only as potential triggers of migraine headaches, whereas rhinology experts have developed clinical guidelines that primarily regard facial pain or pressure, combined with nasal congestion and purulent discharge, as signs of infection within the paranasal sinuses. Such patients are often managed very differently depending on whether they present first to neurology or rhinology, and there is often little collaboration between these specialties.

Some evidence from clinical studies and broader clinical experience point to another explanation, one that requires a distinctive diagnostic and treatment approach. This explanation could lead to a profound shift in thinking and alter recommendations regarding how medical professionals should screen patients, prescribe antibiotic therapy, perform computed tomography (CT), and plan treatment. The poor correlation of sinus CT findings with symptoms, the routine failure of antibiotic and steroid treatment of infectious and inflammatory sinusitis to result in a lasting resolution of symptoms, and a more robust therapeutic response to migraine interventions suggest that rhinosinusitis (RS) symptoms may be more likely to have a neurogenic cause than an infectious one.[1,2] However, this hypothesis needs to be substantiated by more research.

Epidemiology

Each year in the United States, sinusitis affects one in seven adults, and it is diagnosed in 31 million patients. Sinusitis is one of the most common conditions treated by primary care physicians. Migraine affects approximately 12% of the population (Chapter 5). It is not surprising that these common conditions are often misdiagnosed and commonly co-occur. Chronic rhinosinusitis (CRS) patients have a ninefold risk of chronic migraine compared to the general population, with almost 50% of these patients having migraine.[3] The common self-diagnosis, and often the primary care diagnosis, is "sinus headache." This term is discouraged because the majority of these patients, in fact, have episodic migraine in 52%, chronic migraine in 11%, probable migraine in 23%, and RS in only 3%.[4] It is agreed that approximately 90% of "sinus headache" cases are attributable to migraine.

The overall direct cost (outpatient physician visits, prescription medical therapy, and endoscopic sinus surgery) related to CRS is estimated to range between $10 billion and $13 billion per year in the United States. The overall indirect cost related to CRS-related losses in work productivity is estimated to be in excess of $20 billion per year. The cost of migraine is approximately $17 billion annually in the United States. Likely affecting these costs are the delays to diagnosis leading to unnecessary testing and inappropriate treatment, potentially leading to worsening disease. Delay in receiving a diagnosis of migraine,

*The authors thank the staff of Neuroscience Publications at Barrow Neurological Institute for assistance with the chapter preparation.

which is greater than 5 years in the majority of cases, is associated with seeing more specialists, presumably due to the initial specialist not being a neurology specialist.

Pathophysiology

The currently accepted primary mechanism to explain the symptoms of facial pain and pressure, nasal congestion, and nasal discharge is that of a viral or bacterial infection or inflammation within one or more paranasal sinuses. The mechanism underpinning balloon sinuplasty is that the ostia connecting paranasal sinuses to the nasal cavity are too narrow and prone to blockage when their mucosal lining is swollen. When the openings to the sinuses are blocked, the air trapped within the affected sinuses is slowly absorbed, which creates a vacuum that causes pain and pressure.

The proposed mechanism to explain the efficacy of contact point and nerve decompression surgery is that the neuropathic pain is secondary to irritated sensory nerves within the nasal mucosa. The contact between septal and turbinates is reasoned to release neuroinflammatory agents, including substance P, bradykinin, serotonin, and prostaglandins. These agents are believed to change the pain thresholds of the local afferent sensory nerves and the sensory pathways in the central nervous system.

A theoretical model of a centrally driven, spontaneously activated trigeminocervical complex of brainstem nuclei and nociceptive pathways, including the superior salivatory nuclei and the parasympathetic system, is not widely accepted or proven but is anecdotally more consistent with the available diagnostic findings and treatment response. This model is based on a variation of migraine disease. If one appreciates that migraine is a complex and highly variable disorder that primarily increases the sensitivity of pain networks, then it is not surprising that migraine can affect other special sensory systems as well as vascular and immune cells. This variability is due in part to the genetic underpinning of migraine disease. With time, we can expect to find that the loci that program the expression of ion channels, transport proteins, mitochondrial function, and more are shared with many other health conditions and to further clarify the association of dozens of chronic comorbidities with migraine.

Genetic factors are important to the development of migraine, but many epigenetic factors also influence the expression of this hypersensitivity disorder and explain why the natural history of this disease varies widely over the course of a lifetime (Chapter 6). The primary explanation for migraine aura is cortical spreading depression, an "electrical storm" of the central nervous system. It is unknown whether aura is a trigger for the headache phase. The headache phase has a complex pathophysiology that includes activation of the trigeminovascular pain and evidence of neuroinflammation. This neurogenic inflammation is mediated by neuropeptides like substance P and calcitonin gene-related peptide, with possible roles for glial cells, increased vascular permeability, and cytokines; however, there is little research on this issue to date. The phenomenon of central sensitization explains the steady evolution of patients from episodic to chronic migraine and the development of allodynia. Migraine pathophysiology involves an interplay between peripheral mechanisms of trigeminovascular activation of the brainstem and central mechanisms within excitation of ascending pathways. As this increased activity progresses, it becomes persistent and leads to the reorganization of the brain both structurally and functionally. These changes may also explain the emergence of symptom patterns, such as vestibular migraine, brain fog, chronic fatigue, ear pressure, and, perhaps, sinus pain and pressure. Central sensitization is associated with dysautonomia, particularly dysfunction of the parasympathetic system. In particular, we know that the dorsal pons is activated and causes the superior salivatory nucleus to upregulate autonomic information through the cranial nerves, including the vascular system. The hypothesis is that this upregulation of the parasympathetic nerves dilates the venules and activates the secretory cells of the inferior nasal turbinates. Cranial autonomic symptoms occur more commonly in individuals with allodynia and correlate to the presence of central sensitization. The hypothesis is that neuroplastic changes between brainstem nuclei, called the trigeminal-autonomic reflex (Figure 32-1), explain this association and the high rates of sinus symptoms as part of this cranial autonomic phenomenon in migraine. Even if these two models are accepted, they do

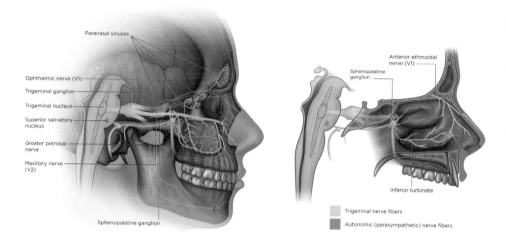

Figure 32-1. Illustrations depicting trigeminal sensory innervation of the mucosa of the paranasal sinuses (left), as well as autonomic nerves to nasal mucus and serous secretory glands and inferior turbinate venules (right). (Reproduced from Godley FA. Sinus Migraine: A costly blindspot in medical care. Research Outreach. 2020.)

not fully explain what appears to be a spontaneous activation of the central nervous system, which the brain interprets as sinus symptoms that vary significantly in duration. An accurate and more nuanced explanation of the pathophysiology of migraine will have to wait for more research findings.

Diagnosis and Clinical Presentation

RS is a term that describes symptomatic inflammation of the paranasal sinuses and nasal passageways. When patients present with sinus complaints, they most commonly report pain and pressure located bilaterally across their forehead, behind their eyes, or within their nose or cheeks, but there can be variations in presentation, including temporomandibular and dental pain. Secondarily, patients complain of nasal obstruction, congestion, blockage, or stuffiness (reported or observed). They also complain of a nasal discharge of thick secretions, either anteriorly as a runny nose or posteriorly as postnasal drip, that are cloudy or discolored, in contrast to the increased clear secretions seen in various forms of rhinitis. There is rarely a fever, but patients may also complain of a sore throat, halitosis, cough, ear pain, headache, or fatigue.

Acute RS (ARS) is defined as a viral or bacterial infection that resolves completely within 4 weeks. Subacute sinusitis is an infection that resolves within 4 to 12 weeks. Recurring ARS describes two to four episodes of acute sinusitis within a year with at least 8 weeks between episodes. CRS describes the persistence of symptoms with variations in the intensity of symptoms.

For headache specialists, the rule of thumb is that if a patient has a headache and computer tomography (CT) findings that indicate a sinus infection or inflammation, such as a swollen mucosa or a cyst, the *International Classification of Headache Disorders*, third edition (ICHD-3) diagnosis is either "11.5.1 Headache attributed to AR" or "11.5.2 Headache attributed to ARS or CRS."[5] The detailed criteria for each of these diagnostic tags depend on endoscopic or CT evidence of an infection (acute or chronic), some link between worsening or improvement of both the infection and headache, and/or more pain on digital pressure over the sinuses.

The 2015 American Academy of Otolaryngology–Head and Neck Surgery Clinical Guidelines base the diagnosis of sinusitis on three key clinical findings: purulent nasal drainage, nasal obstruction, and facial pain and/or pressure for 10 days.[6] During the first 10 days of symptoms, the recommendation is to encourage the use of analgesics, nasal saline irrigations, and nasal steroid spray while avoiding imaging and antibiotic therapy. Further recommendations (see "Treatment" section) are available for ARS and CRS. What is missing from both sets of recommendations is to consider the diagnosis of dysfunction of sensory and autonomic nerves. If it proves true that there is a chronic migraine variant that can create the impression that there is something wrong within the nose and sinuses, several of these guidelines become controversial and could lead to the use of the wrong treatments. For instance, one of the criteria for diagnosing RS is the radiologic finding of sinus mucosal thickening, CT findings that are correlated poorly with sinus symptoms.[7] Furthermore, studies have shown no significant correlations between the sinuses and the location of pain nor between pain severity and disease severity, as confirmed by sinus CT findings.[8] Another way to interpret this issue is to recognize that facial pain and headache are not useful predictors of sinus disease severity. Current recommendations for diagnosing CRS do not acknowledge other etiologies for the finding of mucosal thickening. Mucosal thickening is often a manifestation of an idiopathic inflammatory condition (polyp disease) or allergic rhinitis.

Finally, the finding of intranasal purulent discharge may be less diagnostic than is commonly believed. Only a third of patients with intranasal purulent discharge report facial pain, and the pain correlates with the location of the secretions in only two-thirds of cases. About one-half of adult patients with suspected acute maxillary sinusitis following a viral infection have pus or mucus within the sinus on needle aspiration, and one-third of those with purulence have bacterial pathogen growth in culture.

Most strikingly, many patients have clear paranasal sinuses when complaining of sinus pain or pressure. If pain is removed from the criteria for RS therapy, the specificity of the guidelines improves dramatically, with a nonsignificant decrease in sensitivity. The pain associated with CRS is typically described as throbbing or aching pain located around the eyes, temple, top of the head, or occipital region, which is consistent with migraine. Nasal congestion and purulence are unreliable symptoms for the diagnosis of RS. Autonomic symptoms, particularly turbinate vascular engorgement and spontaneous nasal secretions caused by excessive parasympathetic activity, occur in almost half of those with migraine.

An alternative etiology for RS symptoms is often overlooked. It is possible that the cause of RS symptoms might be neurogenic; therefore, a clinician might consider this diagnosis early in the evaluation of a patient with a suspected sinus infection, even before prescribing antibiotics.

One efficient migraine screening tool is the ID Migraine.[9] This validated questionnaire has only three questions: Do light and sound bother you more when you have a headache? Does a headache limit your daily activities? Do you feel nauseated when you have a headache?

If a patient answers "yes" to at least two of these questions, the patient can be assumed to meet the ICHD-3 criteria for migraine with a sensitivity of 0.84 and a specificity of 0.76. It is a three-item test colloquially referred to as "PIN the diagnosis," with PIN being an acronym for photophobia, impairment, and nausea. This tool could help link headache to migraine, including when migraine affects other parts of the nervous system (ocular or autonomic systems) and is disabling.

Diagnosing a headache of neurogenic etiology in patients who complain of sinus pain and pressure remains challenging because this headache type is unclassifiable by the ICHD-3. Another strategy for identifying patients with migraine disease is to ask about common comorbid diseases, such as fibromyalgia, vertigo, and irritable bowel disease. The comorbidities of temporomandibular joint disorder, chronic cervical pain, and depression and anxiety are associated with normal endoscopy and CT findings in patients with facial pain and/or pressure.

Autonomic symptoms are common in migraine. Nasal congestion is seen in up to one-third of patients in addition to other RS symptoms, like nasal obstruction and rhinorrhea. Migraine patients reporting facial pain are more likely to report RS symptoms. Facial pain or pressure is common in migraine, reported in the majority of cases. Facial pain, which is often initially attributed to RS, is likely to ultimately be diagnosed as migraine or tension-type headache.

Beyond "PIN the diagnosis," osmophobia may be a helpful way to differentiate RS from migraine. Osmophobia has a high positive predictive value for migraine. Hyposmia or anosmia is more predictive of RS, whereas pulsating pain and photophobia are negatively predictive.

Differential diagnoses in the setting of facial pain and RS symptoms should also be considered. In particular, clinicians need to consider trigeminal autonomic cephalgias (see Chapters 14 and 15 for detailed descriptions of diagnosis and management). An important differentiating factor here is that pain is completely unilateral, with prominent ipsilateral cranial autonomic symptoms that can include rhinorrhea and congestion.[5] The duration of attacks can be helpful in diagnosis, with cluster headache being the most common type, involving distinct attacks lasting 15 minutes up to 3 hours, often in recurring patterns within a cluster period lasting weeks or months.

Expert opinion is that patients with headaches who experience facial and RS symptoms need evaluation for both migraine and RS. Attributing facial pain to RS, often colloquially referred to as "sinus headache," is a misnomer that can lead to RS-directed treatment; in reality, approximately 90% of these patients will have migraine, risking a missed treatment opportunity. It is also important to consider that RS and migraine are common conditions that co-occur at high rates in any given patient and who need treatment that is directed at both conditions.

Treatment

Treatment of RS as an infectious condition fails in the vast majority of cases because bacterial infection occurs in only a very small percentage of ARS episodes. The current therapeutic guidelines are based on the 2015 American Academy of Otolaryngology–Head and Neck Surgery Clinical Guidelines, which assume that the symptoms of facial pain, pressure, or fullness and nasal obstruction, combined with the observation of purulent nasal discharge, are caused primarily by a viral or bacterial infection.[6] Therefore, the recommendation is to use conservative measures, including analgesics, topical intranasal steroids, and/or nasal saline irrigation, for the first 7 days after symptom onset. If the patient's condition worsens or fails to improve, a 5- to 10-day regimen of oral antibiotics, such as amoxicillin with or without clavulanate, is typically prescribed. Clinicians should not obtain radiographic imaging for patients who meet diagnostic criteria for ARS unless a complication or alternative diagnosis is suspected. If the first course of antibiotics fails, a change in antibiotics is recommended. The clinical diagnosis should be confirmed with anterior rhinoscopy, nasal endoscopy, or CT findings documenting sinonasal inflammation. The patient should also be assessed for chronic conditions that would modify management, such as asthma, cystic fibrosis, immunocompromised state, and ciliary dyskinesia. Testing for allergies or immune function is optional. Patients with CRS (duration of symptoms ≥12 weeks) should be assessed for sinonasal inflammation. Patients should be evaluated for nasal polyposis as a possible cause of CRS. CRS should be treated with saline nasal irrigation and topical intranasal corticosteroids but not with topical or systemic antifungal therapy. Functional endoscopic sinus surgery (FESS) is indicated for patients with CRS that is unresponsive to therapy and patients with ARS.

There are significant concerns regarding these recommendations. First, the use of one or two courses of antibiotics based solely on a clinical diagnosis is one of the most egregious failures in antibiotic stewardship. Inappropriate use of broad-spectrum antibiotics leads to a selection of resistant strains. A 5-year analysis (2006-2010) revealed that ARS and CRS were the most common diagnoses associated with outpatient antibiotic prescriptions, most of which were for broad-spectrum antibiotics.[10] But the efficacy of this heavy use of antibiotics is doubtful. Patients with RS symptoms who are not treated with antibiotics report symptom resolution at rates comparable to those for patients who are treated with antibiotics. This finding suggests that the added value of antibiotics is small. The suspicion that antibiotics are often inappropriate for treating patients with RS symptoms is reinforced by the finding that a very small percentage of ARS cases treated in the primary care setting are due to bacteria. Unfortunately, despite guidelines that are intended to curtail the use of antibiotics, antibiotic therapy is prescribed to the vast majority of patients with a diagnosis of ARS and more than half of patients with a diagnosis of CRS.

Approximately 350,000 sinus procedures, including FESS, balloon sinuplasty, and a mix of both, called a "hybrid" procedure, are performed annually in the United States to treat CRS. However, the effectiveness of FESS for the relief of headache and/or facial pain and pressure is low. Although the number of FESS procedures performed has remained steady, the use of the newer technique of balloon sinuplasty has increased steadily since U.S. Food and Drug Administration approval in 2005, to over 25,000 cases per year. Balloon sinuplasty is currently performed either as an adjunct procedure to traditional endoscopic sinus surgery or as a stand-alone procedure. To date, no randomized controlled trial has proven that this less invasive but highly reimbursed procedure offers any advantage to the patient.

The use of balloon sinuplasty in patients with normal paranasal sinuses but narrow ostia on CT is of particular concern. In a small prospective, single-blinded randomized controlled study of 34 patients with sinus pressure, there was no significant difference in outcome between those who underwent balloon dilation of the sinus ostia versus those who underwent a sham procedure in which the balloon catheter was dilated in the nasal cavity only.[11] Another study found that nearly 85% of 106 CRS patients who also had migraine (including those with sinus pathology) did not respond to medical and surgical treatment for suspected infection.[12] Still, nearly 70% improved with migraine treatment. Because there is evidence that patients have improved outcomes when treated by a headache specialist, otolaryngologist, and/or orofacial specialist, a rational therapeutic approach for patients with sinus symptoms is to be familiar with the medical care of both infectious and neurogenic RS. These findings also support the notion that better collaboration between neurology and otolaryngology is needed to treat this patient population. Importantly, this information needs to be better distributed to primary care physicians. For further discussion of the optimal treatment of migraine, please see Chapters 7 and 8.

Prognosis

Although a high percentage of patients with RS are treated with antibiotics or surgery, those treatments are often unsuccessful, especially in patients with CRS. Many of these poor outcomes are likely attributable to an incorrect diagnosis or untreated concurrent migraine.

Correct diagnosis of "sinus headache" as migraine leads to excellent treatment response, whereas misdiagnosis leads to high rates of inappropriate investigations and treatments. Patients with migraine that is misdiagnosed may undergo repeated courses of antibiotics or unnecessary surgery. The prognosis can be good in this patient population, but it is vital that all patients with facial pain and/or pressure and RS symptoms are screened for underlying migraine.

Summary

- Sinus pain and/or pressure, nasal congestion, and drippy nose are common complaints, and such patients often first present to primary care.
- The assumption that facial pain and/or pressure is caused by infection or allergies rather than migraine can lead to a misdiagnosis or a delay in diagnosis, inappropriate use of antibiotics, and inappropriate surgery.
- All patients with facial pain and/or pressure and RS symptoms should be screened for migraine using tools like the ID Migraine questions regarding "PIN the diagnosis."
- If migraine is suspected, it is safer to treat the patient for migraine (e.g., with triptan therapy) rather than for an infection.
- When appropriate treatment is used, there is potential for a good prognosis.
- Migraine and rhinosinusitis can coexist, and treatment is occasionally needed for both conditions.

Secondary Headaches

REFERENCES

1. Agius AM, Jones NS, Muscat R. Prospective three-year follow up of a cohort study of 240 patients with chronic facial pain. *J Laryngol Otol.* 2014;128(6):518-526.

2. Ishkanian G, Blumenthal H, Webster CJ, Richardson MS, Ames M. Efficacy of sumatriptan tablets in migraineurs self-described or physician-diagnosed as having sinus headache: a randomized, double-blind, placebo-controlled study. *Clin Ther.* 2007; 29(1):99-109.

3. Aaseth K, Grande RB, Kvaerner K, Lundqvist C, Russell MB. Chronic rhinosinusitis gives a nine-fold increased risk of chronic headache. The Akershus study of chronic headache. *Cephalalgia.* 2010;30(2):152-160.

4. Eross E, Dodick D, Eross M. The sinus, allergy and migraine study (SAMS). *Headache.* 2007;47(2): 213-224.

5. International Headache Society. *The International Classification of Headache Disorders,* 3rd edition. *Cephalgia.* 2018;38(1):1-211.

6. Rosenfeld RM, Piccirillo JF, Chandrasekhar SS, et al. Clinical practice guideline (update): adult sinusitis. *Otolaryngol Head Neck Surg.* 2015;152 (2 Suppl):S1-S39.

7. Bhattacharyya T, Piccirillo J, Wippold FJ 2nd. Relationship between patient-based descriptions of sinusitis and paranasal sinus computed tomographic findings. *Arch Otolaryngol Head Neck Surg.* 1997;123(11):1189-1192.

8. Pokharel M, Karki S, Shrestha BL, Shrestha I, Amatya RC. Correlations between symptoms, nasal endoscopy computed tomography and surgical findings in patients with chronic rhinosinusitis. *Kathmandu Univ Med J (KUMJ).* 2013; 11(43):201-205.

9. Lipton RB, Dodick D, Sadovsky R, et al. A self-administered screener for migraine in primary care: the ID Migraine validation study. *Neurology.* 2003;61(3):375-382.

10. Smith SS, Kern RC, Chandra RK, Tan BK, Evans CT. Variations in antibiotic prescribing of acute rhinosinusitis in United States ambulatory settings. *Otolaryngol Head Neck Surg.* 2013;148(5):852-859.

11. Laury AM, Chen PG, McMains KC. Randomized controlled trial examining the effects of balloon catheter dilation on "sinus pressure"/barometric headaches. *Otolaryngol Head Neck Surg.* 2018;159(1):178-184.

12. Al-Hashel JY, Ahmed SF, Alroughani R, Goadsby PJ. Migraine misdiagnosis as a sinusitis, a delay that can last for many years. *J Headache Pain.* 2013; 14(1):97.

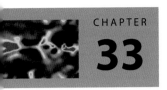

Headache and Eye Disease

*Alison V. Crum, Meagan D. Seay, and Kathleen B. Digre**

It is not surprising that eye disease can be associated with headache, as the trigeminal sensory system responsible for innervating the dura, facial structures, and intracranial arteries also innervates the eye and the orbit (Chapter 4). Therefore, the eye should always be considered a potential factor in the occurrence of headaches (Table 33-1). In addition to this, certain intraocular conditions such as angle-closure glaucoma and scleritis can cause headaches, as well as orbital pathology. Furthermore, ocular conditions like dry eye have the potential to exacerbate underlying migraines and may even be linked to chronic migraine. Although the precise prevalence or incidence of headaches originating from eye disorders remains uncertain, our understanding of the causes of eye pain in ophthalmology and neurology clinics has provided us with valuable insights.

Approach to Patient with Eye Pain

For clinicians who are not ophthalmologists but need to evaluate patients with eye pain, there are certain algorithms or approaches that can be followed to aid in the assessment. Although it is crucial to acknowledge that a comprehensive eye examination by an ophthalmologist is ideal for accurate diagnosis, the following general steps can be considered when evaluating a patient with eye pain.[1,2] It is crucial to assess the urgency of the situation by considering the severity of symptoms, associated findings, and the potential for sight-threatening conditions. If there is any suspicion of a serious condition or if the patient's symptoms worsen or rapidly deteriorate, it is imperative to promptly refer the patient to an ophthalmologist or Emergency Department for further evaluation and management. For a summary of eye diseases causing headache and eye pain, see Table 33-1.

History

Begin by obtaining a detailed history of the patient's eye pain, including its onset, duration, pain characteristics (e.g., sharp, dull, throbbing), associated symptoms (e.g., redness, discharge), aggravating or alleviating factors, and any relevant medical and surgical history of any recent trauma.

Examination of Patient with Eye Pain

In the evaluation of the eye, a systematic approach to the examination is crucial.[1]

Secondary Headaches

*Drs. Crum, Seay, and Digre are supported in part by an unrestricted grant from Research to Prevent Blindness, New York, NY, to the Department of Ophthalmology & Visual Sciences, University of Utah.

Table 33-1. Eye Pain and Headaches Due to Eye Diseases/Conditions

Disease/Condition	Eye Finding	Neurological Finding	Diagnosis	Treatment and Other Comments
Eye Pain with Red Eye— In General Referred to Ophthalmologist				
Dry eye	Redness of eye, decreased tearing	None	Schirmer's testing	Symptomatic treatment with artificial tears, etc. Common cause of eye pain and headache
Angle-closure glaucoma	Red eye, mid-dilated pupil, increased intraocular pressure	Usually none	Measurement of intraocular pressure (referral to ophthalmologist)	Reduction of intraocular pressure (medical and/or surgical)
Refractive error	Often normal	None	Refraction (referral to optometrist/ophthalmologist)	New refraction
Episcleritis/scleritis	Red eye	Usually none	Exam: blanching of vessels with topic sympathomimetic (referral to ophthalmologist)	Steroid drops occasionally
Ocular ischemia	Red eye, trouble with light blindness and night vision	May have vascular risk factors and previous stroke	Diagnosis by imaging of MRI/CT arteriography	Often surgical correction
Decreased Vision and Eye Pain				
Optic neuritis	Pain with eye movements, decreased visual acuity	May have neurological findings	MRI orbit with gadolinium to see enhancement of the optic nerve Blood test: MOG and NMO antibodies	IV steroid treatment
Arteritic AION	Usually headache, rarely eye pain, loss of vision, pale swelling of disc	Pain with chewing food	Blood test: ESR and CRP levels Temporal artery biopsy	Treatment with oral steroids

Disease/Condition	Eye Finding	Neurological Finding	Diagnosis	Treatment and Other Comments
Herpes zoster involvement of eye	Intense pain, red eye, may see vesicles/rash on the face and tip of the nose	Variable, often normal	Clinical diagnosis (check for rash/vesicles)	Acyclovir, IV or oral steroids
Orbital Causes of Eye Pain				
Trochleitis	Pain over the trochlea of superior oblique that can be palpated	Usually none	Physical/eye examination CT imaging sometimes helpful	Oral steroids, steroid injection into trochlea of superior oblique
Dacryoadenitis	Pain over orbit, sometimes red eye, swelling around the eye	Usually none	Physical/eye examination	Oral steroids, occasionally antivirals, antibiotics
IgG4 disease	Proptosis, ache around eye	May have neurological accompaniments if not just orbital	MRI of orbit most helpful Blood test: IgG4 antibodies	Steroid treatment
Thyroid orbitopathy	Proptosis, sometimes red eye	Usually none	Ultrasound of orbit; MRI/CT orbit (findings of thickening of muscles inferior, medial superior, obliques in that order involved)	Endocrine evaluation and sometimes treatment with steroids and monoclonal antibody, teprotumumab
Eye Finding with Neurological Findings				
Painful Horner's syndrome	Ptosis, miosis, occasionally red eye	Look for any face/extremity weakness to suggest arterial dissection Differentials include primary cluster headache or other TAC	MRI of brain and MRA of neck or CTA of neck to diagnose dissection of carotid or vertebral artery and accompanying stroke	Treatment of underlying condition

(Continued)

Secondary Headaches

Table 33-1. Eye Pain and Headaches Due to Eye Diseases/Conditions (*Continued*)

Disease/Condition	Eye Finding	Neurological Finding	Diagnosis	Treatment and Other Comments
Tolosa Hunt—painful ophthalmoplegia	May be normal, sometimes proptosis	Extraocular muscle involvement—usually third nerve	MRI may show enhancement of the cavernous sinus (need to rule out secondary causes, including malignancy)	Oral steroids helpful for pain and cranial neuropathy
IIH or secondary intracranial hypertension)	Usually papilledema; if significant visual field defect—rapid assessment for surgery	May be normal	MRI of brain with CTV or MRV to rule out cerebral venous thrombosis Lumbar puncture: opening pressure	Treat underlying condition, acetazolamide; if visual loss occurs, may need lumbar drain and surgical treatment
Pituitary tumor/apoplexy	Decreased vision, visual field defect, may have cranial neuropathy	Cranial neuropathy (third nerve)	MRI of brain (enlarged pituitary and hemorrhage if apoplexy)	Neurosurgical consultation

AION, anterior ischemic optic neuropathy; CT, computer tomography; CTV, CT venography; CRP, C-reactive protein; ESR, erythrocyte sedimentation rate; IIH, idiopathic intracranial hypertension; MOG, myelin oligodendrocyte glycoprotein; MRI, magnetic resonance imaging; MRV, MR venography; NMO, neuromyelitis optica; TAC, trigeminal autonomic cephalalgia.

Visual Acuity Assessment

Assessment of visual acuity can be performed using a near or distance Snellen chart. For accurate measurement, it is recommended that the patients utilize their glasses or contacts to determine their best corrected visual acuity. In cases where the patient does not have 20/20 vision, employing a pinhole occluder can be valuable in determining potential best corrected visual acuity. If a pinhole occluder is not available, a simple alternative is to create a small hole in a piece of paper and have the patient look through it while reading the eye chart.

Pupillary Examination

It is essential to examine the pupillary light reflex and identify the presence of a relative afferent pupillary defect (RAPD). The swinging flashlight technique is commonly employed to detect an RAPD.

Visual Field Testing

Confrontation visual fields are evaluated by asking the patient to cover one eye and maintain fixation on the examiner's opposite eye, typically positioned around 3 to 5 feet away. The examiner then presents fingers in various quadrants of the visual field, and the patient is asked to count the number of fingers they see. Alternatively, the patient can indicate when they detect movement, such as finger wiggling, in each quadrant, although this technique is less sensitive. For a more sensitive assessment, a red target can be displayed in each quadrant, and the patient can be asked if the quality of the red color appears consistent throughout. Confrontation visual field testing should be conducted separately for each eye.

External Examination

Inspect the external structures of the eye, including the eyelids, conjunctiva, and surrounding tissues, for any sign of conjunctival or eyelid redness, swelling, discharge, or any other abnormalities.

Extraocular Movements

To evaluate the efferent visual system, the patient's ocular range is examined by instructing them to look fully in all nine cardinal gazes. If the patient exhibits an obvious eye misalignment, one eye can be covered, and ocular motility can be assessed for each eye individually (known as ocular ductions) and also for any restrictions, misalignments, nystagmus, or pain with movement.

Funduscopic Examination

With a direct ophthalmoscope or portable nonmydriatic camera, the examiner must look for optic disc swelling or optic disc atrophy.

Ocular Causes of Headache

Dry Eye

Dryness of the ocular surface is a common condition reported by patients, with prevalence estimates ranging from 5% to 50%.[1] It is the most common cause of eye pain in an ophthalmology clinic and is frequently also seen in neurology clinics.[3] Patients often describe various sensations such as "heaviness," "burning," "fatigue," and "scratching." Interestingly, dry eyes can paradoxically manifest as tearing eyes. This counterintuitive phenomenon occurs when the compromised corneal surface fails to maintain a stable tear film, leading to ocular discomfort and reflexive tear production. As a result, patients with dry eyes may present with the unexpected symptom of increased lacrimation, often misconstrued as excessive tearing.

Secondary Headaches

The pathophysiology of this condition involves the altered innervation of the corneal surface by the ophthalmic division of the trigeminal nerve, which lies beneath the corneal epithelium (the outermost layer of the cornea). The cornea possesses the highest density of sensory innervation in the human body. When the tear film evaporates and the corneal epithelium becomes compromised, the exposed nerves transmit pain signals to the brain. In some cases, patients may also exhibit conjunctival redness, which refers to the inflammation of the thin vascular membrane covering the sclera (the white portion of the eyeball). In some cases, there is a dry eye sensation without actual dryness on testing.

Currently, most individuals use computers or screens frequently. Digital-related eye strain occurs when the blink rate decreases while using screens, as opposed to conversation or less visual attention requiring tasks. This allows for evaporation of the tear film and dryness. Dry eye can coexist with or be caused by various disorders. Here are some notable examples:

1. Migraine: Patients with chronic migraines may experience dry eye symptoms along with abnormalities in corneal nerves.[4] Dry eye disease can also exacerbate migraine.

2. Parkinsonism: This condition, characterized by infrequent blinking, eyelid retraction, or a fixed stare, can contribute to the evaporation of the protective tear film that covers the cornea.

3. Benign essential blepharospasm: Patients with this disorder often exhibit a triad of symptoms, including frequent blinking or spasms, dryness, and light sensitivity. Treating blepharospasm with botulinum toxin alone may not alleviate eye discomfort or headaches if dry eyes and photophobia are left unaddressed.

4. Sjögren's syndrome/autoimmune disorders: Sjögren's syndrome commonly presents with severe dry eyes and dry mouth. It is frequently observed in patients with other autoimmune disorders. Interestingly, individuals with Sjögren's syndrome also have an increased incidence of migraines.

5. Prior refractive surgery: Patients who have undergone procedures like Lasik or photorefractive keratectomy (PRK) may experience dry eye symptoms as a result of the surgery.

These coexisting or causative disorders highlight the multifactorial nature of dry eye and the importance of considering underlying conditions when managing the condition.

The treatment of dry eyes encompasses addressing underlying causes or diseases. Symptomatic treatment involves the utilization of over-the-counter, preservative-free artificial tear drops or lubricating eye drops, which can be administered as necessary throughout the day. Furthermore, applying warm compresses to the eyes, engaging in blinking exercises, employing a humidifier in environments with dry or air-conditioned spaces, and avoiding eye irritants such as smoke or allergens are recommended. Wearing protective glasses and practicing proper eyelid hygiene are also beneficial. In cases where these measures prove insufficient, a referral to an ophthalmologist may be necessary for the prescription of medications tailored to the specific needs of the patient.

Angle-Closure Glaucoma

Angle closure, although not commonly encountered, is not an infrequent occurrence. It arises from the obstruction of fluid drainage within the eye.[1] Contributing factors include genetically inherited anatomical structures, advancing age, and an eyeball size characterized by hyperopia or farsightedness. Symptoms may encompass visual halos, cloudy vision, redness of the eye, and pupillary mydriasis with poor reaction. During examination, it is imperative to assess for narrowed angles by directing a flashlight across the pupil and observing for the presence of a shadow. Notably, medications commonly prescribed for migraine treatment, such as topiramate, tricyclic antidepressants, serotonin reuptake inhibitors, antihistamines, and anticholinergics, have the potential to induce angle closure. Vigilance regarding this potential complication is of utmost importance. In such cases, promptly referring the patient to an ophthalmologist for appropriate treatment is essential (Figure 33-1).

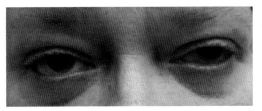

Figure 33-1. A 49-year-old female with no history of migraines presented with intermittent dilated pupil and nighttime headaches. She was treated for migraines in the emergency room. A month later, she was admitted for posterior reversible encephalopathy syndrome after stopping her antihypertensive medications. Examination revealed a fixed dilated pupil on the left side, along with reduced visual acuity (20/50) compared to the right eye (20/20). Intraocular pressures were elevated in the left eye (50 mm Hg) compared to the right eye (20 mm Hg). She was diagnosed with angle-closure glaucoma. Treatment with pressure-lowering drops and iridotomy normalized the pressure and resolved the dilated pupil. Antihypertensive medications were restarted, and she had no further episodes of dilated pupil or headaches.

Astigmatism/Presbyopia/Refractive Errors

Incorrect prescriptions for eyeglasses can lead to headaches in individuals.[2] One particular issue arises from unaddressed changes in astigmatism that occur over time, as these changes are not accounted for in an updated prescription. Consequently, eye strain and headaches can develop. When patients find themselves squinting to read a text on a computer/tablet/phone or at a close reading distance, their eyes may inwardly rotate or undergo accommodation to achieve focus. This accommodation alters the shape of the lens within the eye, resulting in eye strain, discomfort, and potentially triggering or exacerbating headaches, including primary headache conditions. In such cases, an evaluation by an optometrist or ophthalmologist would prove advantageous in determining the appropriate course of action.

Inflammatory Disorders of the Sclera and Its Coverings

Scleritis and episcleritis are inflammatory conditions affecting the sclera and its surrounding tissues, and they have been associated with headaches.[1] These disorders typically manifest as unilateral and painful processes. The diagnosis of scleritis or episcleritis is typically established through various methods, including ultrasound of the orbit, clinical examination conducted by an ophthalmologist, and in some cases, even a magnetic resonance imaging (MRI) scan revealing enhanced scleral findings. The underlying cause of these conditions is often attributed to autoimmune factors. Treatment for scleritis and episcleritis is primarily provided by ophthalmologists, and it may lead to the improvement of associated headaches.

Ocular Ischemia

Although uncommon, this condition is of great significance due to its association with an elevated risk of stroke.[1] It arises when there is a constriction of the carotid artery, impairing the blood flow to the ophthalmic artery. Patients typically experience ocular pain, and there may be accompanying redness. Headache can also manifest as a symptom.[1] Clinical diagnosis is primarily based on the presence of specific symptoms, such as light-induced amaurosis (visual loss triggered by light) and difficulties with night vision. Imaging techniques such as computed tomography angiography (CTA) or magnetic resonance angiography (MRA) of the head and neck are employed to visualize any stenosis in the affected arteries. Patients with suspected ocular ischemia require emergent referral to a stroke specialist and treatment directed at the underlying cause for appropriate treatment.

Secondary Headaches

Optic Nerve Disease

Optic neuritis is characterized by varying degrees of eye pain upon movement and a decrease in vision in the affected eye, and can manifest with headache.[1] It can manifest as an idiopathic condition or be associated with multiple sclerosis and other autoimmune causes, including myelin oligodendrocyte glycoprotein (MOG) and neuromyelitis optica (NMO), among others. MRI of the orbits, often performed with gadolinium contrast, frequently reveals abnormal contrast enhancement of the optic nerve. The diagnostic workup for optic neuritis may involve laboratory studies to assess for MOG and NMO, as well as cerebrospinal fluid analysis to check for the presence of oligoclonal bands. Treatment involves proper diagnosis and often acute treatment with intravenous steroids.

Arteritic anterior ischemic optic neuropathy, most commonly caused by giant cell arteritis, primarily affects older individuals, typically over the age of 50, with a higher incidence in those over the age of 70 (see also Chapter 22). Symptoms may include headache and eye pain.[1] Diagnosis can be made by identifying optic nerve swelling or through elevated markers such as erythrocyte sedimentation rate (ESR) or C-reactive protein (CRP). Immediate treatment with steroids, followed by a temporal artery biopsy, is essential in managing this condition (Chapter 22).

Orbital Causes of Headache

Trochleitis

Trochleitis is an inflammatory syndrome affecting the trochlea, which is a collagenous sheath responsible for housing the tendon of the superior oblique muscle.[1] Inflammation of the trochlea can be objectively visualized on MRI scans, specifically when interpreted by experienced neuroradiologists who are specifically looking for this condition. Alternatively, orbital ultrasonography can also be utilized to identify signs of trochleitis. Subjectively, patients may experience tenderness upon palpation in the superomedial corner of the eye socket. The symptoms reported by patients typically include a dull, aching pain, which may be accompanied by intermittent stabbing pains. Treatment options for trochleitis consist of administering steroid injections at the trochlea or prescribing oral steroids and nonsteroidal anti-inflammatory drugs (NSAIDs).

Dacryoadenitis

Inflammation of the lacrimal gland, situated in the superolateral aspect of the orbit, can elicit severe pain and potentially lead to headaches.[1,5,6] Patients typically present with a visibly swollen superolateral eye socket, resembling facial or orbital cellulitis due to the swift and pronounced edema. Subjectively, the pain is described as intense, deep, and persistent, most likely attributed to the acute and rapid edema affecting the lacrimal gland and its surrounding tissues. While viral causes are the most prevalent, other etiologies such as sarcoidosis, IgG4-related disease, bacterial infections, and tumors should also be considered. A timely referral to an ophthalmologist is paramount in managing this condition. Diagnostic imaging, utilizing techniques such as CT scan or ultrasound, may be employed to aid in accurate diagnosis. Treatment often involves the administration of indomethacin and/or oral steroids, which have shown efficacy in alleviating symptoms.[6] Gradual tapering of steroid dosage is typically recommended, and if the underlying cause is viral, the condition is self-limiting and resolves over time.

IgG4-Related Disorder

Immunoglobulin G4 (IgG4) disease is an immune-mediated systemic condition that can initially manifest in the eye socket.[1,6] Although the antibodies themselves do not appear to be problematic, their production is believed to be a response to cytokines released during autoimmune stimulation. The most common presentation involves proptosis, which refers to the forward movement of the eyeball within the eye socket, accompanied by persistent, aching pain. Orbital signs may include eyelid swelling, lacrimal gland enlargement, or diffuse orbital pain and swelling. In adults, IgG4 disease can manifest unilaterally or bilaterally. Imaging techniques such as MRI or CT scans may reveal thickening or stranding of intra- and extraconal tissues, as well as enhancement of various orbital structures. Treatment is usually immunosuppression starting with steroids, but other treatments may be needed.

Thyroid Orbitopathy

Thyroid antibodies have the potential to stimulate insulin growth factor receptors present in orbital tissues, including fat cells and muscle cells. This stimulation leads to fibroblast proliferation and subsequent production and deposition of glycosaminoglycans within the orbital tissues. The resulting swelling and fibrosis can occur rapidly and are associated with symptoms such as soreness, eye pain, pain upon eye movement, and potentially headache.[1] To assess the severity and activity of thyroid eye disease, clinicians may utilize a clinical activity grading score. The disorder can also cause rapid onset of double vision, limited eye muscle movements (referred to as ductions), eyelid swelling, and eyelid retraction. Thyroid eye disease most commonly occurs alongside elevated levels of thyroid hormones; however, it can also be associated with hypothyroid or even euthyroid states. Treatment primarily involves managing the underlying thyroid disease, focusing on normalization of thyroid hormone levels.

Summary

- A careful history and examination will help identify the anatomic cause of eye pain and headache.
- When there is no clear anatomical source of eye pain, an evaluation by an ophthalmologist is important.
- When there is loss of vision, it is important to have the patient seen by an ophthalmologist.
- Disorders that cause red eyes are usually inflammatory and should be evaluated by an ophthalmologist.
- Dry eye is important to treat and it participates in migraine; even the corneal nerves are changed in chronic migraine.
- Some causes of eye pain should be treated emergently, such as acute angle closure, ocular ischemic syndrome, and giant cell arteritis.

REFERENCES

1. Lee MS, Digre KB. *A Case-Based Guide to Eye Pain: Perspectives from Ophthalmology and Neurology.* Springer; 2018.
2. Digre KB, Friedman DF. Headache and eye pain. In: Albert DM, Miller JW, Azar DT, Young LH, eds. *Albert & Jakobiec's Principles & Practice of Ophthalmology.* 4th ed. Springer; 2022.
3. Bowen RC, Koeppel JN, Christensen CD, et al. The most common causes of eye pain at 2 tertiary ophthalmology and neurology clinics. *J Neuroophthalmol.* 2018;38:320-327.
4. Kinard KI, Smith AG, Singleton JR, et al. Chronic migraine is associated with reduced corneal nerve fiber density and symptoms of dry eye. *Headache.* 2015;55:543-549.
5. Ringeisen AL, Harrison AR, Lee MS. Ocular and orbital pain for the headache specialist. *Curr Neurol Neurosci Rep.* 2011;11:156-163.
6. Ronquillo Y, Patel BC. Nonspecific Orbital Inflammation. StatPearls. Treasure Island (FL) ineligible companies. Disclosure: Bhupendra Patel declares no relevant financial relationships with ineligible companies. StatPearls Publishing. Copyright © 2023, StatPearls Publishing LLC.; 2023.

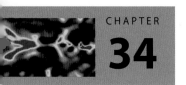

CHAPTER
34

Headache in Temporomandibular Disorders*

Marcela Romero-Reyes and James Hawkins

Temporomandibular disorders (TMD) are an orofacial pain diagnostic subcategory that encompasses a group of over 30 musculoskeletal diagnoses involving the temporomandibular joint (TMJ), the muscles of mastication, and their associated structures.[1,2] According to the Diagnostic Criteria for TMD (DC/TMD), the most prevalent TMD conditions associated with pain include muscle disorders such as myalgia and myofascial pain, disorders affecting the TMJ such as arthralgia, and headache attributed to TMD.[3] Headache attributed to TMD is classified as a secondary headache.

Epidemiology

TMD affect approximately 5% of the population in the United States on an annual basis, with an average incidence of 4%.[2,4] TMD negatively impacts life-sustaining and enhancing activities such as eating, breathing, talking, expressing emotion (e.g., smiling), and intimate interactions. The impact of TMD has been highlighted in a comprehensive report published in 2020 by the National Academies of Science, Engineering, and Medicine titled *The National Academies Collection: Reports funded by National Institutes of Health*, in *Temporomandibular Disorders: Priorities for Research and Care*, which provides recommendations to improve TMD care, education, and research.[1] TMD is more commonly observed in women, with a prevalence two to four times higher than in men. The OPPERA project (Orofacial Pain: Prospective Evaluation and Risk Assessment) conducted research to identify risk factors associated with the development of chronic TMD.[5] These factors include, but are not limited to, jaw trauma, parafunctional habits (e.g., teeth grinding or clenching), psychological variables, and genetic predisposition. TMD patients often have more chronic overlapping pain conditions (COPC), or comorbidities, including migraine and tension-type headache (TTH), fibromyalgia, irritable bowel syndrome, low back pain, and vulvodynia.[6]

Pathophysiology

This relationship between TMD and primary headaches extends beyond the interconnected anatomical structures and involves a shared sensitization pathway, which may explain why the presence of TMD can increase the prevalence and worsen symptoms of primary headache disorders (Figure 34-1). The calcitonin gene-related peptide (CGRP) may also be involved in TMD pathophysiology, as well as in the exacerbated phenotype of TMD and migraine comorbidity. This relationship may explain why the presence of TMD may influence the overall nociceptive input and exacerbate trigeminovascular activation, and in a clinical context, may accelerate progression to chronic migraine.[7] Furthermore, there may be a bidirectional pathway of sensitization, as the presence of migraine may be a

*The authors would like to thank Dr. Simon Akerman, Department of Neural and Pain Sciences, University of Maryland, Baltimore, School of Dentistry, for his assistance with Figure 34-1.

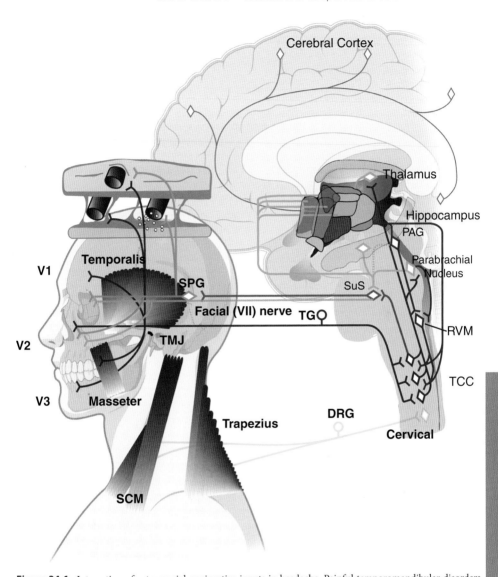

Figure 34-1. Interaction of extracranial nociceptive inputs in headache. Painful temporomandibular disorders may influence headache disorders. Headache, particularly migraine, is largely mediated by the V1 distribution or C1-C2 distribution (neck), and felt intracranially, as a consequence of activation of nociceptive trigeminal afferents innervating the intracranial dural vasculature. Pain arising from extracranial structures innervated by the mandibular (V3) branch of the trigeminal nerve such as the temporomandibular joint (TMJ) and muscles of mastication (including the masseter and the temporalis) may influence activation of the dural-trigeminovascular system and potentially exacerbate headache symptomatology. Likewise, dural-trigeminovascular activation may influence symptomatology of extracranial structures but this relationship needs to be explored further. Convergent nociceptive inputs from cervical musculature (including sternocleidomastoid and trapezius) also contribute to TMD and headache pain. TMJ, temporomandibular joint; TG, Trigeminal Ganglion; TCC trigeminocervical complex; VI, ophthalmic branch of the trigeminal nerve; V2, maxillary branch of the trigeminal nerve; V3, mandibular branch of the trigeminal nerve; C1- C2, regions of the cervical spinal cord; DRG, Dorsal root ganglion; SCM, sternocleidomastoid; PAG, ventrolateral periaqueductal gray; RVM, rostral ventromedial medulla; SPG, Sphenopalatine ganglion; SuS, superior salivatory reflex. (Reproduced with permission from Romero-Reyes M, Klasser G, Akerman S. An Update on Temporomandibular Disorders (TMDs) and Headache. *Curr Neurol Neurosci Rep.* 2023;23(10):561-570.)

predictor of new onset TMD.[8] Genetic predisposition may also influence TMD and headache onset and progression in some patients.[5] On the other hand, dental factors such as malocclusion, once thought to play a significant role in the development and persistent of TMD, have been shown to have minimal influence in the etiology of TMD.[1]

Diagnosis and Clinical Characteristics

TMD pain is most often reported in the jaw, face, temples, ears, and pre-auricular areas. Common symptom(s) include pain and/or limitation with TMJ biomechanics involved with chewing and mouth opening, as well as a sensation of jaw "locking" during mouth opening or closing.

TMD often mimics the symptomatology of TTH. TMD may also cause a headache. Headache caused by TMD is considered a secondary headache and is classified by the third edition of the *International Classification of Headache Disorders* (ICHD-3), code 11.7 as "Headache attributed to temporomandibular disorder." Clinicians need to be aware that TMD commonly coexist with primary headache disorders, especially with tension-type headache and migraine, and that this comorbidity may influence patient outcomes.

A brief TMD screening questionnaire may be utilized by the medical provider to promptly identify TMD symptoms in a headache patient. While more comprehensive and validated screening tools are available, the following questions may be useful to include during medical history taking:

1. Do you feel pain in your jaw?
2. Do you experience pain or stiffness in your jaw on awakening?
3. Do you have pain when you open your mouth, yawn, and/or chewing your food?

It is common to associate parafunctional habits such as diurnal clenching and grinding the teeth together (bruxing) with TMD. These may initiate or perpetuate TMD symptoms in some persons, but not all. Including a question regarding the presence of these habits can be useful during medical history (e.g., do you clench or grind your teeth during the day? do you know if you clench or grind your teeth during the night?). Nocturnal bruxism may increase the risk of primary headache disorders, but this relation is still controversial.[9]

Clinically, assessment of pain on mouth opening, as well as discomfort on palpation of the TMJs, masseter, and temporalis muscles is important. Intraoral palpation of the temporal tendon is also recommended, as temporal tendonitis can commonly mimic headache. During examination, it is important to be aware that approximately 33% of the general population has a TMJ noise (click, pop) on jaw movement.[2] This noise alone is common and may indicate a disc-condyle discoordination, known as TMJ disc displacement, and is not cause for concern unless pain or jaw movement limitation are also present. If TMD symptoms are present, particularly with chewing, the patient should initially be evaluated by their general dentist, as pain coming from diseased teeth can mimic both TMD and headache, as well as other neurological entities such as trigeminal neuralgia.

Treatment

The natural history of TMD demonstrates a tendency to improve over time,[10,11] and therefore management should be conservative, reversible, founded in evidence-based therapies, and tailored to the specific diagnosis and needs of the patient. Initial therapy includes education about the diagnoses and factors that may be perpetuating their condition. Next, self-management strategies focused on minimizing oral parafunction behaviors (e.g., clenching, gum chewing) and teaching the patients how to maintain their jaw in a position of rest are emphasized. Soft diet, avoiding hard, chewy, and crunchy foods, and regular application of moist heat to the masticatory muscles, as well as gentle jaw stretches, can also be beneficial.

While adaptive patients may respond well to the conservative care options listed above, other patients may need additional care. Further management provided by an orofacial pain specialist may include other nonpharmacological approaches such as an oral appliance or nightguard therapy, but only in cases when nocturnal parafunctional habits such as clenching or bruxing are found to be perpetuating symptoms. Pharmacological modalities including nonsteroidal anti-inflammatory drugs (NSAIDs), muscle relaxants, antidepressants, and trigger point injection therapy may also prove useful. The use of onabotulinum toxin A injection therapy has been shown to be effective in refractory cases and when severe parafunctional activity is present; however, this use is off-label (Chapter 43). Currently, onabotulinum toxin A is not FDA approved for the management of TMD and should not be used as first line of management.

For patients with TMD presenting with COPCs (fibromyalgia, irritable bowel syndrome, headache, neck pain, etc.), sleep disturbance, psychosocial distress, and a history of negative life events, a biopsychosocial approach to management is optimal.[2] Therefore, this group is often best cared for utilizing a holistic, multidisciplinary approach that spans medicine, dentistry, and multiple allied health professions. In patients with comorbid headache and TMD, the healthcare provider should consider working closely with a dentist who is board certified in orofacial pain to address these overlapping conditions, as well as other appropriate team members that may benefit the patient. This may include, but is not limited to, physical therapy with a professional skill in craniofacial and cervical therapeutics, pain psychology, and sleep medicine. It is important to recognize the comorbidity between primary headache disorders and TMD. Effective management of both conditions with a multidisciplinary approach will provide optimal patient outcomes and assist in minimizing the risk of headache chronification.

Prognosis

Approximately 50% of patients improve within 6 months of developing a TMD, while the other half have persistent pain.[5] Progression to a chronic TMD depends largely on the degree of central sensitization and associated comorbidities a patient presents with.[12] Therefore, the headache clinician should ensure perpetuating factors are addressed by the patient's healthcare team to optimize prognosis.

Summary

- TMD include over 30 musculoskeletal diagnoses related to the TMJ, masticatory muscles, and associated structures.
- Patients with headache disorder are at increased risk of developing a TMD, and TMD patients are at risk for developing headache disorders, particularly migraine.
- Screening for TMD is essential for patients with headache disorders.
- Patients with a headache and TMD may be at greater risk for having additional comorbid pain and psychosocial disorders.
- Multidisciplinary management team including a dentist who is board certified in orofacial pain is important for the care of patients with comorbid migraine and TMD.

Disclaimers

The views of this article reflect the results of a review of the literature and expertise of the authors and do not necessarily reflect the official policy or position of the Department of the Navy, Department of Defense, Uniformed Services University of the Health Sciences, nor the U.S. Government.

"I am (Dr. James Hawkins) a military service member or federal/contracted employee of the United States government. This work was prepared as part of my official duties. Title 17 U.S.C. 105

provides that 'copyright protection under this title is not available for any work of the United States Government.' Title 17 U.S.C. 101 defines a U.S. Government work as work prepared by a military service member or employee of the U.S. Government as part of that person's official duties.

Neither I nor any member of my family have a financial arrangement or affiliation with any corporate organization offering financial support or grant monies for this research, nor do I have a financial interest in any commercial product(s) or service(s) I will discuss in the presentation or publication."

REFERENCES

1. National Academies of Sciences, Engineering, and Medicine; Health and Medicine Division; Board on Health Care Services; Board on Health Sciences Policy; Committee on Temporomandibular Disorders (TMDs): From Research Discoveries to Clinical Treatment. In: Yost O, Liverman CT, English R, Mackey S, Bond EC, eds. Temporomandibular Disorders: Priorities for Research and Care. Washington (DC): National Academies Press (US); 2020.

2. Klasser GD, Romero-Reyes, M. (ed.). *Orofacial Pain: Guidelines for Assessment, Diagnosis, and Management.* 7th ed. Chicago: Quintesssence Publishing; 2023.

3. Schiffman E, Ohrbach R, Truelove E, et al. Diagnostic criteria for temporomandibular disorders (DC/TMD) for clinical and research applications: recommendations of the international RDC/TMD Consortium Network* and Orofacial Pain Special Interest Group†. *J Oral Facial Pain Headache.* 2014;28(1):6-27.

4. Slade GD, Fillingim RB, Sanders AE, et al. Summary of findings from the OPPERA prospective cohort study of incidence of first-onset temporomandibular disorder: implications and future directions. *J Pain.* 2013;14(12 Suppl):T116-T124.

5. Slade GD, Ohrbach R, Greenspan JD, et al. Painful temporomandibular disorder: decade of discovery from OPPERA studies. *J Dent Res.* 2016;95(10):1084-1092.

6. Slade GD, Greenspan JD, Fillingim RB, Maixner W, Sharma S, Ohrbach R. Overlap of five chronic pain conditions: temporomandibular disorders, headache, back pain, irritable bowel syndrome, and fibromyalgia. *J Oral Facial Pain Headache.* 2020;34:s15-s28.

7. Akerman S, Romero-Reyes M. Preclinical studies to dissect the neural mechanism for the comorbidity of migraine and temporomandibular disorders (TMD): the role of CGRP. *Br J Pharmacol.* 2020;177(24):5555-5568.

8. Tchivileva IE, Ohrbach R, Fillingim RB, Greenspan JD, Maixner W, Slade GD. Temporal change in headache and its contribution to the risk of developing first-onset temporomandibular disorder in the orofacial pain: prospective evaluation and risk assessment (OPPERA) study. *Pain.* 2017;158(1):120-129.

9. Teruel A, Romero-Reyes M. Interplay of oral, mandibular, and facial disorders and migraine. *Curr Pain Headache Rep.* 2022;26(7):517-523.

10. Fillingim RB, Slade GD, Greenspan JD, et al. Long-term changes in biopsychosocial characteristics related to temporomandibular disorder: findings from the OPPERA study. *Pain.* 2018;159(11):2403-2413.

11. Ohrbach R, Dworkin SF. Five-year outcomes in TMD: relationship of changes in pain to changes in physical and psychological variables. *Pain.* 1998;74(2-3):315-326.

12. Costa YM, Conti PC, de Faria FA, Bonjardim LR. Temporomandibular disorders and painful comorbidities: clinical association and underlying mechanisms. *Oral Surg Oral Med Oral Pathol Oral Radiol.* 2017;123(3):288-297.

*International Association for Dental Research.
†International Association for the Study of Pain.

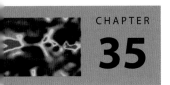

Headache and Sleep

Shayna Y. Sanguinetti and Adelene Jann

Sleep is a vital mechanism for maintaining homeostasis, particularly for the brain. On average, a person spends approximately one-third of their life asleep. Sleep is regulated by the circadian rhythm, controlled by the suprachiasmatic nucleus (SCN) in the hypothalamus.[1] The mechanisms of sleep are also utilized by processes implicated in headaches. This close relationship between sleep and headache disorders is well established. Although specific headache disorders, such as hypnic headache (Chapter 17), have been described for decades, recent research has shed light on the brain pathways that explain these connections more comprehensively. Understanding the connection between sleep and headache is crucial for clinicians to address underlying issues that affect both. By exploring these relationships, clinicians can develop more comprehensive and effective treatment strategies for patients with sleep and headache disorders.

Primary Headaches and Sleep

Sleep is an important factor in the pathophysiology of various primary headache disorders, including migraine, cluster headache, hypnic headache, and tension-type headache (TTH). The association between sleep and headache has been observed and described for over a century. Primary headache disorders have been found to occur predominantly during specific stages of sleep, particularly rapid eye movement (REM) sleep.

Migraine

Individuals with migraine often rely on sleep as a means of relieving pain, with many reporting resolution of migraine after sleep. However, excessive or insufficient sleep can also trigger headaches.[5] Individuals with migraines experience poor sleep quality, and report increased frequency of attacks in association with poor sleep (Chapter 5). Moreover, individuals with migraine are at increased risk for developing insomnia, which in turn can increase the intensity, frequency, and even lead to chronic headache development.[6] Many times, treatment of migraine is also aimed at improving the quality of sleep.

Migraine often occurs during REM sleep or excessive amounts of stage III and IV sleep. Interestingly, cortical spreading depression (CSD) can also prolong NREM sleep.[8] CSD has also been shown to modulate the trigeminovascular system including brainstem nuclei that are involved in arousal. Alterations in the thalamocortical circuits may lead to alterations in sleep patterns. Neuropeptides such as pituitary adenylate cyclase-activating polypeptide (PACAP) may play a role in sleep mechanisms. PACAP is a vasodilatory peptide that is released during headaches, particularly migraine, and is widely expressed throughout the trigeminovascular system. It is implicated in light entrainment in the pons, increasing REM sleep, crossing the blood–brain barrier to act on central sites to induce sleep alterations.[8]

Cluster Headache

Cluster headache and chronic paroxysmal hemicrania tend to occur during the REM cycle of nocturnal or diurnal sleep.[3] Clinical evidence supports the belief that there is a close relationship between circadian rhythm and the timing of cluster headaches (Chapter 14). Attacks can occur on a seasonal or yearly basis, and during a particular time of day or night for any given individual. The highest frequency of cluster headache occurs around the winter or summer solstice, where there is either increasing or decreasing exposure to daylight.[5] Studies have shown that there are alterations in the secretion of melatonin, cortisol, prolactin, and thyrotropin among other hormones in patients with cluster headaches. In addition, there is increased activation of the anteroventral hypothalamus during a cluster attack. This is an area which contains the pacemaker neurons of the SCN.[5]

Tension-Type Headache

TTH is the most common primary headache, and evidence suggests a bidirectional relationship between TTH and sleep (Chapter 13). Lack of sleep, oversleeping, or sleep disruption are common triggers for TTH reported by patients. The relationship between daily stress and length of sleep, whether short or long periods of sleep, was associated with increased headache intensity.[11] Sleep affects the ability to handle stress and regulate mood, leading to exacerbation of headaches. Stress, obesity, comorbid psychiatric illness, and sleep disturbance are risk factors for chronification of TTH.[11] In contrast to other headache types, TTH is not strongly associated with a specific sleep stage. As in other chronic musculoskeletal pain conditions, chronic TTH can lead to decreased total sleep time, slow wave sleep, increased nocturnal awakenings and movements, and perceived decrease in overall sleep quality.[7]

Hypnic Headache and Exploding Head Syndrome

Hypnic headache is a primary headache disorder that occurs only during sleep and is typically seen in individuals over the age of 60. These headaches are known to occur at the same time every night with striking consistency (Chapter 17).[3] Another primary headache disorder, exploding head syndrome, also occurs exclusively during transition between sleep and wakefulness. This disorder is characterized by a loud, sudden explosion-like sound that can be jolting.[7] Although hypnic headache and exploding head syndrome are more commonly described in adults, there are also case reports of these disorders occurring in children.[8] There is an intimate relationship between sleep and these two conditions. It may be related to the increased disturbance in sleep-wake cycles in the elderly as the number of cells in the SCN decreases with age.[5] This also leads to the reduction in melatonin production as seen in other headache disorders.

Sleep Disorders and Headache

Several medical conditions and diseases that disrupt sleep, such as anxiety, depression, and sleep-related breathing disorders, are associated with an increased risk of headache.[3]

Obstructive Sleep Apnea

Obstructive sleep apnea (OSA) is characterized by abnormal breathing during sleep, which is caused by a blocked or partially blocked airway, leading to frequent oxygen desaturations and arousals from sleep. Approximately 30% to 70% of patients with sleep apnea experience morning headaches.[9] The cerebrovascular effects resulting from hypoxia and hypercapnia during sleep are likely the etiology of these headaches.[7] There is an increased incidence of OSA in patients with cluster headache. OSA can trigger cluster headache within a few hours of sleep onset.[8] It is recommended that patients should be screened for sleep apnea during headache evaluation to determine if they would benefit from treatment, particularly if headaches occur exclusively during sleep. Treatment of OSA, particularly with positive airway ventilation, often results in resolution of associated headaches.[5,6]

Restless Leg Syndrome

Restless leg syndrome (RLS) is the most common sleep-related movement disorder, causing disruption of sleep onset. Patients experience uncomfortable sensation in the legs, primarily with rest or inactivity, partially relieved by movement. The prevalence of RLS in the general population ranges between 5% and 14.3%, whereas the prevalence of RLS among patients with migraine is significantly higher, ranging from 13.7% to 25%. Studies have shown that RLS is associated with higher migraine severity, increased occurrence of photophobia, phonophobia, nausea, dizziness, migraine-related disability, anxiety, and depression.[2]

Parasomnias

Parasomnias are another group of sleep disorders that are strongly associated with headache. Parasomnias include complex movements, perceptions, behaviors, emotions, and autonomic activity that occur at the transition from wake to sleep, during sleep, or arousal from sleep, and may affect sleep quality.[4] Children with headaches are more likely to sleep-talk, have nightmares, and sleepwalk. This finding extends into adolescence. Adults with migraine are more likely to report a history of childhood somnambulism (sleepwalking) compared to other headache types (33% vs. 5%). In contrast, there is a higher risk of migraine in adult patients diagnosed with somnambulism. Dream-enacting behavior is present almost twice as often in patients with migraine than in those without migraine and is associated with higher pain-related disability and lower sleep quality.[12]

Summary

- There is a complex neuroanatomical and neurobiological relationship between headache and sleep.
- This relationship is bidirectional: sleep disturbances may worsen headache and frequent headache leads to poor sleep.
- Sleep disturbances are often reported as a trigger in primary headache disorders such as migraine, cluster headache, and TTH.
- Secondary causes of sleep disturbance such as OSA should be evaluated as they can exacerbate headache.
- Sleep disorders such as restless leg syndrome and parasomnias are common in patients with headache.
- Treating underlying sleep disorders and improving sleep quality is likely to also improve headache conditions.

REFERENCES

1. Abrahamson E, Leak R, Moore R. The suprachiasmastic nucleus projects to posterior hypothalamic arousal systems. *Neuroreport.* 2001;12:435-440.
2. Chen PK, Fuh JL, Chen SP, Wang SJ. Association between restless legs syndrome and migraine. *J Neurol Neurosurg Psychiatry.* 2010;81:524-528.
3. Dodick DW, Eross EJ, Parish JM. Views and perspectives: clinical, anatomical, and physiologic relationship between sleep and headache. *Headache.* 2003;43:282-292.
4. Tiseo C, Vacca A, Felbush A, et al. Migraine and sleep disorders: a systematic review. *J Headache and Pain.* 2020;20:126-139.

Secondary Headaches

5. Fernandez-Matarrubia M, Cuadrado ML, Sánchez-Barros CM, et al. Prevalence of migraine in patients with restless legs syndrome: a case-control study. *Headache*. 2014;54:1337-1346.

6. Holland PR. Headache and sleep: shared pathophysiological mechanisms. *Cephalalgia*. 2014;34(10):725-744.

7. Johnson K, Ziemba A, Garb J. Improvement in headaches with continuous positive airway pressure for obstructive sleep apnea: a retrospective analysis. *Headache*. 2013;53:333-343.

8. May A, Goadsby P. The trigeminovascular system in humans: pathophysiologic implications for primary headache syndromes of the neural influences on the cerebral circulation. *J Cereb Blood Flow Metab*. 1999;19:115-127.

9. Ohayon M, O'Hara R, Vitiello M. Epidemiology of restless legs syndrome: a synthesis of the literature. *Sleep Med Rev*. 2012;16:283-295.

10. Pirizada A, Almeneessier A, BaHammam AS. Exploding head syndrome: a case series of undiagnosed hypnic parasomnia. *Case Rep Neurol*. 2020;12:348-358.

11. Rains J, Davis R, Smitherman T. Tension-type headache and sleep. *Curr Neurol Neurosci Rep*. 2015;15:1-9.

12. Suzuki K, Miyamoto T, Miyamoto M, et al. Dream-enacting behavior is associated with impaired sleep and severe headache-related disability in migraine patients. *Cephalalgia*. 2013;33:868-878.

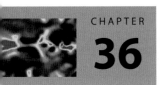

Headache and Hormones

36

Jelena M. Pavlovic and Niki Holtzman-Hayes

Among primary headache disorders, migraine has the highest prevalence and socio-economic burden, particularly afflicting women at a threefold greater rate than men. It stands as the leading cause of years lived with disability among women of reproductive age. Migraine often fluctuates predictably across reproductive milestones in women, including puberty, pregnancy and lactation, and perimenopause and menopause. These clinical observations have long been linked to the role of ovarian hormones in migraine pathophysiology. Women experience the highest burden of migraine during menstruation and perimenopause, the times of marked hormonal fluctuations, necessitating a nuanced approach to management during these phases. This underscores the importance of understanding the hormonal mechanisms underlying the preponderance of migraine in females in order to better elucidate the presentation and treatment of the most common disabling headaches in women throughout the lifespan.[1] The *International Classification of Headache Disorders,* third edition (ICHD-3), provides diagnostic criteria that categorize perimenstrual attacks into two distinct diagnoses: pure menstrual migraine (PMM) and menstrually related migraine (MRM).

This chapter will focus on the discussion of migraine occurrence in relation to hormones across the menstrual cycle and the naturally occurring hormonal changes across the lifespan focusing on perimenopause and menopause. The discussion regarding migraine presentation and treatment during pregnancy and lactation can be found in Chapter 48.

Menstrual Migraine

Epidemiology

About two-thirds of women experience perimenstrual migraine attacks, characterized by headaches that occur in close temporal association with menses. PMM is a rare disorder affecting less than 10% of women, while MRM tends to be common, affecting about half of women with migraine. Risk factors for perimenstrual migraine attacks include early menarche, premenstrual syndrome, longer menstrual bleeding, and dysmenorrhea.[2]

Pathophysiology

The estrogen withdrawal theory, first postulated in the 1970s, suggests that falling estrogen levels trigger migraine attacks while high estrogen levels tend to be protective. In particular, the naturally occurring decline in estrogen preceding menstruation (late luteal phase of the cycle) is implicated as the driver of perimenstrual migraine attacks. Interestingly, migraine risk is relatively low during the ovulatory phase of the menstrual cycle despite dynamic changes in estrogen and progesterone during that time. This could be attributed, in part, to the faster rate of estrogen decline in the late luteal phase that is unique to women with migraine. This phase-specific accelerated decline has been suggested to impact susceptibility to perimenstrual migraine attacks rather than focusing solely on absolute estrogen levels. The abrupt withdrawal of estrogen's inhibitory effects on various pain pathways likely acts as a trigger of perimenstrual migraine by lowering the migraine threshold.[3,4] Additional contributors to perimenstrual migraines include the release of prostaglandins around menses, the decline in magnesium and serotonin levels, and dysfunction of the endogenous opioid pathways during the perimenstrual interval. In particular, estrogen modulates serotonin transmission enhancing its synthesis while reducing degradation. Abrupt drops in estrogen lead to serotonin deficiency, disinhibiting trigeminal vascular activation and in that way causing migraine activation. Estrogens also suppress neurogenic inflammation by inhibiting the release of calcitonin gene-related peptide (CGRP), substance P, prostaglandins, and proinflammatory cytokines but the precise relationships between estrogen levels and these mediators of neuroinflammation are not yet understood.[3]

In addition to estrogen, roles of other reproductive hormones such as progesterone and oxytocin have been considered in migraine pathogenesis, but the evidence for their involvement is limited.[4] Progesterone withdrawal coincides with declining estrogen levels prior to menses but studies indicate that it does not directly contribute to migraine occurrence.[3] A recently put forth theoretical model proposes that estrogen balances proinflammatory/promigraine factors like CGRP against anti-inflammatory/antimigraine factors like oxytocin. Therefore, the decline in estrogen prior to menstruation would allow pro-migraine effects to dominate by disinhibiting trigeminal excitability and pain signaling thus decreasing the pain threshold and leading to migraine occurrence.[3,4]

Clinical Characteristics and Diagnosis

For both PMM and MRM, a clear temporal association between migraine attacks and menstruation should be verified for at least two out of three cycles using a headache diary or calendar for both diagnoses. For PMM, attacks have to occur exclusively during the perimenstrual days −2 to +3 (where +1 is the first day of bleeding). While the occurrence of attacks during the perimenstrual window and at other times of the cycle confirms MRM diagnosis. Prospective headache diaries need to be kept for the diagnosis to be confirmed as they are more reliable than retrospective patient recall, though patient recall is often used in clinical practice for the purpose of diagnosing patients with PMM or MRM and guiding appropriate treatment.[2] Within both diagnostic subtypes, perimenstrual attacks tend to be longer in duration, more severe, and more refractory to treatment compared to nonmenstrual attacks. Perimenstrual attacks are also rarely associated with aura and, therefore, women who have PMM tend to have aura much less frequently than women with MRM with estimates of 16% of women with MRM having migraine with aura compared to only 6% of women with PMM.

Treatment

While perimenstrual migraine attacks are particularly debilitating, causing a great burden to women with migraine, no therapies to date have been specifically approved for MRM, with the current guidelines suggesting that traditional acute and preventive treatments for migraine be used in the treatment of women who experience perimenstrual attacks. These traditional acute and preventive treatment approaches are discussed in Chapters 7 and 8, respectively.

With respect to the treatment of perimenstrual attacks, a mini-prophylaxis concept has been developed. This concept refers to short-term prevention therapies that occur specifically around the time of anticipated perimenstrual attacks. The goal is to prevent acute migraine medication overuse by reducing attack frequency, severity, and associated symptoms of perimenstrual attacks. Successful implementation depends on collaborative efforts between patients and clinical providers to identify the days of highest attack risk in relation to menses. Patients should be asked to keep a daily headache diary with particular focus placed on the days of bleeding and the occurrence of headaches in relation to the onset of bleeding.[1,2,5] A number of small clinical trials have evaluated therapies aimed at preventing perimenstrual attacks focusing on both traditional acute migraine treatments and hormonal treatments.[4,5] Long-acting triptans, NSAIDs, and magnesium have all been studied as nonhormonal options for mini-prophylaxes of perimenstrual attacks given about 3, 5, or 7 days prior to menses through the first few days of bleeding itself. In general, triptans taken two times per day effectively reduced menstrual attacks by about 50%, and are recommended as the first-line acute treatment.[1,5] Frovatriptan 2.5 mg has the longest half-life compared to other triptans and has demonstrated efficacy in menstrual migraine with sustained relief and reduced recurrence of migraine attacks. Naproxen sodium 500 mg taken twice daily prior to the onset of bleeding was superior to placebo in decreasing MRM frequency, duration, and severity. Magnesium supplementation starting seven days prior to the onset of menses until 3 days into menses also decreased the number of migraine days and reduced pain severity compared to placebo.[5]

Recently developed novel therapies targeting CGRP provide overall highly effective acute and preventive migraine treatments, and have been postulated to be effective in MRM, but the evidence is currently limited.[1,3-5] Overall, though there are a number of new treatment approaches to perimenstrual attacks, rigorous clinical trials are still needed to validate the efficacy and safety of novel therapies for the treatment of perimenstrual migraine specifically.

Treatment of Menstrual Migraine with Hormones

Hormonal treatments have been extensively used in treatment of migraine in general and treatment of menstrual migraine in particular. They are most widely used as contraceptive agents, referred to as combined hormonal contraceptives (CHCs) that are available in different regimens and administration routes to improve convenience and adherence. They can also help manage gynecological conditions associated with migraine, making them popular among women with migraine. However, the effects of CHCs on migraine can vary with some women experiencing aggravation, improvement, or no change in migraine symptoms with CHCs. Starting CHCs can even trigger migraine in certain cases. The hormone-free interval in CHCs is identified as a vulnerable period for migraine, and strategies like using transdermal estrogen or shortening the interval have been studied and show efficacy.[4,5] Women with migraines have unrestricted contraceptive choices, but accurate diagnosis and consideration of the impact of different methods on migraines are crucial.[6]

Contraceptive Pills and Risk Factors

Migraine with aura is considered a risk factor for ischemic stroke. Similarly, the use of any estrogen-containing compounds increases the risk of stroke in all patients regardless of migraine. In CHC users with migraine with aura, studies indicate this risk is further elevated, with the additional vascular risk factor of smoking conferring the highest risk for ischemic stroke. As a result, even low-dose estrogen-containing CHCs have long been considered contraindicated in patients with migraine with aura due to concern for increased stroke risk. Studies support a dose-related effect of estrogen in CHC such that lower estrogen-containing compounds confer a lower risk of stroke.[7,8]

A 2022 case-control study performed at the Cleveland Clinic[7] examined stroke risk in women with migraine diagnosis on varying estrogen doses of CHC. The study differentiated between both low- and high-dose ethinyl estradiol (EE) CHCs and migraine with and without aura. Though overall stroke risk was low, the risk was higher in those with a diagnosis of migraine.[7] Importantly, migraine with aura did not independently increase stroke risk compared to migraine without aura. Higher-dose EE CHCs were associated with higher stroke risk in both cases and controls. This study calls for counseling and shared decision-making regarding the use of estrogen-containing CHCs in all patients with migraine, regardless of aura.[7] Clinicians must bear in mind the critical point that venous and arterial thrombotic risks are higher in pregnancy than in the use of any contraceptive. Lower-dose EE CHC can mitigate stroke risk in women with migraine. Overall, CHCs increase the risk of stroke independently from migraine, particularly in patients with concomitant traditional vascular risk factors. Studies on CHC in migraine and migraine with aura are scarce, and those that exist are consistently underpowered, having poorly addressed stroke risk in patients with migraine using CHC.[8]

Secondary Headaches

Progesterone-Only Versus Estrogen-Containing Pills

Cardiovascular risk associated with CHCs is attributable to the estrogen component due to its effects on the coagulation cascade. Thus, progesterone-only contraceptive pills, subdermal implants, intrauterine devices, and depot injections have been deemed safe in terms of cardiovascular and stroke risk in patients with migraine with or without aura.[5,9] These formulations can be especially useful in patients with migraine and other conventional cardiovascular/stroke risk factors. Observational studies suggest progesterone-only OCPs can be associated with a reduction in migraine days.[9] However, progesterone-only contraceptive pills are less effective for pregnancy prevention, and the risk of stroke in migraine, especially in the absence of other vascular risk factors, is low. To date, no studies have specifically evaluated the risk of ischemic stroke in progesterone-only birth control of any type for patients with migraine.

Headache During Perimenopause and Menopause

The perimenopausal transition represents a stage of particular vulnerability for worsening migraine symptoms in women. During perimenopause, women experience irregular menstrual cycles and fluctuations in estrogen and progesterone levels as ovarian function declines. It has been reported that perimenopausal women suffer more frequent, longer lasting, and more intense migraine attacks compared to the premenopausal period.[10] Furthermore, up to 60% of women with migraine report an exacerbation of headaches during the menopausal transition.[10] The erratic hormonal fluctuations characteristic of perimenopause are believed to underlie increased migraine susceptibility due to estrogen withdrawal, reduced estrogen stability, and falling progesterone levels. Migraine improvement eventually occurs in a majority of women as they fully transition into menopause.[10] However, the period of hormone instability during perimenopause can last for several years and represents a challenging stage of high migraine burden for many women.[1,6,10] Understanding the factors associated with perimenopausal-related migraine worsening and developing effective management strategies for this population remains an important research and clinical priority.

The onset of menopause often signals an improvement in migraine symptoms in the majority of women as the estradiol fluctuations believed to trigger migraine attacks in premenopausal women stabilized after ovarian senescence.[1,10] Population-based studies indicate that approximately two-thirds of women with migraine experience complete migraine remission or significant improvement during the menopausal transition further providing evidence for the pivotal role of estrogen withdrawal in migraine pathogenesis.[1,3,4] Migraine persists after menopause in about 15% to 20% of women who report either no change or even worsening in migraine frequency following menopause.[10] Therefore, postmenopausal women can require ongoing migraine management which can be challenging due to medication side effects, comorbidities, and lack of evidence-based guidelines in this population.[10] Use of hormone therapy in symptomatic postmenopausal women appears safe but does not consistently improve migraine.[5,6,9,10] As women with migraine experience a higher burden of vasomotor motor symptoms, they may benefit from hormone therapy treatment, while keeping doses low to minimize cardiovascular risk.[10]

Further research is needed to determine optimal management for migraine persisting after menopause as well as the risk factors for migraine chronification in this stage. For women with risk factors, such as aura, obesity, and cardiovascular risk factors, nonhormonal approaches are preferable for both perimenopausal and menopausal treatment. Patients and providers must weigh migraine relief against potential medication side effects and vascular events, while taking into consideration existing comorbidities and individual cardiovascular risk factors. Overall migraine management during the perimenopausal and postmenopausal stages requires an individualized approach with attention to a woman's physiological changes, migraine characteristics, and other comorbidities with particular emphasis on cardiovascular risk profile.

Summary

- Migraine predominantly impacts women, with hormonal shifts increasing susceptibility to attacks during menstruation and perimenopausal hormonal changes.
- The ICHD-3 categorizes perimenstrual attacks into PMM and MRM.
- Mini-prophylaxis with frovatriptan or naproxen, initiated around anticipated perimenstrual attacks, may effectively reduce migraine frequency, severity, and duration.
- Migraines generally improve after menopause due to hormone stabilization.
- In users of estrogen-containing pills with migraines with aura, the risk of stroke is elevated, especially when combined with the vascular risk factor of smoking.
- Progesterone-based contraceptives are considered safe for migraine patients in terms of cardiovascular and stroke risks.

REFERENCES

1. Pavlović JM. Headache in women. *Continuum (Minneap Minn)*. 2021;27(3):686-702.
2. Vetvik KG, MacGregor EA. Menstrual migraine: a distinct disorder needing greater recognition. *Lancet Neurol*. 2021;20(4):304-315.
3. Krause DN, Warfvinge K, Haanes KA, Edvinsson L. Hormonal influences in migraine: interactions of oestrogen, oxytocin and CGRP. *Nat Rev Neurol*. 2021;17(10):621-633.
4. Nappi RE, Tiranini L, Sacco S, De Matteis E, De Icco R, Tassorelli C. Role of estrogens in menstrual migraine. *Cells*. 2022;11(8):1355.
5. Ornello R, De Matteis E, Di Felice C, Caponnetto V, Pistoia F, Sacco S. Acute and preventive management of migraine during menstruation and menopause. *J Clin Med*. 2021;10(11):2263.
6. MacGregor EA. Menstrual and perimenopausal migraine: a narrative review. *Maturitas*. 2020;142:24-30.
7. Batur P, Yao M, Bucklan J, et al. Use of combined hormonal contraception and stroke: a case-control study of the impact of migraine type and estrogen dose on ischemic stroke risk. *Headache*. 2023;63(6):813-821.
8. Sheikh HU, Pavlovic J, Loder E, Burch R. Risk of stroke associated with use of estrogen containing contraceptives in women with migraine: a systematic review. *Headache*. 2018;58(1):5-21.
9. Sacco S, Merki-Feld GS, Ægidius KL, et al. Effect of exogenous estrogens and progestogens on the course of migraine during reproductive age: a consensus statement by the European Headache Federation (EHF) and the European Society of Contraception and Reproductive Health (ESCRH). *J Headache Pain*. 2018;19:76.
10. Pavlović JM. The impact of midlife on migraine in women: summary of current views. *Womens Midlife Health*. 2020;6:11.

Secondary Headaches

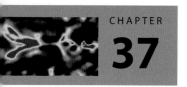

Headache Due to Psychiatric Disorder

Jane Lee and Noah Rosen

Headaches and mental disorders are the leading causes of disease burden throughout the world. There is a strong association between psychiatric disorders and primary as well as secondary headaches. However, a causal relationship may exist between a new or significantly worsening headache and psychiatric disorder. Headache attributed to psychiatric disorder is included in the third edition of the *International Classification of Headache Disorders* (ICHD-3).[1]

Epidemiology

According to the Global Burden of Disease Study in 2019 (GBD 2019) for psychiatric diseases, there were 970.1 million reported cases of mental disorders worldwide, and mental disorders ranked the second leading cause of years lived with disability.[2] A similar analysis for headache disorders reported that 52% of the studied populations suffered from different types of headaches, and migraine alone ranked as the second leading cause of disability.[3] Moreover, many studies reported a positive association between mental disorders and headaches. For instance, Breslau et al. reported that there is a bidirectional association between depression and migraine.[4] In American Migraine Prevalence and Prevention (AMPP) study, population with depression or generalized anxiety was associated with poor treatment optimization.[5] Despite many studies showing positive associations, there are limited studies exploring causal relationship between the disorders. In addition, the disuse of standardized screening tools to diagnose headaches due to psychiatric disorders leads to a lack of diagnosis and unclear prevalence.[6] With some effort to adhere to the standardized guidelines for the diagnosis, clinicians will better understand and be able to manage headaches due to psychiatric disorders.

Pathophysiology

The exact pathophysiology of pain transmission in the setting of psychiatric disorders is unclear. However, there is a growing recognition that serotonin and norepinephrine act as the main mediator of descending pain pathways as well as in mood regulation. Any dysregulation or imbalance of serotonin and norepinephrine due to depression, for example, may contribute to persistent headache. There is additional evidence supporting the role of cerebral inflammation from glial cell activation in the pathophysiology of both conditions.

The primary anatomical regions involved in depression as well as other mood disorders include the subcortical limbic brain areas including the amygdala, hippocampus, and dorsomedial thalamus. Decreased hippocampal volumes have been noted in depression. However, frontal cortical areas, as well as the prefrontal cortex, have emerged as regions consistently involved in major depressive disorders. Other regional changes have been identified in the parietal lobe, thalamus, caudate, pallidum, putamen, and temporal lobes.[1,2] This truly suggests mood is a circuit engaging multiple areas. Similarly, headache disorders also engage many of the same pathways. Pain is a complex network also engaging frontal and prefrontal lobes, as well as deep limbic structures.[7] Serotonin dysfunction has been implicated in the pathophysiology of anxiety and depression in primary headache disorders such as migraine and tension-type headache, and provide the basis for comorbidity of these diseases.[8]

Diagnosis and Clinical Presentation

In 2004, headache secondary to psychiatric disorders as a diagnostic term first appeared in the second edition of the *International Classification of Headache Disorders* (ICHD-2). ICHD-2 established that such disorders involve a new headache in the context of an active psychiatric disorder as defined by the Diagnostic and Statistical Manual of Mental Disorders (DSM-IV). It is similarly outlined in the most recent version of classification, ICHD-3. Headaches attributed to somatization and psychotic disorders are listed under section 12 of the classification. Under the appendix section A12, headaches attributed to other psychiatric disorders are listed. These diagnoses are diagnoses of exclusion and should be made when no other ICHD-3 diagnosis better accounts for the headaches and only when a causal relationship between the new onset headache and a psychiatric disorder is found.

No specific quality of pain, location, duration, or associated features has been established for headaches attributed to psychiatric disorders. The presentation may be unique, or it may appear similar to other primary headaches. In considering epidemiology of other disorders associated with psychiatric condition, it may be worth noting that these may occur in conjunction with other headache syndromes.

Somatization Disorder

Headaches attributed to somatization disorder require establishing the diagnosis of a somatic disorder. Somatic disorders are diagnosed when there are multiple unexplained physical symptoms before the age of 30 without other known medical conditions. Somatic symptoms should include all of the following: at least four pain symptoms from different anatomical sites, at least two gastrointestinal symptoms other than pain, at least one sexual symptom other than pain, and at least one pseudoneurological symptom not limited to pain (conversion symptoms such as impaired coordination or balance, paralysis, or localized weakness). In order to make the diagnosis of a headache attributable to somatization disorder, there needs to be a new headache or worsening quality of preexisting headache in conjunction with the aforementioned symptoms. If a headache is already present, it should fluctuate in severity with the other somatic symptoms attributed to the somatic disorder. Similarly, if the headache improves, then it should do so in conjunction with the remission of other somatic symptoms.

Psychotic Disorder

Headaches attributed to psychotic disorder involve delusions that patient holds which explains the reason for the headache. Similar to other diagnoses in this area, the headache should develop at the time of or in conjunction with the onset of delusion. As an alternative, if headache resolves after remission of the delusion, the diagnosis may also be used appropriately.

Other Psychiatric Disorders

Headaches attributed to other psychiatric disorders such as depressive disorder, separation anxiety disorder, panic disorder, specific phobia, social anxiety disorder, generalized anxiety disorder, bipolar disorder, or post-traumatic stress disorder involve headaches exclusively in the presence of aforementioned psychiatric disorders with known diagnoses according to DSM-5 criteria. Establishing a temporal association is important, and elucidating whether symptoms fluctuate together is essential.

Psychiatric Comorbidity in Patients with Headache

When the above criteria are not met, the preexisting primary headache and psychiatric disorders must be diagnosed separately. While they may still have significant impact on the individual and occur comorbidly, they cannot be considered a singular condition. In addition, the diagnosis is also established if the headache improves after effective treatment or spontaneous remission of the psychiatric disorder.

Treatment and Prognosis

As in many medical diagnoses, headache due to psychiatric origin is best managed in multidisciplinary settings. The first challenge is often recognizing the condition and ensuring that patients are appropriately referred to expert evaluation with a psychiatrist and/or a psychologist. A diagnostic interview remains the gold standard for establishing diagnoses. While there are some screening scales that may be utilized, they do not serve the same purpose as an appropriate live evaluation. Once an accurate diagnosis is made, it is possible to treat the condition directly, whether through pharmacological or nonpharmacological intervention. There is little evidence established in determining the effective first-line treatment. One may either approach the situation by trying to find a single medication that may be used for both psychiatric disorders and headache, or it may be reasonable to choose the best option for both conditions. For example, for depression, traditional antidepressants, such as tricyclic antidepressants, and noradrenaline reuptake inhibitors (SNRIs) can be used to address both mood instability and migraine or tension-type headache. However, a tricyclic antidepressant may not be the best choice to control mood despite its potential dual purpose. For bipolar disorders, valproic acid may be a treatment of choice as it addresses both mania and migraine. Tricyclic antidepressants may increase the risk of a manic episode in individuals with bipolar disorder. For anxiety disorders, antidepressants and cognitive behavioral therapy can be used.[8]

Addressing a headache attributed to somatization requires a more intensive model where collaborative care with patient and provider, self-management, and cognitive behavioral therapies work together. Insight into the condition is important and may take a long period to establish. Collaborative care can help highlight the importance of patient–provider relationship in that it may contribute to the patient feeling better understood and improve adherence to treatment plans. Such supportive evaluation and careful assessment allow patients to identify their triggers, recognize obstacles to feeling better, and build better coping mechanisms. This will guide patients to plan day-to-day responsibilities of confronting their chronic illnesses. Many literature support such patient-centered approach in initial evaluation and adding on pharmacologic as well as cognitive behavioral therapy to improve physical symptoms that arise from psychological issues.[9-11]

Summary

- Psychiatric disorders and headaches are highly prevalent in the general population.
- Limited research has been conducted on the prevalence of headaches attributed to psychiatric disorders, mainly due to challenges in establishing a causal relationship.
- The pathophysiology of headache in psychiatric disorders likely involves complex networks including serotonin and norepinephrine dysregulation.
- The headaches of psychiatric origin require the presence of psychiatric illnesses and the presence of headache only during worsening of psychiatric episodes.
- Treatment requires a multidisciplinary approach that focuses on managing the primary psychiatric illness to alleviate headaches.

REFERENCES

1. Headache Classification Committee of the International Headache Society (IHS). *The International Classification of Headache Disorders,* 3rd edition. *Cephalalgia.* 2018;38(1):1-211.

2. GBD 2019 Mental Disorders Collaborators. Global, regional, and national burden of 12 mental disorders in 204 countries and territories, 1990-2019: a systematic analysis for the global burden of disease study 2019. *Lancet Psychiatry.* 2022;9:137-150.

3. Stovner LJ, Hagen K, Linde M, et al. The global prevalence of headache: an update, with analysis of the influences of methodological factors on prevalence estimates. *J Headache Pain.* 2022;23:34.

4. Breslau N, Lipton RB, Stewart WF, Schultz LR, Welch KM. Comorbidity of migraine and depression: investigating potential etiology and prognosis. *Neurology.* 2003;60(8):1308-1312.

5. Serrano D, Buse DC, Manack Adams A, Reed ML, Lipton RB. Acute treatment optimization in episodic and chronic migraine: results of the American Migraine Prevalence and Prevention (AMPP) study. *Headache.* 2015;55(4):502-518.

6. Kim BK, Cho SJ, Kim BS, et al. Comprehensive application of *the international classification of headache disorders* third edition, beta version. *J Korean Med Sci.* 2016;31:106-113.

7. Oakes P, Loukas M, Oskouian RJ, Tubbs RS. The neuroanatomy of depression: a review. *Clin Anat.* 2017;30(1):44-49.

8. Vaidiya N, Welch KM. Headache attributed to psychiatric disorder. In Olesen J, ed. *The Headaches.* Philadelphia, PA: Linppincott Williams & Wilkins; 2006.

9. Gonzales GR. Central pain: diagnosis and treatment strategies. *Neurology.* 1995;45(Supp 9): S11-S16.

10. Edwards T. The treatment of patients with medically unexplained symptoms in primary care; a review of literature. *Ment Health Fam Med.* 2010;7:209-221.

11. Lipchik GL, Smitherman TA, Penzien DB, Holroyd KA. Basic principles and techniques of cognitive-behavioral therapies for comorbid psychiatric symptoms among headache patients. *Headache: The Journal of Head and Face Pain.* 2006;46: S119-S132.

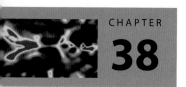

Headache and Dysautonomia

38

Karissa Arca

Autonomic dysfunction, also known as dysautonomia, is a common cause of headache or may coexist with primary or secondary headache disorders. However, it is often underrecognized due to the limited availability of autonomic testing and specialists in the field. One type of dysautonomia, postural orthostatic tachycardia syndrome (POTS), is relatively common and is strongly associated with migraine. The autonomic nervous system (ANS) comprises central and peripheral components. The central autonomic network (CAN) consists of several key areas of the brain, including the anterior and midcingulate cortex, insular cortex, amygdala, hypothalamus, periaqueductal gray, parabrachial nucleus, nucleus of the solitary tract, ventrolateral medulla, and medullary raphe. These areas of the brain are responsible for regulating visceral activity such as gastrointestinal, genitourinary, respiratory, and cardiac functions, as well as maintaining homeostasis.[1] The ANS is divided into the parasympathetic and sympathetic nervous systems, both of which consist of preganglionic neurons located in the brainstem (parasympathetic), intermediolateral cell column in the thoracolumbar spinal cord (sympathetic), and sacral spinal cord (parasympathetic). Postganglionic neurons innervate various effector organs such as the lacrimal and salivary glands, pupils, heart, bladder, adrenal medulla, sweat glands, and gut, utilizing neurotransmitters such as norepinephrine or acetylcholine, among others.[1] Blood pressure is regulated by the baroreflex which modulates heart rate and vascular tone. The nucleus tractus solitarius (NTS) regulates sympathetic and parasympathetic tone, thereby controlling blood pressure. Damage to the afferent portion of the baroreflex can result in severe blood pressure lability with hypertensive crises, as well as orthostatic hypotension, tachycardia, and bradycardia. Conversely, failure of the efferent portion of the baroreflex can result in orthostatic hypotension.[1]

Epidemiology

The prevalence of POTS is not well established, primarily due to the absence of robust epidemiologic studies. However, it is estimated to affect at least 0.2% to 1% of the population in the United States.[2] Among individuals with POTS, headache is a commonly reported symptom, with a prevalence ranging from 41% to 96%. These headaches can be either primary, such as migraine, or secondary, as seen in spontaneous intracranial hypotension (SIH). However, many studies only report "headache" without specifying the type.

In a recent meta-analysis, the pooled prevalence of migraine in individuals with POTS was reported to be 36.8%.[2] Unfortunately, information on the epidemiology of migraine in other forms of dysautonomia is not currently available.

Proposed Pathophysiology of Headache-Related Autonomic Dysfunction

There is still much to be learned about the pathophysiology of headache associated with autonomic disorders. The CAN is integral to this understanding. POTS has traditionally been viewed as a disorder that affects the peripheral ANS, except for postconcussive autonomic dysfunction. However, findings of cerebral hypoperfusion in patients with POTS suggest that the CAN may also be affected.[3] The pathophysiology of migraine, particularly its premonitory phase, is intricately linked to the CAN. This connection may shed light on the high comorbidity between migraine and disorders of the ANS.

Epidural venous hypotension may provide a potential link between hypovolemic POTS and orthostatic headache, particularly in those that have no neuroimaging signs of a CSF leak. It has been proposed that low pressure in the inferior vena cava, which may be due to a hypovolemic state, will drive the flow of spinal fluid into the epidural space and veins, following a pressure gradient.[4] Connective tissue disorders such as benign joint hypermobility and Ehlers Danlos syndrome that are prevalent in patients with POTS may increase the risk for this phenomena.

Clinical Presentation of Autonomic Disorders and Associated Headache

When evaluating a patient with headache, symptoms that may indicate the presence of an autonomic disorder as an exacerbating factor or cause of the headache include the location of the head pain (e.g., coat-hanger distribution), aggravation of headache when in an upright position with significant improvement or resolution when supine, the presence of new daily persistent headache (NDPH), and other symptoms of either orthostatic intolerance or autonomic dysfunction that coincide with the onset or worsening of headache.

POTS is defined as a sustained postural rise in heart rate of at least 30 beats per minute in adults and 40 beats per minute in children and adolescents, over a period of 10 minutes. To meet consensus criteria for POTS, orthostatic hypotension must be absent, and the patient must also exhibit symptoms of orthostatic intolerance such as lightheadedness, palpitations, breathlessness, presyncope, or syncope, which are relieved by assuming a seated or supine position. The symptoms must be present for at least 6 months, and other potential causes or mimics of postural tachycardia must be ruled out.[5] POTS is a heterogenous disorder that can coexist with several other medical conditions, including autoimmune and connective tissue diseases, Ehlers-Danlos syndrome, migraine, and autism spectrum disorder. It may also develop as a consequence of viral or bacterial infections or concussion. On the other hand, several disorders may mimic POTS, including anemia, thyroid dysfunction, mastocytosis, adrenal dysfunction, catecholamine-secreting tumors, and panic disorder.[6] Moreover, POTS linked to cerebrospinal fluid (CSF) leak has also been reported.[4] In a retrospective study of pediatric patients with POTS, five different types of headache were reported in 114 patients: migraine (43%), nonspecific headache (22%), chronic daily headache (14%), NDPH (4%), and orthostatic headache (2%).[7] While POTS is more common in individuals with chronic migraine, the manifestation of orthostatic headache may warrant additional investigation for SIH. POTS and SIH can both present with orthostatic/postural headache. While there are limited studies that offer a detailed description of headache in POTS, the prevalence of orthostatic headache appears to be higher in SIH.[4] The overlapping symptomatology of orthostatic/postural headache in POTS and SIH can pose a diagnostic challenge, and these conditions can coexist. The lack of extensive research on the relationship between POTS and SIH means that there are no distinct headache features that aid in differentiating the two conditions.

Headache associated with orthostatic hypotension is included in the appendix of the third edition of the *International Classification of Headache Disorders* (ICHD-3). This headache typically involves the occiput, neck, and shoulders in a "coat-hanger" distribution. Headache must occur in the upright position and resolve in the supine position.[8] Orthostatic hypotension is defined as a persistent decrease of systolic blood pressure of at least 20 mm Hg and diastolic blood pressure of 10 mm Hg within 3 minutes after standing with associated symptoms of orthostatic intolerance.[5] Autonomic disorders like autonomic neuropathy or multiple system atrophy are not always the underlying cause of orthostatic hypotension; it can also occur due to hypovolemia, medication effect, and cardiac conditions. It has been suggested in one study that a greater degree of orthostatic hypotension correlates with a higher frequency of neck pain.[9] While ischemia of the neck muscles has been a long-standing hypothesis for headache in orthostatic hypotension, it is likely more complex and involves perivascular nociceptors in the posterior fossa.[4]

Baroreflex failure and autonomic dysreflexia can both result in episodes of hypertension and associated headache. Baroreflex failure occurs when there is damage to any part of the afferent baroreflex pathway, often due to neck surgeries, trauma, or radiation. Blood pressure lability occurs acutely when it is the result of trauma or surgery, or in a delayed fashion in the setting of head/neck radiation. In this disorder, headache can occur in the setting of hypotension or hypertension, though hypertensive episodes are more characteristic of baroreflex failure. The specific headache features are not well characterized but physical or mental stressors, including physical exertion, may be triggers.[4]

Autonomic dysreflexia is a condition that occurs in patients with spinal cord injuries at or above T6 which results in impaired communication between ascending and descending autonomic neurons.[4] The specific headache phenotype associated with this condition is recognized in the ICHD-3 and occurs as a sudden-onset headache associated with systolic blood pressure ≥ 30 mm Hg and/or diastolic pressure is ≥ 20 mm Hg from baseline.[8] The location of the head pain is variable, but quality tends to be throbbing. Other associated symptoms include anxiety, diaphoresis and flushing above the level of the spinal cord injury, and pallor below the level of injury. Blood pressure spikes tend to occur due to bowel or bladder fullness or pain.[4]

Diagnosis of Autonomic Disorders

Accurate diagnosis of an autonomic disorder requires a detailed history outlining orthostatic symptoms, as well as symptoms affecting other organ systems under the control of the ANS. A review of the ANS should include a query of dry eyes and mouth, blurred vision when adjusting to ambient light, dysphagia, abdominal bloating, early satiety, diarrhea, constipation, urinary retention, orthostatic lightheadedness, presyncope, syncope, and dry or itchy skin. A thorough neurologic examination should be conducted for all patients, with specific areas of attention including pupillary responses to light, detailed sensorimotor evaluation for signs of peripheral neuropathy, assessment of joint hypermobility using the Beighton scale, and orthostatic vitals.

When an underlying autonomic disorder is suspected based on the patient's history and exam, a diagnosis can be confirmed with various tests of the ANS. The most comprehensive test is the autonomic reflex screen (ARS), which measures postganglionic sympathetic sudomotor, cardiovagal, and cardiac adrenergic function. This four-part test involves iontophoresis of acetylcholine to retroactively stimulate a sweat response, deep breathing to measure inspiratory and expiratory changes in heart rate, measurements of heart rate and blood pressure responses to the Valsalva maneuver, and during 10-minute head-up tilt at 70°. Depending on the patient's clinical presentation, a combination of diagnostic tools may be used to better understand the extent and severity of autonomic dysfunction, as well as the origin (central or peripheral). The pattern of findings can also help determine the underlying cause of autonomic dysfunction, though this also requires additional laboratory evaluations. Laboratory evaluations are performed to identify a secondary cause of autonomic dysfunction, though the etiology can also be idiopathic. In POTS, it is important to rule out mimics as described previously. Recommended laboratory evaluations for POTS are found in articles listed in the References. Overall, the laboratory evaluation should be tailored to the patient's clinical presentation.

Treatment

There are several lifestyle measures that are recommended as the foundation of treatment for autonomic disorders with symptoms of orthostatic intolerance. For the treatment of orthostatic intolerance, the following measures are recommended: water intake of 2.5 to 3 L daily (half containing electrolytes), salt (NaCl) intake up to 10 g daily, use of compression garments and physical countermeasure maneuvers to prevent venous pooling, sleeping at an incline with the head of bed elevated, and a regular exercise routine including resistance training and aerobic reconditioning.[6] Some of these measures, excluding exercise and sleeping at an incline, may also improve symptoms of orthostatic headache due to SIH in a subset of patients.

Pharmacotherapy may be necessary for some patients with autonomic disorders to reduce symptoms of orthostatic intolerance. In patients with postural tachycardia, the goal is to lower heart rate, increase blood volume or vascular tone, and alleviate central and/or peripheral sympathetic tone. Patients with orthostatic hypotension will benefit from increased blood volume and medications that augment sympathetic tone. Beta-blockers are the main pharmacologic category of medications used to lower heart rate, but ivabradine, which exhibits its effect at the sinoatrial node, may be preferable in some patients to avoid the potential blood pressure-lowering effects of beta-blockade. In patients with POTS and migraine, beta-blockers may reduce migraine frequency and severity; however, the doses with established efficacy for migraine prevention are higher than what is recommended for the treatment of POTS. Augmenting blood pressure with an alpha-1 agonist such as midodrine or mineralocorticoid such as fludrocortisone should improve or resolve headache due to orthostatic hypotension. These medications can cause side effects such as headache, and it should be noted that pharmacological blood pressure augmentation can result in supine hypertension, which may also cause headache and require dose adjustments to prevent hypertensive complications.[6]

Prognosis

Autonomic disorders are typically chronic and may be progressive in nature. POTS is a chronic and fluctuating condition, and long-term prognosis has not been well studied. While some data suggests that patients tend to improve over time, this is not the case for all individuals and requires further investigation. The prognosis for headache in patients with POTS is even less understood, especially since headache may be primary or secondary in nature. Chronic migraine in patients with POTS may be more refractory to treatment. However, anecdotally, some patients may experience improvement in headache once orthostatic intolerance is better controlled. Earlier recognition of POTS as a potential etiology for orthostatic headache can significantly improve treatment outcomes and quality of life for patients.

Summary

- Migraine pathophysiology is innately linked to the CAN which may explain its association with disorders of the ANS.
- Orthostatic headache is more common in patients with SIH but may also be a prominent symptom in POTS.
- Baroreflex failure and autonomic dysreflexia can result in hypertensive attacks with associated headache.
- Treatment for POTS and other disorders of orthostatic intolerance should start with lifestyle measures.
- In patients with POTS and migraine, the use of low-dose beta-blockers may be preferred to treat both conditions.

REFERENCES

1. Benarroch EE. Physiology and pathophysiology of the autonomic nervous system. *Continuum (Minneap Minn)*. 2020;26(1):12-24.
2. Ray JC, Pham X, Foster E, et al. The prevalence of headache disorders in postural tachycardia syndrome: a systematic review and meta-analysis of the literature. *Cephalalgia: An International Journal of Headache*. 2022;42(11-12):1274-1287.
3. Blitshteyn S. Is postural orthostatic tachycardia syndrome (POTS) a central nervous system disorder? *J Neurol*. 2022;269(2):725-732.

Secondary Headaches

4. Iser C, Arca K. Headache and autonomic dysfunction: a review. *Curr Neurol Neurosci Rep.* 2022;22(10):625-634.

5. Freeman R, Wieling W, Axelrod FB, et al. Consensus statement on the definition of orthostatic hypotension, neurally mediated syncope and the postural tachycardia syndrome. *Auton Neurosci.* 2011;161(1-2):46-48.

6. Vernino S, Bourne KM, Stiles LE, et al. Postural orthostatic tachycardia syndrome (POTS): state of the science and clinical care from a 2019 National Institutes of Health Expert Consensus Meeting - Part 1. *Auton Neurosci.* 2021;235:102828.

7. Staples A, Thompson NR, Moodley M. Pediatric-onset postural orthostatic tachycardia syndrome in a single tertiary care center. *J Child Neurol.* 2020;35(8):526-635.

8. Headache Classification Committee of the International Headache Society (IHS) *The International Classification of Headache Disorders*, 3rd edition. *Cephalalgia.* 2018;38(1):1-211.

9. Bleasdale-Barr KM, Mathias CJ. Neck and other muscle pains in autonomic failure: their association with orthostatic hypotension. *J R Soc Med.* 1998;91(7):355-359.

PART IV

Facial Pain and Cranial Neuralgias

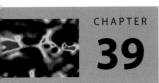

CHAPTER

39

Trigeminal Neuralgia

Hossein Ansari and Lars Bendtsen

Neuralgia, by definition, manifests as a transient paroxysmal episode characterized by electric, shock-like pain. When neuralgia occurs within the distribution of the fifth cranial nerve or trigeminal nerve, it is termed trigeminal neuralgia (TN), colloquially known as "tic douloureux."[1] TN is a debilitating neuropathic pain disorder. The pain associated with TN can exhibit an unpredictable pattern of remission, with periods lasting for months or even years, especially during the initial stages of the disease and among younger individuals.

Epidemiology

Prevalence of TN in the general population ranges from 0.03% to 0.3%.[2] This wide range of prevalence is likely attributed to diagnostic uncertainty surrounding TN and variations in diagnostic criteria used by different subspecialties. In 90% of cases, symptoms begin after age 40.[2] Incidence progressively increases with age, from 17.5 per 100,000/year between 60 and 69 years of age up to 25.6 per 100,000/year after age 70. The average age of onset was reported to be 53 to 57 years.[3] It has female predominance with 3:1-2. There are no reports of racial or geographic differences accounting for TN incidence. Familial cases of TN are even rarer, comprising about 1% to 2% of all cases. Certain patient populations are at higher risk for TN development. As far as neurological disorders are concerned, it is well documented that the incidence of TN in multiple sclerosis (MS) patients is higher than that within the general population. Overall, 2% to 8% of TN patients have MS, which is 20-fold higher than in the general population. Bilateral TN in patients with MS is more common compared to other types of TN.[4]

Pathophysiology

The trigeminal nerve (CN V) originates from pons and has three divisions: ophthalmic (V1), maxillary (V2), and mandibular (V3) (Chapter 4). It provides sensory innervation to most of the face, gums, and both motor and sensory supply to the muscles of mastication.

It is important to note that areas such as the posterior third of the scalp, the outer ear (excluding the tragus), and the skin overlying the angle of the mandible are not innervated by the trigeminal nerve. The area of the pons where the trigeminal nerve originates is called the trigeminal entry zone (TEZ), which has a rich vasculature. The superior cerebellar artery, anterior inferior cerebellar artery, vertebral artery, and petrosal vein are adjacent to the TEZ, and often come into contact with it. As individuals age, structural changes in the brain, such as sagging, may occur, leading to potential compression of the nerve at the TEZ by adjacent arteries or veins. If compression is severe or prolonged, injury to myelin sheath at the TEZ can ensue, and the nerve may even experience displacement or morphological changes including atrophy. Compression of trigeminal nerve at TEZ by one of the aforementioned vessels is referred to as a "classical" TN.

Since the most common risk factor for this vascular compression is age, "classical" TN is most common in people over the age of 40.[5] In the area of compression, demyelination plus dysmyelination and subsequent remyelination occurs. The injury to the myelin sheath causes ectopic impulse generation, which leads to electric shock attacks, known as "neuralgia." TEZ is the area that peripheral Schwann cell myelination to central oligodendroglia myelination transition takes place. This is probably the reason for TEZ susceptibility to pressure by adjacent blood vessels. The fibers that form the trigeminal nerve are classified into nociceptive fibers (myelinated Aδ and unmyelinated C fibers) and low-threshold mechanoreceptors (Aα and Aβ fibers).[6] In the trigeminal nerve, the proportion of unmyelinated/myelinated fibers is much lower, compared to spinal nerves. Ephaptic connections between demyelinated Aβ and Aδ fibers might provide the mechanism for touch-evoked pain, which is clinically known as a "cutaneous" trigger (see next section). On the contrary, injury to the myelin sheath can occur due to other causes, including compression by tumors (meningioma, acoustic neuroma, epidermoid cyst), vascular pathologies (arteriovenous malformation or a saccular aneurysm), or due to a noncompression etiology like demyelination disorders, resulting in "secondary" TN. When there is no vascular compression or secondary etiology identified in patients with TN, it is classified as "idiopathic" TN. Classical and idiopathic TN are sometimes collectively referred to as "primary" TN. With the advancement in imaging modalities, some cases currently classified as "idiopathic" TN may be classified as secondary TN in the future. Molecular mechanisms of TN are largely unknown. Proinflammatory cytokines (e.g., IL-1beta, TNF-alpha) may play a role in immune response and sensitization of trigeminal ganglion neurons, potentially linking inflammation to pain reactions and explaining earlier vascular compression susceptibility in autoimmune disorders and younger TN onset.

Clinical Characteristics, Classification, and Diagnosis

Diagnosis of TN is clinical. A comprehensive assessment involving a detailed history, preferably using a standard questionnaire, and neurological as well as orofacial examination allows physicians to establish the diagnosis before ordering additional tests or imaging.

Abrupt onset and termination of each paroxysm are distinctive symptoms. Pain attacks are often triggered by innocuous stimuli, including even a "gentle touch." This "stimulus-evoked attack" is characteristic of TN with high diagnostic value.[7] The lack of "cutaneous trigger" should question the diagnosis of TN. Other common triggers include talking, eating, chewing, washing the face, brushing teeth, shaving, a cool breeze, blowing the nose, kissing, and sometimes hot or cold beverages. Most patients have several triggers, both intraoral and extraoral, which usually correspond to the area of pain.

Pain attacks can occur several times per day, depending on triggers. The frequency, duration, and severity of pain often vary considerably over time with periods with full or partial remission and other periods with intense pain. Up to 50% of patients report persistent and constant underlying pain between their paroxysmal attacks.[3] This persistent pain is much less intense compared to paroxysmal attacks and is often described as a dull, burning pain rather than sharp, electric shock-like. Therefore, the *International Classification of Headache Disorders*, third edition (ICHD-3), classifies the classical and idiopathic TN into two subtypes: TN, purely paroxysmal, and TN, with concomitant continuous pain (see Box 39-1).[8] The International Association for the Study of Pain (IASP) has its own classification for TN. Although this classification differs from ICHD in format, the two classifications are

Box 39-1. ICHD-3 Diagnostic Criteria for TN

Recurrent paroxysms of unilateral facial pain in the distribution(s) of one or more divisions of the trigeminal nerve, with no radiation beyond, and fulfilling criteria B and C:

A. Pain has all of the following characteristics:
  1. *Lasting from a fraction of a second to 2 minutes*
  2. *Severe intensity*
  3. *Electric shock-like, shooting, stabbing or sharp in quality*
B. Precipitated by innocuous stimuli within the affected trigeminal distribution[4]

C. Not better accounted for by another ICHD-3 diagnosis

Classical TN

TN developing without apparent cause other than neurovascular compression:

I. **Purely paroxysmal:** Classical TN without persistent background facial pain
II. **With concomitant continuous pain:** Classical TN with persistent background facial pain

Idiopathic TN

TN with neither electrophysiological tests nor MRI showing significant abnormalities:

I. **Purely paroxysmal:** Pain-free between attacks in the affected trigeminal distribution
II. **With concomitant continuous pain:** Concomitant continuous or near-continuous pain between attacks in the affected trigeminal distribution

similar with regard to the clinical characteristics required for diagnosis. The presence of any red flags in the history and exam should question the diagnosis of TN (see Box 39-2). Due to possible overlap with other neuropathic and neuralgiform headache and orofacial pain disorders, TN might be mistaken with the other conditions (see Box 39-3 for differential diagnosis).

Box 39-2. Red Flags in the Diagnosis of TN

Absence of cutaneous trigger

Abnormal neurological finding(s) like diplopia or papilledema

Age of onset less than 40 years (except for secondary TN)

Bilateral symptoms (except for TN due to MS)

Pain radiates outside of trigeminal distribution

Prominent sensory symptoms (tingling or numbness) of trigeminal nerve

Presence of photophobia and phonophobia

Poor response to therapeutic dose of carbamazepine/oxcarbazepine

Prominent ipsilateral autonomic symptoms like lacrimation, nasal congestion

Pain associated with photophobia and phonophobia

Pain associated with vertigo, tinnitus, or hearing loss

Pain attacks lasting >2 minutes

Presence of objective facial muscle spasm

Pain exclusively localized to V1

Facial Pain and Cranial Neuralgias

Box 39-3. Differential Diagnosis of TN

Other cranial neuralgia, e.g., glossopharyngeal neuralgia, nervus intermedius neuralgia

Trigeminal autonomic cephalalgia, particularly SUNT/SUNA subtypes

Painful trigeminal neuropathy, e.g., post–herpetic neuralgia

Trigeminal neuropathy due to autoimmune disorders, e.g., Sjogren syndrome

Dental disorder, e.g., traumatic trigeminal neuropathy, pulpitis

Temporomandibular joint disorder

Salivary gland disorders, e.g., infection or stone

Paranasal sinus pathology

Persistent idiopathic facial pain

Primary stabbing headache

After the "clinical diagnosis" of TN has been made, further investigations for clarifying the TN type (classical, idiopathic, or secondary) need to be pursued, since these three forms of TN may be clinically indistinguishable (Figure 39-1). Evaluation of TN might involve clinicians in diverse fields of medicine, including neurology, neuroradiology, neurosurgery, dentistry, maxillofacial surgery, and specialists in pain medicine. MRI is the modality of choice for evaluation of TN, which can be performed with or without gadolinium contrast (Chapter 2). However, what is important is doing high-resolution MRI with dedicated protocol for evaluation of cranial nerve V. This protocol is called "Steady-State Free Precession" (SSFP).[9] SSFP sequences are often referred to by their vendor-specific acronyms:

- Fast Imaging Employing Steady-State Acquisition (FIESTA), *GE Healthcare*
- Constructive Interference Steady State (CISS), *Siemens Healthcare*

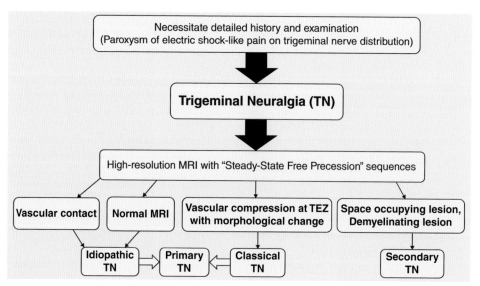

Figure 39-1. Summary of diagnostic steps of trigeminal neuralgia with three subtypes: classical, idiopathic and secondary.

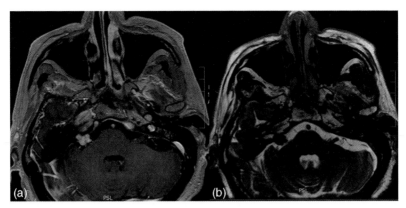

Figure 39-2. MRI brain with contrast of 79-year-old male with right-sided TN. (a) Homogenously enhancing mass on the right cerebellopontine angle, more likely a meningioma, schwannoma, or other rarer tumors. (b) FIESTA sequences reveal that the caudal part of this tumor is causing some pressure on the inferior aspect of TEZ, which is the cause of this patient's TN.

MRI sections as thin as 1 mm can be taken in a coronal plane without any skips in between the images. By using this method, the imaging of the entire course of the trigeminal nerve can be obtained, and the offending vessel causing potential compression can be identified. MRI can be done using either 3.0 Tesla (T) or 1.5 T MRI, but neurovascular compression is more clearly delineated with the 3.0 T resolution. Since for some of the secondary TN, like tumors, gadolinium contrast is needed (Figure 39-2), we recommend doing high-resolution, three-dimensional (3D) MRI in patients with TN including the following sequences:

1. T2-weighted (coronal, axial, and sagittal views);
2. Time-of-flight (TOF) and MR angiography (MRA); and
3. T1-weighted images with gadolinium.

This is standard protocol for TN, which has proved to be reliable in detecting vascular contact versus compression of TEZ to differentiate between classic, idiopathic, and secondary TN. Sometimes 3D TOF MRA is another useful sequence, which can help visualize the offending vessels; therefore, it is recommended as part of the standard trigeminal nerve MRI protocol in most institutions. It is critical that ordering providers be familiar with the stared protocol, since as discussed above, this is different from a regular brain MRI. More importantly, the interpretation of MRI should be done with physicians who are familiar with this protocol, since neurovascular contact or even slight compression is a normal finding. Neurovascular compression, which causes TN, is often associated with displacement or morphological change of the trigeminal nerve (Figures 39-3 and 39-4). If MRI is contraindicated, CT scan with contrast can help to rule out tumor or vascular malformation (such as arteriovenous malformation). In addition, electrophysiological studies (trigeminal reflexes) can be helpful, for example, abnormal trigeminal evoked potentials are more likely associated with an increased risk of secondary TN.

Treatment

When we outline the treatment plan for patients with TN, several factors must be taken into consideration. These include the type of TN, age, general health conditions and underlying disorders, the patients' other medication use, severity of disease, and finally, patient preference.

In general, pharmacologic treatment is the first line in primary TN.[12,13] However, threshold for procedural treatment is lower in classical TN, depending on patients' choice and availability of well-trained physicians to perform the procedures. On the other hand, treatment of secondary TN, based on the etiology, varies.

Facial Pain and Cranial Neuralgias

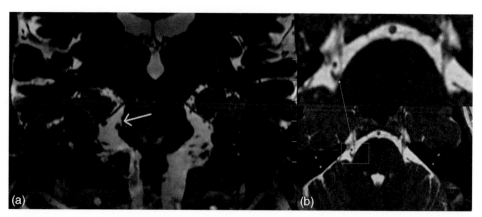

Figure 39-3. A 57-year-old female with classical right TN. (a) Coronal FIESTA MRI shows compression of right trigeminal nerve by superior cerebellar artery with deformity of the nerve (arrow). (b) Axial FIESTA MRI of the same patient, with magnification of TEZ (rectangle), shows compression and displacement of trigeminal nerve (arrow).

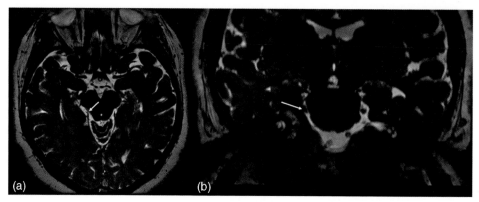

Figure 39-4. FIESTA MRI of a 35-year-old female with right-sided TN. (a) Axial image: arrow shows the abutment of the root exit zone of the right trigeminal nerve by a collateral vein extending from the right inferior petrosal sinus. (b) Coronal image: The vein appears to contour the lateral margin of the proximal right trigeminal nerve (arrow).

Pharmacologic Treatment

The most commonly used medications for treatment of TN are anticonvulsant drugs, which potentially block the "sodium channel."[10] Carbamazepine is highly effective in reducing TN pain symptoms, and the onset of effects on pain paroxysms is generally very rapid. In fact, a lack of response to carbamazepine is regarded as an indicator that warrants caution when diagnosing TN (see Box 39-2). It is noteworthy to note that while a positive response to carbamazepine is suggestive of TN, it does not conclusively confirm the diagnosis, as this medication can also be efficacious in treating various other neuropathic pain conditions. In order to reduce any side effects and increase patient adherence, carbamazepine should be started at a low dose, and the dose is gradually increased until it controls the pain. It controls pain for most people in the early stages of the disease. However, in patients with Asian ancestry, prior to commencing carbamazepine therapy, it is recommended to conduct HLA-B*15:02 allele testing, as the presence of this allele is associated with an elevated risk of developing toxic epidermal necrolysis or Stevens-Johnson syndrome.[11] Effective dose of carbamazepine for TN normally ranges between 200 and 1800 mg, which can be taken in two, three, or four divided doses, based on the type of the available product. Carbamazepine use can be associated with various hypersensitivity reactions, spanning from mild maculopapular exanthemas to severe conditions such as Stevens-Johnson syndrome and toxic epidermal necrolysis. In addition, common side effects of carbamazepine can be drowsiness, dizziness, ataxia, double vision, and nausea. It is also important to note that hyponatremia, renal toxicity, and hepatic toxicity are potential adverse effects of this medication.

Oxcarbazepine, another "sodium channel" blocker with a chemical structure similar to carbamazepine, but with different metabolism, is being increasingly used as first-line therapy for TN, particularly due to lack of auto-induction property, plus a shorter and narrower half-life. In addition, oxcarbazepine has fewer side effects and is generally better tolerated. Possible side effects include double vision and dizziness. It can also cause hyponatremia, which sometimes occurs faster than with carbamazepine. It should also be avoided in patients with HLA-B*15:02 allele. Dose range of oxcarbazepine for TN is normally between 300 and 2400 mg but sometimes higher. Similar to carbamazepine, oxcarbazepine also needs to be titrated slowly and used in two to four divided doses per day depends on the type of available product (short-acting or extended release).

In case of insufficient efficacy or side effects it is recommended to switch between carbamazepine and oxcarbazepine, since efficacy and tolerability of the two drugs can differ from patient to patient. In this circumstance, the ratio is 2:3. For example, 400 mg of carbamazepine is equipotent to 600 mg of oxcarbazepine.

Beside "sodium channel" blockers, potential "calcium channel" blockers, like gabapentin and pregabalin, have been shown to be effective in controlling the pain of TN. These agents are considered as second-line treatment and are usually used in patients who did not tolerate first-line treatment, either as monotherapy or as add-on treatment. Similar to oxcarbazepine and carbamazepine, these medications also need to start slowly and titrate up. An effective dose of gabapentin for TN is between 600 and 3600 mg per day. Most patients need at least 900 mg to be effective and doses higher than 3600 mg are rarely tolerated. Therefore, in practice, a dose range would be between 900 and 3600 mg. This needs to be taken in three to four divided doses, unless the patient is using an extended release formulation of gabapentin which can be taken once daily. Effective dose of pregabalin for TN ranges between 150 and 600 mg per day in two to three divided doses. Common side effects of these two drugs are relatively similar and include tiredness, somnolence, dizziness, gastrointestinal symptoms, balance issue, and peripheral edema. In addition, they can increase the appetite and cause weight gain which can sometimes be a major limiting factor for using this medication.

Other agents that show to be effective in TN include:

- Lamotrigine: It is an antiepileptic agent with sodium channel blockage property. Recommended dose for TN is 100 to 400 mg per day (with slow titration) in two divided doses. Common side effects are rash, tiredness, dizziness, ataxia, and nausea.

- Fosphenytoin. A recent prospective study demonstrated that intravenous fosphenytoin, 20 mg per kilo bodyweight as loading, followed by short-term oral phenytoin, 5 mg per kilo bodyweight, is effective for acute exacerbations in most patients.[10] Long-term treatment with oral phenytoin is rarely used because of side effects.

- Baclofen is a muscle relaxant, which with the dose of 15 to 100 mg, in three divided doses, has been effective in some TN patients. Side effects include dizziness, sedation, and dyspepsia.

- Medication which blocks calcitonin gene-related peptide (CGRP) or its receptor, including monoclonal antibodies or oral agents (gepants), has been reported effective in case series. However, a recent placebo-controlled trial clearly demonstrated that erenumab, which blocks the CGRP receptor, has absolutely no effect in TN.[12]

- Clonazepam had been used during the acute phase of TN pain and titration of main therapy.

- Other antiepileptics like valproic acid and topiramate have not been shown to be effective and therefore are not recommended.

Facial Pain and Cranial Neuralgias

Procedural/Surgical Treatment

It has been suggested that before surgery is offered, carbamazepine and oxcarbazepine should be tested, with the best of these drugs then combined with either gabapentin, pregabalin, or lamotrigine. Decision on referral should also take into account possible degree of neurovascular compression and patient preference.[13,14] There are no sham-controlled or comparative trials on any interventional or surgical procedures in TN patients. These treatments can be divided into destructive and nondestructive procedure:

1. Destructive procedures:

   a. Invasive destructive procedures: These procedures involve controlled lesioning of the trigeminal ganglion or root (distracting), thereby interrupting the pain transmission signals to the brain. Four main destructive procedures are:

      - Rhizotomy with thermo-coagulation uses an electrode to apply heat to damage the nerve fibers.

      - Chemical injection involves injecting the chemical glycerol into the trigeminal nerve.

      - Mechanical balloon compression: Balloon compression involves inserting a tiny balloon to the point of location of nerve fibers and then inflate the balloon to damage the trigeminal nerve fibers.

      - Peripheral neurectomy and nerve block have been performed on peripheral branches of the trigeminal nerve like the supraorbital, infraorbital, lingual, and the alveolar nerves. This can be accomplished by alcohol injection, incision, cryotherapy, or radiofrequency lesioning. There are very sparse data on efficacy of these procedures. Due to destruction of nerve fibers, complications like postoperative dysesthesia, corneal numbness, sensory loss in trigeminal nerve distribution, and anesthesia dolorosa can occur following these procedures. Since these complications sometimes could be even worse than the TN pain, use of these procedures needs to be the last option.

   b. Noninvasive destructive procedures (Radiosurgery): This procedure involves using radiosurgery instrumentation wherein a highly concentrated dose of ionizing radiation is delivered to a precise target at the trigeminal nerve root. The radiation creates a lesion near the nerve root, thereby interrupting the pain signals from transmission to the brain. The formation of the lesion can be slow, and hence the pain relief using this procedure is delayed by up to several weeks or months. Similar to invasive procedures, complications like facial sensory loss and paresthesia can occur although with lower incidence plus no evidence of anesthesia dolorosa has been reposted in this procedure. Since this is one of the least invasive procedures, it can be repeated in patients who have a recurrence of pain.

2. Nondestructive procedures: Microvascular decompression (MVD) is one of the most common procedures used to treat TN. This is beneficial for patients with TN, where vascular compression, with nerve displacement or morphological change of the nerve root (based on MRI), is the cause.[15] This involves craniotomy and posterior fossa exploration for identifying and moving the blood vessel that is compressing the trigeminal nerve. A soft cushion is then inserted between the nerve and the vessel to allow the nerve to recover, which eventually relieves the pain. The first prospective study performed by independent observers recently demonstrated high efficacy of MVD with 86% of patients having good outcome after 2 years' follow-up. In most patients, this procedure can result in sustained pain relief for greater than 10 years. The long-term effectives of MVD seems to be less in patients with venous compression and therefore utility of MVD in these patients is controversial. Though MVD is the most effective procedure, it is also the most invasive. Some of the complications associated with it are decreased hearing, cerebellar hematoma, cerebrospinal fluid (CSF) leaks, infarction, and

facial weakness. It is believed to be the most effective long-term surgical treatment available currently for patients with TN and, therefore, in patients with classical TN, it should be offered as first-line procedural option. Utility of MVD in patients with idiopathic TN is not well established and is not recommended as a first-line treatment option.

Other nondestructive procedures: Botulinum toxin injections can be beneficial for some patients, who are refractory to medical therapy or who cannot tolerate medical therapy due to its side effects.[16] There is no standard protocol or dose for it. In practice, doses ranging between 25 and 100 units have shown efficacy. Injections are mostly subcutaneous and transdermal rather than intramuscular, which injects in the grid pattern. Facial asymmetry and aesthetic complications are the most common issues associated with this injection. Since injection for TN is very different from injection for migraine and there is no standard protocol, injection technique and dosage will be a major determining factor in its success rate.

Prognosis

The course of TN is variable. It usually does have cycles of recurrences and remissions. Some patients may have severe pain for episodes lasting weeks or months, followed by pain-free intervals. Spontaneous prognosis is not known, but it has been demonstrated that the prognosis is good after 2 years of treatment when patients are managed by TN specialists with approximately 50% of patients having the burden of pain reduced by more than 50%.[17]

Summary

- TN is a severely painful condition that can cause a high degree of disability.
- Prevalence of TN is approximately 0.15% with symptoms often starting at age 50-60 or perhaps better with the fifties.
- TN may be caused by dysmyelination of the nerve by compression from a vessel or a tumor or by multiple sclerosis leading to ectopic nerve impulses perceived by the patient as electric shock like pains.
- Accurate diagnosis relies on a detailed patient history, thorough examination, and appropriate imaging.
- TN diagnosis is based on the presence of recurrent and shortlasting paroxysms of severe electric shock-like pains in one side of the face triggered by innocous stimuli.
- Effective management of TN include pharmacological therapies mainly sodium channel blocker anti-epileptics and surgical modalities mainly microvascular decompression and destructive procedures.

REFERENCES

1. Ashina S, Robertson CE, Srikiatkhachorn A, et al. Trigeminal neuralgia. *Nat Rev Dis Primers*. 2024;10(1):39.
2. De Toledo IP, Conti Réus J, Fernandes M, et al. Prevalence of trigeminal neuralgia: a systematic review. *J Am Dent Assoc*. 2016;147(7):570-576.e2.
3. Lambru G, Zakrzewska J, Matharu M. Trigeminal neuralgia: a practical guide. *Pract Neurol*. 2021;21(5):392-402.
4. Solaro C, Brichetto G, Amato MP, et al. The prevalence of pain in multiple sclerosis: a multicenter cross-sectional study. *Neurology*. 2004;63(5):919-921.
5. Yadav YR, Nishtha Y, Sonjjay P, Vijay P, Shailendra R, Yatin K. Trigeminal neuralgia. *Asian J Neurosurg*. 2017;12(4):585-597.
6. Love S, Coakham HB. Trigeminal neuralgia: pathology and pathogenesis. *Brain*. 2001;124(Pt 12):2347-2360.

7. Maarbjerg S, Benoliel R. The changing face of trigeminal neuralgia: a narrative review. *Headache*. 2021;61(6):817-837.

8. Headache Classification Committee of the International Headache Society (IHS). *The International Classification of Headache Disorders*, 3rd edition. *Cephalalgia*. 2018; 38:1-211.

9. Hitchon PW, Bathla G, Moritani T, Holland MT, Noeller J, Nourski KV. Predictability of vascular conflict by MRI in trigeminal neuralgia. *Clin Neurol Neurosurg*. 2019;182:171-176.

10. Andersen ASS, Heinskou TB, Asghar MS, et al. Intravenous fosphenytoin as treatment for acute exacerbation of trigeminal neuralgia: a prospective systematic study of 15 patients. *Cephalalgia*. 2022;42(11-12):1138-1147.

11. Dean L. Carbamazepine Therapy and *HLA* Genotype. 2015 Oct 14 [updated 2018 Aug 1]. In: Pratt VM, Scott SA, Pirmohamed M, Esquivel B, Kattman BL, Malheiro AJ, editors. Medical Genetics Summaries [Internet]. Bethesda (MD): National Center for Biotechnology Information (US); 2012.

12. Schott Andersen AS, Maarbjerg S, Noory N, et al. Safety and efficacy of erenumab in patients with trigeminal neuralgia in Denmark: a double-blind, randomised, placebo-controlled, proof-of-concept study. *Lancet Neurol*. 2022;21(11):994-1003.

13. Cruccu G, Di Stefano G, Truini A. Trigeminal neuralgia. *N Engl J Med*. 2020;383:754-762.

14. Bendtsen L, Zakrzewska JM, Abbott J, et al. European Academy of Neurology guideline on trigeminal neuralgia. *Eur J Neurol*. 2019;26(6):831-849.

15. Bendtsen L, Zakrzewska JM, Heinskou TB, et al. Advances in diagnosis, classification, pathophysiology, and management of trigeminal neuralgia. *Lancet Neurol*. 2020;19(9):784-796.

16. Zhang H, Lian Y, Ma Y, et al. Two doses of botulinum toxin type A for the treatment of trigeminal neuralgia: observation of therapeutic effect from a randomized, double-blind, placebo-controlled trial. *J Headache Pain*. 2014;15:65.

17. Heinskou TB, Maarbjerg S, Wolfram F, et al. Favourable prognosis of trigeminal neuralgia when enrolled in a multidisciplinary management program: a two-year prospective real-life study. *J Headache Pain*. 2019;20(1):23.

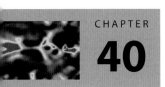

CHAPTER

40

Persistent Idiopathic Facial Pain

Audrey L. Halpern

Persistent idiopathic facial pain (PIFP), formerly termed atypical facial pain, is characterized as chronic facial pain without evidence of structural or other specific causes of pain, and without neurologic deficit, although hypesthesia has been described.[1] It is considered a neuropathic pain syndrome, and treatment considerations generally fall under this category.

Epidemiology

PIFP is more common in women than in men (75-90% of patients), and occurs most commonly between the ages of 30 and 60, with mean age of onset of 40. Population lifetime prevalence is 0.03%. The incidence of PIFP is 4.4 (95% CI: 3.2-5.9) per 100,000 person-years.[2] It may be underrecognized and underdiagnosed. There is a high comorbidity with other forms of headache (43%), migraine (26%), chronic pain (32%), and depression (30%).[3]

Pathophysiology

The abnormal central pain processing has been suggested to be involved in the pathophysiology of PIFP. Activation of the ipsilateral spinal trigeminal nucleus (SpV) occurs in PIFP. Anatomic changes in the area, including gray matter volume reduction, especially pars oralis of SpV using T1-weighted MRI have been demonstrated.[4] Functional MRI of brain during painful stimulation of the trigeminal nerve in patients with PIFP shows increased activation of SpV as compared to control subjects indicating the potentially important role of the SpV as a pain generator in PIFP.[5] The quantitative sensory testing (QST) using thermal stimuli evaluates the function of the small myelinated Aδ and unmyelinated C fibers. Together with neurophysiologic recordings, it increases the sensitivity to detect the trigeminal neuropathy that may underlie facial pain symptoms. Neurophysiologic testing and thermal QST have demonstrated differences in subjects with PIFP when compared to peripheral trigeminal neuropathic pain. Nevertheless, some subjects with PIFP did demonstrate abnormalities in QST, suggesting that there may be different subtypes and, in fact, neurophysiologic testing and QST may help to identify peripheral involvement.[6]

Some features of PIFP are similar to some features of complex regional pain syndromes, including spread beyond a standard nerve distribution and potentially a disproportionate response to mild injury. This would therefore incriminate established mechanisms in typical traumatic neuropathy and other factors, as in complex regional pain syndrome.[7] Neurovascular compression on MRI imaging in PIFP patients may be present but found in equal proportions on both the symptomatic and asymptomatic side. It does not appear that neurovascular compression is the underlying pathophysiology for PIFP.[3]

Facial Pain and Cranial Neuralgias

Clinical Presentation and Diagnosis

The pain of PIFP is poorly localized, achy, dull, pressure, stabbing, or burning, and does not follow a peripheral nerve distribution.[1] PIFP can present a diagnostic challenge due to overlapping symptoms with other disorders, including secondary etiologies. The differential diagnosis includes both primary and secondary disorders involving the face, such as migraine, trigeminal neuralgia (TN), trigeminal autonomic cephalalgias (TACs), central post-stroke pain, temporomandibular joint (TMJ) disorder, traumatic injury, and demyelinating, inflammatory, infectious, and neoplastic diseases.

The character of the pain and the lack of specific nerve distribution clearly differentiate this disorder from TN. The lack of autonomic features differentiates it from TACs; and the duration and pattern of the pain and the pain character differentiate it from neuralgiform headaches and facial pain such as short-lasting unilateral neuralgiform headache with conjunctival injection and tearing (SUNCT), short-lasting unilateral neuralgiform headache with cranial autonomic symptoms (SUNA), and TN. The pain often spreads from one division of the trigeminal nerve to another, and is not typically triggered by touch. There are often sensory complaints associated (>50%), and can be bilateral (13-40%).[3,7] Secondary causes of pain, such as dental issues, trauma, and infection, should be investigated and ruled out. PIFP is a diagnosis of exclusion in the absence of any pathology. The neurological examination should be within normal limits. Diagnostic brain imaging is often needed, and attention to the course of the trigeminal nerve should be indicated. Contact of trigeminal nerve with vascular structures is not typically associated with PIFP. Dental procedures have often already been performed and are not necessarily indications of dental pathology. In fact, many patients have been evaluated by a dentist and are unsure of the order in which the pain developed. Of the patients with PIFP, 99.3% (149/150) had primarily consulted a dentist due to their pain syndrome.[8]

Diagnostic criteria are found in third edition of the *International Classification of Headache Disorders* (ICHD-3) and require the pain to be present for more than 3 months, at least 2 hours per day.[1] The pain may have been initiated by minor trauma, but persists despite the normal healing of the initiating pathology. This may represent a diagnostic dilemma when considering the possible diagnosis of painful post-traumatic trigeminal neuropathy (PTTN) which may rest on a continuum with PIFP.[7] See Box 40-1 for ICHD-3 criteria for PIFP.

Box 40-1. ICHD-3 Diagnostic Criteria for Persistent Idiopathic Facial Pain

Persistent facial and/or oral pain, with varying presentations but recurring daily for more than 2 hours/day over more than 3 months, in the absence of clinical neurological deficit.

A. Facial and/or oral pain fulfilling criteria B and C.
B. Recurring daily for >2 hours/day for >3 months.
C. Pain has both of the following characteristics:
   1. Poorly localized and not following the distribution of a peripheral nerve.
   2. Dull, aching, or nagging quality.
D. Clinical neurological examination is normal.
E. A dental cause has been excluded by appropriate investigations.
F. Not better accounted for by another ICHD-3 diagnosis.

Treatment

No randomized controlled trials on the treatment of PIFP have been conducted. Pharmacologic treatment is the primary method of treatment and is based on the treatment of neuropathic pain syndromes in general. In addition, behavioral approaches are an important adjunct, and referral to pain psychologist early on may be helpful. Other noninvasive, complementary, or body therapies, including diet and exercise, may be helpful especially when adding stress-coping strategies. Hypnosis was helpful in a small study of 41 patients.[9]

Anticonvulsants and antidepressants are the mainstay of pharmacotherapy, and combination therapy may provide added benefit.[2] Best recommendations include tricyclic antidepressants (amitriptyline, doxepin), duloxetine, venlafaxine, and anticonvulsants (gabapentin, pregabalin). Lamotrigine, topiramate, carbamazepine, oxcarbazepine, phenytoin, and others have been used.[2,7] Use of nonsteroidal anti-inflammatory drugs and acetaminophen for the treatment of PIFP lack supportive data, and opioids are not recommended.

Interventional treatments may be attempted, but there is insufficient evidence to support these treatments as first line. Pulsed radiofrequency of the sphenopalatine ganglion (SPG) after therapeutic response to SPG block has been shown to be effective in one small study.[10] Limited studies of botulinum toxin, a combination of botulinum toxin injections and pulsed radiofrequency treatment of the infraorbital nerve, CT-guided trigeminal ganglion neurolysis combined with SPG, percutaneous trigeminal nerve stimulation (TNS), and repetitive transcranial nerve stimulation (rTMS) have been reported to have potential benefit.[7,10] Cannabinoids have been studied in patients with neuropathic pain and may be helpful.[11]

There is now evidence that dental procedures should not be performed without finding dental pathology. Dental procedures pose risk of developing chronic pain or even spread of pain ipsilaterally or contralaterally.[2] In addition, there is no role for vascular decompression surgery. Occipital nerve blocks have not been effective.

Prognosis

PIFP is a chronic condition with only a small percentage of patients achieving remission. Some patients do find relief. Response to pharmacotherapy is generally observed in fewer than 15% of patients.[8] Long-term follow-up revealed that remission in patients with PIFP was 16.0% in contrast to 37.1% in TN patients.[8] Of those in remission, 1/3 reported that medication instigated remission, 1/3 reported remission after PT or a procedure, and 1/3 reported spontaneous remission. Of the remaining 84% of PIFP patients who were still reporting pain, 65.6% of patients reported pain-free intervals in contrast to 92.3% of patients with TN.[3]

Summary

- PIFP is a distinct neuropathic pain condition with an uncertain underlying pathophysiology.
- It is important to carefully evaluate and rule out secondary causes, as well as consider dental or traumatic history, which can complicate the diagnosis of PIFP.
- Vascular compression of the trigeminal nerve is not associated with PIFP.
- Treatment for PIFP should focus on neuropathic pharmacotherapies and include behavioral or psychological support, considering the chronic nature of the condition.
- There is insufficient evidence to recommend invasive interventional treatments as first-line therapies for PIFP.

Facial Pain and Cranial Neuralgias

REFERENCES

1. Headache Classification Committee of the International Headache Society (IHS). *The International Classification of Headache Disorders*, 3rd edition. *Cephalalgia*. 2018;38:1-211.

2. Ziegeler C, Beikler T, Gosau M, May A. Idiopathic facial pain syndromes: an overview and clinical implications. *Dtsch Arztebl Int*. 2021;118:81-87.

3. Maarbjerg S, Wolfram F, Heinskou TB, et al. Persistent idiopathic facial pain: a prospective systematic study of clinical characteristics and neuroanatomical findings at 3.0 Tesla MRI. *Cephalalgia*. 2017;37:1231-1240.

4. Wilcox SL, Gustin SM, Macey PM, Peck CC, Murray GM, Henderson LA. Anatomical changes at the level of the primary synapse in neuropathic pain: evidence from the spinal trigeminal nucleus. *J Neurosci*. 2015;35:2508-2515.

5. Ziegeler C, Schulte LH, May A. Altered trigeminal pain processing on brainstem level in persistent idiopathic facial pain. *Pain*. 2021;162:1374-1378.

6. Forssell H, Tenovuo O, Silvoniemi P, Jääskeläinen SK. Differences and similarities between atypical facial pain and trigeminal neuropathic pain. *Neurology*. 2007;69:1451-1459.

7. Benoliel R, Gaul C. Persistent idiopathic facial pain. *Cephalalgia*. 2017;37:680-691.

8. Ziegeler C, Brauns G, May A. Characteristics and natural disease history of persistent idiopathic facial pain, trigeminal neuralgia, and neuropathic facial pain. *Headache*. 2021;61:1441-1451.

9. Zakrzewska JM. Chronic/persistent idiopathic facial pain. *Neurosurg Clin N Am*. 2016;27:345-351.

10. Weiss AL, Ehrhardt KP, Tolba R. Atypical facial pain: a comprehensive, evidence-based review. *Curr Pain Headache Rep*. 2017;21:8.

11. Boychuk DG, Goddard G, Mauro G, Orellana MF. The effectiveness of cannabinoids in the management of chronic nonmalignant neuropathic pain: a systematic review. *J Oral Facial Pain Headache*. 2015;29:7-14.

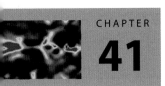

CHAPTER

41

Occipital Neuralgia

Paul G. Mathew

According to the third edition of the *International Classification of Headache Disorders* (ICHD-3), occipital neuralgia (ON) is a paroxysmal pain disorder that can involve the greater occipital nerves (GON), lesser occipital nerves (LON), and/or third occipital nerves (TON) in a unilateral or bilateral distribution.[1] Like most neuralgias, ON typically has a severe intensity with a shooting, stabbing, or sharp quality, which can last a few seconds to minutes. In addition, dysesthesia/allodynia in response to innocuous stimulation of the scalp and/or hair is often present in the distribution of the affected nerves.[1]

Epidemiology

The incidence and prevalence of ON are not well elucidated as ON tends to be underdiagnosed, which may be due to multiple reasons including clinicians being unfamiliar with this diagnosis, the patients only discussing certain symptoms of their clinical presentation that are not necessarily suggestive of ON, and/or the clinician assuming that all symptoms are due to another coexisting headache disorder, such as migraine. ON as the chief complaint and/or ON occurring in the absence of another headache diagnosis is uncommon. In a study conducted at the University of Southern California involving 35 patients presenting with ON, 20 also had a diagnosis of migraine.[2] When comparing the patients with ON, there was no significant difference in terms of age, sex, or ethnicity between patients with and without migraine. The patients with migraine and ON tended to have significantly more pain traveling to the scalp, scalp tenderness, and paresthesias than patients with isolated ON.[2] In a retrospective study conducted at the Cambridge Health Alliance Headache Center/Harvard Medical School, among 800 patients (648 females) presenting with a chief complaint of headache, 195 patients had a diagnosis of ON.[3] Isolated ON was present in 15.38% ($n = 30$) of patients. Multiple regression analysis demonstrated that the odds of ON were higher in patients with chronic migraine compared to episodic migraine (adjusted odds ratio = 2.190 [95% confidence interval: 1.364-3.515]), even when adjusted for significant covariates. Although not generalizable to a primary care or general neurology clinic, these data suggest that ON is a highly prevalent headache disorder, occurring in up to 25% of patients presenting for evaluation at a headache subspecialty clinic.[3]

Pathophysiology

The GON originates from the dorsal ramus at the level of C2, and courses between the inferior capitis oblique and semispinalis capitis. Although there can be anatomical variants, the GON subsequently tends to pierce through deep cervical fascia, the semispinalis capitis muscle in most cases, the aponeurotic fibrous layer of the trapezius, and the sternocleidomastoid as it courses past the superior nuchal line toward the apex, at times traversing the occipital artery.[4] The LON originates from the ventral rami of the C2 and C3 spinal nerves, travels along the posterior margin of the sternocleidomastoid, and like the GON, pierces deep cervical fascia as it ascends with branching to innervate the mastoid, lateral occiput, and portions of the ipsilateral ear.[4] In one study, 45% of subjects had contact between the LON and occipital artery.[5] The TON originates from the superficial medial branch of the dorsal ramus of the C3 spinal nerve. As the TON ascends, small branches innervate the midline as the nerve pierces the splenius capitis, trapezius, and semispinalis capitis before ultimately terminating around the superior nuchal line.[4]

The GON, LON, and TON have tortuous courses, and the adjacent structures can contribute to nerve compression/irritation that can result in ON. ON can be triggered by whiplash injuries such as sports trauma or a motor vehicle accident. In other cases, trivial trauma and/or microtrauma in the form of years/decades of poor posture can trigger ON. In clinical practice, sedentary occupations, such as those that involve heavy computer use, can be a risk factor for ON.[3]

Clinical Presentation and Diagnosis

The ICHD-III diagnostic criteria for ON are detailed in Box 41-1, which requires a response to occipital nerve blocks (ONBs) to confirm the diagnosis[1] (see Chapter 44). In addition to a routine neurological examination, evaluating for an occipital Tinel's sign can be useful in a patient with suspected ON. An occipital Tinel's evaluation is performed by tapping along the skull base from mastoid to mastoid. In a patient with ON, percussion will often elicit pain/tingling in the distribution of the affected nerve. In cases of GON and TON involvement, the pain/paresthesias will radiate toward the apex. In the case of lesser occipital nerve involvement, the pain/paresthesias will radiate toward the ipsilateral ear/temple. Up to 75% of patients with ON can have a positive occipital Tinel's sign on examination.[3] A positive occipital Tinel's sign should radiate in the distribution of the nerve, and not

---

Box 41-1. ICHD-3 Diagnostic Criteria for ON

Unilateral or bilateral paroxysmal, shooting or stabbing pain in the posterior part of the scalp, in the distribution(s) of the GON, LON, and/or TON, sometimes accompanied by diminished sensation or dysesthesia in the affected area and commonly associated with tenderness over the involved nerve(s):

A. Unilateral or bilateral pain in the distribution(s) of the GON, LON, and/or TON and fulfilling criteria B-D

B. Pain has at least two of the following three characteristics:
   1. Recurring in paroxysmal attacks lasting from a few seconds to minutes
   2. Severe in intensity
   3. Shooting, stabbing, or sharp in quality

C. Pain is associated with both of the following:
   1. Dysesthesia and/or allodynia apparent during innocuous stimulation of the scalp and/or hair
   2. Either or both of the following:
      a) Tenderness over the affected nerve branches
      b) Trigger points at the emergence of the greater occipital nerve or in the distribution of C2

D. Pain is eased temporarily by local anesthetic block of the affected nerve(s)

E. Not better accounted for by another ICHD-3 diagnosis

trigger holocephalic pain, which would be more suggestive of an acute migraine. In clinical practice, patients often note that certain neck movements, like looking over one's shoulder while driving, can trigger an ON attack. Assessment of the neck's passive range of motion including flexion, extension, rotation, and lateral flexion can be useful, as these maneuvers can at times provoke an ON attack, which provides further confirmation of the diagnosis.

Treatment

When ON is suspected, ONBs are both diagnostic and therapeutic. ONBs involve the injection of an anesthetic agent in the scalp along the course of the occipital nerves (see Chapter 44). In clinical practice, there is great variability in how ONBs are performed in terms of the size of the needle (gauge and length), the anesthetic agent(s), the use of steroids, the patient's physical position during the procedure, the point of needle insertion, and extent of needle advancement into the scalp. The most commonly used anesthetics are lidocaine, bupivacaine, or a combination of these medications. The most commonly used steroids are triamcinolone acetonide, dexamethasone, and methylprednisolone. Training and experience tend to guide how a particular injector performs ONBs.[6] In a retrospective study, 41 patients (34 female) diagnosed with probable ON received 6 mL ONBs consisting of 5.5 mL of 0.75% bupivacaine and 0.5 mL of triamcinolone acetonide (20 mg).[7] The ONBs were being performed in order to confirm the diagnosis of ON, as a response to nerve blocks is required to shift the diagnosis from probable ON to ON. Patients with bilateral ON received bilateral ONBs with a total injection volume of 12 mL. Among the patients, 29 had bilateral ON and 14 had unilateral ON. Duration of benefit was defined as complete remission of lancinating pain at the time of their follow up appointment(s). Among the 41 patients there was an average duration of benefit of 206.95 days with a range of 4 to 840 days. These duration of benefit data do not reflect the actual duration of benefit as they are based on follow-up appointment data rather than when/if the patient experienced an actual recurrence of lancinating pain. A possible mechanism of action that may explain this long duration of benefit is that larger volume injections may generate hydrodynamic pressure that induces expansion of tissue planes, resulting in decompression of the affected nerves.[7] It has been suggested in the literature that nerve compression can play a role in the genesis of different headache disorders, including ON.[8,9] In patients who are averse to receiving injections or have inadequate relief ONBs, other treatment strategies should be considered. In terms of pharmacologic treatment, neuropathic medications can be effective, and commonly used agents include gabapentin, pregabalin, carbamazepine, amitriptyline, nortriptyline, and duloxetine.[10] As with many pain conditions that can involve a musculoskeletal component, physical therapy can effectively complement any medication regiment. In refractory cases, radiofrequency ablation and occipital nerve stimulation could be considered.[9] Another option for the treatment of refractory ON is occipital nerve decompression surgery.[11] Occipital nerve decompression surgery is typically performed by a plastic surgeon, and can target multiple occipital nerves in the case of both unilateral and bilateral ON in a single procedure. Surgical intervention should only be considered in cases of failed best medication management including a combination of medications, large volume ONBs (preferably multiple cycles), and physical therapy.

Prognosis

The prognosis for ON is generally good in clinical practice, but many cases require a combination of ONBs, medication, and physical therapy for optimal improvement. Refractory cases may require more aggressive treatment including radiofrequency ablation, occipital nerve stimulation, and occipital nerve decompressions surgery. Adequate treatment of ON can often result in the improvement of the frequency, intensity, and response to medications of any coexisting headache disorders, such as migraine.

Facial Pain and Cranial Neuralgias

Summary

- ON is a common, but highly underdiagnosed.

- ON often develops in patients with preexisting headache disorders, and chronic migraine is the most common comorbid headache disorder.

- ONBs are part of the diagnostic criteria of ON and can be therapeutic.

- ONBs that utilize larger injection volumes may be exerting larger amounts of tissue dissecting pressure resulting in longer-lasting benefit.

- Pharmacologic treatment for ON typically involves the use of antiepileptic and antidepressant medications, including gabapentin, pregabalin, carbamazepine, amitriptyline, nortriptyline, and duloxetine.

- In cases of ON that are refractory to medication, physical therapy, and ONBs, radiofrequency ablation, occipital nerve stimulation, and occipital nerve decompression surgery can be considered.

REFERENCES

1. Headache Classification Committee of the International Headache Society (IHS). *The International Classification of Headache Disorders*, 3rd edition. *Cephalalgia.* 2018;38(1):1-211.

2. Sahai-Srivastava S, Zheng L. Occipital neuralgia with and without migraine: difference in pain characteristics and risk factors. *Headache.* 2011;51:124-128.

3. Mathew PG, Najib U, Khaled S, Krel R. Prevalence of occipital neuralgia at a community hospital-based headache clinic. *Neurol Clin Pract.* 2021;11(1):6-12.

4. Kemp WJ, Tubbs RS, Cohen-Gadol AA. The innervation of the scalp: a comprehensive review including anatomy, pathology, and neurosurgical correlates. *Surg Neurol Int.* 2011;2:178.

5. Lee M, Brown M, Chepla K, et al. An anatomical study of the lesser occipital nerve and its potential compression points: implications for surgical treatment of migraine headaches. *Plast Reconstr Surg.* 2013;132(6):1551-1556.

6. Blumenfeld A, Ashkenazi A, Napchan U, et al. Expert consensus recommendations for the performance of peripheral nerve blocks for headaches—a narrative review. *Headache.* 2013; 53(3):437-446.

7. Mathew PG, Najib U, Khaled S, Krel R. One and Done: A Case Series of Large Volume Occipital Nerve Blocks for the Treatment of Occipital Neuralgia. American Academy of Neurology Annual Meeting, Philadelphia, PA, May 2019, American Headache Society Annual Scientific Meeting, Philadelphia, PA, July 2019.

8. Mathew PG. A critical evaluation of migraine trigger site deactivation surgery. *Headache.* 2014;54(1):142-152.

9. Mathew PG, Cooper W. The diagnosis and management of posttraumatic headache with associated painful cranial neuralgias: a review and case series. *Curr Pain Headache Rep.* 2021;25(8):54.

10. Dougherty C. Occipital neuralgia. *Curr Pain Headache Rep.* 2014;18(5):411.

11. Jose A, Nagori SA, Chattopadhyay PK, Roychoudhury A. Greater occipital nerve decompression for occipital neuralgia. *J Craniofac Surg.* 2018;29(5): e518-e521.

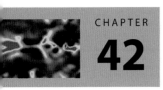

CHAPTER

42

Other Painful Lesions of the Cranial Nerves and Other Facial Pain

Abby Metzler and Madisen Janssen

In this chapter, disabling painful lesions of the cranial nerves and facial pain are discussed. The clinical and anatomical features, triggers, and associated factors of these syndromes are summarized in Table 42-1.

Glossopharyngeal Neuralgia

Glossopharyngeal neuralgia (GN) is a rare pain condition. GN accounts for 0.2% to 1.3% of all cranial neuralgias, 100 times less common than trigeminal neuralgia. GN predominantly affects patients over 50 years of age and, unlike trigeminal neuralgia, has no predilection for gender.[1]

GN is characterized by brief, paroxysmal attacks of severe, unilateral, stabbing, or electrical pain involving the ear, base of tongue, or tonsillar fossa that may radiate up toward the angle of the jaw, sparing the auricular or pharyngeal regions. GN attacks can be provoked by swallowing, talking, coughing, and yawning.[1] The classic symptoms of GN localize to the path and innervation of the glossopharyngeal nerve (CN IX), which exits the brainstem at the level of the medulla, passes through jugular foramen, proceeds under the styloid and the hyoglossus muscle to innervate the posterior tongue, oropharynx, upper pharynx, medial tympanic membrane, mastoid air cells, carotid body, and sinus. Approximately 2% of patients with GN experience an association between the onset of the pain and a vagal response with syncope, bradycardia, hypotension, or cardiac dysrhythmia.[1] This phenomenon is brought on by a branch of the glossopharyngeal called Hering's nerve, which innervates afferents of the chemoreceptors on the carotid body and baroreceptors of the carotid sinus, as well as visceral sensory branches, resulting in irritation of the vagus nerve.[1] In addition to a neurologic history and examination, a thorough intraoral and neck examination should be completed, and further otorhinolaryngology evaluation and imaging may be considered if suspicious for vascular lesion.

For the treatment of GN, see the next section. Most cases of GN have spontaneous resolution, and medications can be helpful in achieving remission. Almost 50% of patients achieve symptom relief in less than 24 months, with 74% of patients reporting spontaneous remission.[1]

Nervus Intermedius Neuralgia and Painful Nervus Intermedius Neuropathy

Nervus intermedius neuralgia (NIN) presents as painful paroxysmal attacks in the deep auditory canal, with radiation to the parieto-occipital region, and occasional involvement of the soft palate or angle of the mandible, but spares the tongue.[2] NIN is thought to be caused by irritation of the nervus intermedius, a branch of the facial nerve (CN VII),

265

Facial Pain and Cranial Neuralgias

Table 42-1. Facial Pain Syndromes Comparison

Syndrome Name with Acronym	Classical Features	Distribution of Pain	Triggers	Associations/Treatments	Nerves Involved
Glossopharyngeal neuralgia	Paroxysmal attacks of severe unilateral stabbing or electrical pain	Ear, base of tongue, pharynx, tonsillar fossa, may radiate up to angle of the jaw (spares the auricular or pharyngeal region)	Swallowing (especially cold items), talking, coughing, yawning	Vagal response	Glossopharyngeal nerve (CN IV), with involvement of Hering's nerve
Nervus intermedius neuralgia	Paroxysmal attacks of deep pain, classically "stabbing"	Auditory canal (external: ear/acoustic meatus, lateral tympanic membrane), radiation to the parieto-occipital, rare involvement of the soft palate or angle of the mandible (spares the tongue)	Light touch or cold wind	Tinnitus, bitter tastes, excess salivation, dizziness, facial flushing, sweating, sensory sensitivity	Nervus intermedius, a peripheral part of CN VII
Painful nervus intermedius neuropathy	Constant burning pain (contrasted to the paroxysmal frequency and stabbing pain in NIN)	Same as NIN	Can develop from Ramsay Hunt syndrome, a zoster infection of the geniculate ganglion	Sensory deficit around the ear and auricle	Nervus intermedius a peripheral part of the facial nerve (CN VII)
Painful optic neuritis	Headache with unilateral or bilateral eye pain that is exacerbated by eye movements with central visual deficits; vision impairments preceded by headache	Ocular, retroocular, periorbital, or frontal head pain. Unilateral or bilateral eye pain	Demyelination flare	Increased risk of developing multiple sclerosis	CN II, III, IV, VI
Ischemic ocular motor nerve palsy	Headaches with ocular pain; cranial nerve ocular palsy can be described as intermittent binocular diplopia, ptosis	Unilateral frontal head pain, ocular eye pain	Cardiovascular risk factors (obesity, diabetes, hyperlipidemia, older age)	Microvascular ischemia secondary to diabetes, classically causes peripheral nerve injury, that is, pupil sparing	CN II, III, IV, VI (CN III most commonly by microvascular ischemia)

Syndrome Name with Acronym	Classical Features	Distribution of Pain	Triggers	Associations/Treatments	Nerves Involved
Tolosa-Hunt syndrome	Periorbital headache with temporal association with unilateral cranial nerve deficits and evidence of cavernous sinus inflammation	Periorbital unilateral head pain may cause pain in CN III, IV, VI, and sympatics	Granulomatous inflammatory disease, viral infection	CSF evidence of viral infection and radiographic evidence for inflammation in the cavernous sinus; treatment with glucocorticoids	Cavernous sinus (internal carotid artery, CN VI, III, IV, ophthalmic/ maxillary division of the CN V) sometimes sympathetics
Raeder's syndrome	A burning headache pain that worsens with eye movements and presents with ipsilateral Horner's syndrome (ptosis, myosis yet with preserved sweating)	Unilateral trigeminal division, VI distribution, that covers the top of the head, forehead, nose, and right below the eyes	Carotid aneurysm/ dissection, Herpes zoster, sinusitis, otitis media, fibromuscular dysplasia	Also called "painful Horner syndrome" or "paratrigeminal oculosympathetic syndrome"; treatment with glucocorticoids	Oculosympathetics, CN V (trigeminal division, VI)
Recurrent painful ophthalmoplegic neuropathy	Transient unilateral headache with subsequent development of ipsilateral paresis of 2-3 different ocular motor nerves days after the onset of headache	Transient unilateral migraine-like headache	Inflammatory	Affects young children, male predilection; most commonly affected CN: III; treatment with glucocorticoids, may consider indomethacin or IVIG if demyelinating etiology	CN III, VI, IV

(Continued)

Table 42-1. Facial Pain Syndromes Comparison (*Continued*)

Syndrome Name with Acronym	Classical Features	Distribution of Pain	Triggers	Associations/Treatments	Nerves Involved
Neck-tongue syndrome	Rapid onset of a severe head and neck pain with abnormal sensations or posturing of the ipsilateral tongue	Unilateral, sharp, stabbing, severe pain in the upper neck and occipital lasting seconds to minutes	Sudden head movements, compression or irritation of C2	Jaw pain, anterolateral neck pain, choking sensation, ear pressure, trapezius pain, dysarthria, congestion, sialorrhea, lingual pseudoathetosis/paralysis, ulnar paresthesias, and retroauricular numbness	Upper C2 and lingual nerve
Burning mouth syndrome	A burning dysesthesia of the mouth, recurring daily for >2 hours/day, and >3 months, without clinically evident any oral/dental causative lesions	Burning dysesthesia of the oral mucosa	Psychosocial	Predilection for females, specifically peri- and postmenopausal; comorbid association with psychosocial and psychiatric disorders; treatment with anti-inflammatory topicals and behavior modification	V and VII (sensory function of the facial and trigeminal cranial nerves)

CN, cranial nerve; CSF, cerebrospinal fluid; C2, cervical nerve 2; IVIG, intravenous immunoglobulin; NIN, nervus intermedius neuralgia.

which can be due to a variety of conditions causing otalgia. The symptoms correlate to the nerve innervation of the concha of the external ear, external acoustic meatus, and lateral tympanic membrane. Patients with NIN may also experience tinnitus, dysgeusia, sialorrhea, lacrimation, dizziness, flushing, diaphoresis, and sensory sensitivity.

In contrast to the intermittent stabbing pain of NIN, painful nervus intermedius neuropathy (PNIN) is a syndrome of constant burning pain with sensory deficits around the ear and auricle. PNIN is a potential consequence of Ramsay Hunt syndrome (RHS), a herpes zoster infection of the geniculate ganglion causing facial paresis.[3]

The pathophysiology of NIN and PNIN is thought to be due to vascular compression and possibly inflammation. Secondary causes to consider include Bell's palsy, dental disorders, myofascial pain, temporomandibular joint dysfunction, nasopharyngeal carcinoma, prior herpes zoster, and rarely demyelination or tumors at the cerebellopontine angle.[3]

Common treatments for NIN, PNIN, and GN include neuropathic pain medications, antiseizure medications, and membrane stabilizers: carbamazepine, oxcarbazepine, gabapentin, pregabalin, duloxetine, amitriptyline, and topical anesthetics. For refractory cases of GN, microvascular decompression, denervation, intracranial nerve sectioning, or radiofrequency ablation have shown effectiveness.[2] For facial palsy associated with PNIN, a short course of high-dose prednisolone was found to be an effective treatment in case studies.[3]

Painful Optic Neuritis

Painful optic neuritis (PON) presents as retroocular headache and central visual impairment. The unilateral or bilateral pain is classically exacerbated by eye movement.

The diagnosis of PON relies on imaging to confirm, typically with gadolinium-enhanced magnetic resonance imaging (MRI) revealing optic nerve enhancement. PON is most commonly caused by demyelinating diseases, such as multiple sclerosis (MS). The optic neuritis treatment trial (ONTT), a longitudinal study assessing patients with ON without definitive MS, investigated the 10-year risk and later the 15-year risks of developing MS after an initial episode of acute optic neuritis.[4] The 10-year risk of developing MS after an episode of acute ON without MRI lesions is considered very low, increasing to a substantial level if one or more typical MRI lesions were present.[4] The reported probability of developing MS, within 15 years of onset of optic neuritis, has been calculated to be 50%, with a strong correlation to presence of nonenhancing MRI lesions at baseline.[4]

PON typically self-resolves, though treatment with steroids is standard for hastening recovery of vision by reducing optic nerve inflammation and for pain management.

Ischemic Oculomotor Nerve Palsy

Ischemic oculomotor nerve palsy (IOMNP) presents as a unilateral frontal headache with associated eye pain, exam showing ocular nerve palsies, with a history of cardiovascular and metabolic risk factors. IOMNP is associated with obesity, advanced age, hypertension, diabetes, and coronary artery disease.[5]

Of the associated cranial nerve palsies, third nerve palsy occurs most frequently, with microvascular ischemia as the most common cause (such as occurs with poorly controlled diabetes). Recall that these third nerve palsies are typically pupil-sparing due to parasympathetic fibers' orientation farther from the ischemic blood supply.

Depending on the examination of these patients, a differential diagnosis may include aneurysmal compression (the posterior communicating artery most commonly), giant cell arteritis, myasthenia gravis, trauma, or demyelination. Laboratory workup should include hemoglobin A1c, lipid panel, and then inflammatory markers and antibody testing may be considered. If there is pupillary involvement with a third nerve palsy, it is imperative to obtain vascular imaging to assess for aneurysmal compression.

IOMNP is most often self-limiting, and the goal of treatment is secondary prevention and symptomatic management, with eye patch, opaque lens, or prism for diplopia.

Tolosa-Hunt Syndrome

Tolosa-Hunt syndrome (THS) presents as periorbital unilateral headache, temporally associated ipsilateral cranial nerve deficits, evidence of a viral infection in the cerebral spinal fluid, and ipsilateral cavernous sinus inflammation radiographically. THS is a granulomatous inflammatory condition, characterized by infiltration of lymphocytes and plasma cells surrounding the cavernous sinus, with occasional extension into the superior orbital fissure. This unilateral periorbital or orbital pain is associated with unilateral involvement of cranial nerves III, IV, VI, and sometimes involves sympathetic innervation to the pupil. Contrast-enhanced brain MRI is often helpful to rule out structural lesions.

High-dose glucocorticoids are the first-line treatment for THS since it is an inflammatory condition, and successful treatment with glucocorticoids is thought to be both diagnostic and therapeutic. Corticosteroid treatment typically improves the periorbital headache pain within 48 hours and the cranial nerve dysfunction in about 14 days, but the range can be 2 to 8 weeks.[6]

Raeder's Syndrome

Painful Horner's and paratrigeminal syndrome, or Raeder's syndrome (RS), is rare but should be considered if a patient presents with constant, burning, unilateral headache in the distribution of the ophthalmic division of the trigeminal nerve (V1). In this syndrome, the V1 pain worsens with eye movement and examination reveals an ipsilateral Horner's syndrome with preserved facial sweating, manifesting as symptoms of ipsilateral oculosympathetic paresis with trigeminal nerve involvement.

RS can be a recognized complication of multiple conditions, such as carotid aneurysms or dissections (above the carotid bifurcation typically), fibromuscular dysplasia, pituitary adenomas, malignancy, herpes zoster, sinusitis, migraine, trauma, hypertension, and chronic otitis media.[7] Considering this broad range of potential causes, vascular radiographic analysis with contrast is recommended, with treatment guided by the underlying etiology and symptomatic management with analgesia.[7]

Recurrent Painful Ophthalmoplegic Neuropathy

Recurrent painful ophthalmoplegic neuropathy (RPON) presents as a transient unilateral headache with subsequent ipsilateral paresis of multiple ocular motor nerves days after the headache. The most commonly affected cranial nerve is oculomotor, followed by abducens, then trochlear.[8] RPON is a rare condition, with an estimated disease prevalence of 0.7 per million people, with a male predominance, and is generally thought to occur in children, though numerous adult case reports have been documented.[8] In about 30% of patients, contrast MRI reveals enhancement of cisternal segments of correlated cranial nerves, and in childhood cases, this enhancement occurs in up to 60%.[8]

In distinguishing RPON from THS, RPON does not typically involve the trigeminal nerve, which, in contrast, is often affected by the cavernous sinus processes of THS. Additionally, it has been reported that gadolinium uptake in the oculomotor nerve and intraneural enhancement on MRI is seen in those diagnosed with RPON, but not in THS.[8] Considering the overlapping presentations, it has been theorized that there is a common pathophysiology, as both conditions are thought to be inflammatory, and demonstrate a response to anti-inflammatory treatments.

RPON is typically self-resolving and most patients make a full recovery, though the ophthalmoplegia symptoms commonly outlast the headache.[9] A few case reports have described patients with multiple attacks that subsequently develop persistent deficits, as well as a few isolated cases with residual cranial nerve impairment, though rare.[9]

The treatment for RPON is corticosteroids, with a perceived benefit seen in as soon as 2 days in 54% of patients.[9,10] There are a few cases demonstrating benefit with indomethacin, and for refractory cases or clinical suspicion for demyelinating etiology or IVIG.[10]

Neck-Tongue Syndrome

Neck-tongue syndrome is defined by the rapid onset of severe, unilateral upper neck and occipital pain, triggered by sudden head movement, and associated with abnormal sensations or posturing of the ipsilateral tongue. The pain is classically sharp and stabbing, lasting seconds to minutes. Epidemiological data reports have calculated a prevalence estimation for adults to be 0.22%.

Compression causes irritation to the second upper cervical nerve (C2), as it travels along the inferior oblique capitis muscles and the atlantoaxial joint is a proposed pathophysiology. It has also been suggested that facet joint subluxation of the atlas of C1 and axis of C2, occurring during axial rotation, may cause compression of the C2 nerve root resulting in the pain and dysesthesia of the tongue through a hypoglossal anastomosis to the lingual nerve. A variety of other conditions have been identified as potential causes including spondylosis, arthritis, ligamentous laxity, trauma, and Chiari malformations. Finally, considering overlapping clinical presentation with vertebrobasilar or carotid artery insufficiency, transient ischemic attacks, and migraine, it is essential to evaluate for vascular etiology.

The treatment for NTS is multimodal and can involve manual therapy, bracing, postural exercises, as well as neuropathic agents, antiepileptics, antidepressants, anti-inflammatories, muscle relaxants, anesthetic injections, and rarely surgical intervention.

Burning Mouth Syndrome

Burning mouth syndrome (BMS) is characterized by a burning dysesthesia of the oral mucosa, recurring for 2 or more hours daily, for more than 3 months.[11] This condition has a predilection for peri- and postmenopausal women, is rare in patients under 30, and has an association with psychosocial and psychiatric disorders.[11] BMS is not well understood and likely multifactorial in etiology, including infection, hyposalivation, medication-induced, and systemic conditions (Sjögren's syndrome, diabetes).

There are a few theories on the pathogenesis of BMS. The development of an abnormal interaction between the sensory function of the facial and trigeminal cranial nerves may permit the development of high-density papillae fungiform growth on the tongue increasing a predisposition for regional burning pain.[12] Additionally, the hyperactivity of the sensory and motor aspects of the trigeminal nerve may be due to a damped inhibition of the central pain pathways.[12]

Treatment for BMS requires a multidisciplinary approach with the combination of systemic medications, anesthetic and anti-inflammatory topicals (capsaicin cream and benzydamine mouthwash), as well as behavioral modifications.[12] Specific medications to consider include antidepressants, sialogogues, antiepileptics, and some reports suggest a benefit with hormone replacement therapy in postmenopausal women.[12]

Summary

- Painful lesions of cranial nerves and facial pain syndromes are rare.
- For the evaluation of cranial nerves and facial pain syndromes, a comprehensive history, neurological examination, and investigations to rule out secondary causes are essential.
- Many rare facial pain syndromes have overlapping features, with most including neuropathic pain descriptions, with a paroxysmal pattern, affecting a specific nerve or nerve branch distribution.

Facial Pain and Cranial Neuralgias

- Treatment includes management of underlying conditions or associated syndromes, and symptomatic treatment.

- Medications for symptomatic management are antiepileptics, membrane stabilizers, drugs for neuropathic pain, and anti-inflammatory medications.

- Topical anesthetics and nerve block injections may also be considered, and surgical intervention is reserved for refractory cases.

REFERENCES

1. Rushton JG, Stevens JC, Miller RH. Glossopharyngeal (vagoglossopharyngeal) neuralgia: a study of 217 cases. *Arch Neurol.* 1981;38(4):201-205.
2. Tubbs RS, Steck DT, Mortazavi MM, Cohen-Gadol AA. The nervus intermedius: a review of its anatomy, function, pathology, and role in neurosurgery. *World Neurosurg.* 2013;79(5):763-767.
3. Yentür EA, Yegül I. Nervus intermedius neuralgia: an uncommon pain syndrome with an uncommon etiology. *J Pain Symptom Manage.* 2000;19(6):407-408.
4. The Optic Neuritis Study Group. Multiple sclerosis risk after optic neuritis: final optic neuritis treatment trial follow-up. *Arch Neurol.* 2008;65(6):727-732.
5. Kobashi R, Ohtsuki H, Hasebe S. Clinical studies of ocular motility disturbances: Part 2. Ischemic ocular motor nerve palsy risk factors. *Jpn J Ophthalmol.* 1997;41(2):115-119.
6. Çakirer S. MRI findings in Tolosa–Hunt syndrome before and after systemic corticosteroid therapy. *Eur J Radiol.* 2003;45(2):83-90.
7. Murnane M, Proano L. Raeder's paratrigeminal syndrome: a case report. *Acad Emerg Med.* 1996;3(9):864-867.
8. Liu Y, Wang M, Bian X, et al. Proposed modified diagnostic criteria for recurrent painful ophthalmoplegic neuropathy: five case reports and literature review. *Cephalalgia.* 2020;40(14):1657-1670.
9. Levin M, Ward TN. Ophthalmoplegic migraine. *Curr Pain Headache Rep.* 2004;8(4):306-309.
10. Gelfand AA, Gelfand JM, Prabakhar P, Goadsby PJ. Ophthalmoplegic "migraine" or recurrent ophthalmoplegic cranial neuropathy: new cases and a systematic review. *J Child Neurol.* 2012;27(6):759-766.
11. Aravindhan R, Vidyalakshmi S, Kumar MS, Satheesh C, Balasubramanium AM, Prasad VS. Burning mouth syndrome: a review on its diagnostic and therapeutic approach. *J Pharm Bioallied Sci.* 2014;6(Suppl 1):S21-S25.
12. Grushka M, Epstein JB, Gorsky M. Burning mouth syndrome and other oral sensory disorders: a unifying hypothesis. *Pain Res Manag.* 2003;8(3):133-135.

PART V

Special Treatments and Procedures

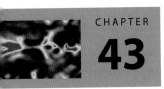

Onabotulinum Toxin Injections for Headache

Alexander Mauskop, Sait Ashina, and Andrew Blumenfeld

Botulinum toxin is an endotoxin that occurs naturally as a product of *Clostridium* bacteria.[1] The toxin cleaves a protein in the nerve terminal termed synaptosomal-associated protein of 25 kDa or SNAP-25 which results in an inability of vesicles to release chemicals that produce muscle contraction and pain transmission. Acetylcholine is the neurotransmitter released by nerve terminals, which attaches to a receptor on the muscle and produces contraction of that muscle. After being injected into the muscle, botulinum toxin enters the terminal part of a motor axon and prevents the release of acetylcholine. This effect persists for 3 to 6 months. The release of acetylcholine always returns to normal even after repeated injections of botulinum toxin into the same muscle over a period of many years. At very low doses, the toxin is effective in treating conditions of increased muscle tone including spasticity and dystonia. In addition, botulinum toxin also blocks the release of neurotransmitters and neuropeptides in sensory nerve terminals. There are seven different types of botulinum toxin (A-G). Onabotulinumtoxin type A or onabotulinumtoxinA is the most widely used toxin in clinics. OnabotulinumtoxinA (Botox®) has been approved for clinical use by the U.S. Food and Drug Administration (FDA) since 1989.

Indications for Headache Conditions

Currently only onabotulinumtoxinA is approved for the preventive treatment of chronic migraine. The FDA approval for chronic migraine treatment in 2010 was based on the safety and efficacy of onabotulinumtoxinA demonstrated in the pivotal phase III Research

Evaluating Migraine Prophylaxis Therapy (PREEMPT) trials.[2] Off-label, onabotulinumtoxinA has been used for the management of frequent episodic migraines, tension-type headaches, hemicrania continua, trigeminal neuralgia, cluster headaches, new daily persistent headaches, nummular headaches, postcraniotomy headache, and other primary and secondary headaches.

Mechanism of Action in Migraine

The mechanism of action of onabotulinumtoxinA in prevention of chronic migraine is not fully understood. The injection sites that are used for migraine align closely with the sensory nerves that supply the head and neck. These nerves are unmyelinated, and the toxin is able to enter them along their entire course. OnabotulinumtoxinA cleaves soluble N-ethylmaleimide-sensitive fusion attachment protein (SNAP-25) in sensory and motor nerve endings.[3] This results in inhibition of exocytosis. OnabotulinumtoxinA decreases exocytosis of proinflammatory and excitatory neurotransmitters and neuropeptides such as calcitonin gene-related peptide (CGRP), and glutamate from primary afferent fibers that transmit nociceptive signal to central nervous system. OnabotulinumtoxinA also decreases the insertion of transient receptor potential cation channel subfamily V (TRPV1 and TRPA1) into the membranes of nociceptive neurons. Thus, onabotulinumtoxinA blocks the development of peripheral and central sensitization.[3]

Precautions and Contraindications

Contraindications include hypersensitivity to any botulinum toxin preparation or any of the components in the formulation and infection at the injection site.[4] The spread of toxin is possible and may cause swallowing and breathing difficulties and can lead to death. It is important to seek urgent and immediate medical evaluation if the patient experiences respiratory, speech, or swallowing difficulties. These remote effects are very rare and have not been reported in chronic migraine trials. The risk is higher in young children. Caution is advised when treating patients with coexistent neuromuscular disorders due to the risk of worsening weakness. This means that a lower dose might be appropriate for some patients.

Practical Issues

The current FDA approval is only for the treatment of chronic migraines. Besides documenting the presence of chronic migraines, almost all insurance companies in the United States require that patients fail two or three oral preventive migraine medications such as beta-blockers, antidepressants, and epilepsy drugs before treatment with onabotulinumtoxinA is covered. The documentation of a positive response to treatment before the reauthorization of the continued treatment is also required. The effect of onabotulinumtoxinA on the release of neurotransmitters and neuropeptides takes several days to occur and tends to last about 12 weeks. Improvement typically takes 2 weeks to begin. There may be a continued decline in the frequency of attacks throughout the 12 weeks. With repeated treatments, continued improvement has been seen in observational studies for up to 2 years. Besides a reduction in frequency, patients often report a decline in pain severity, improved response to abortive drugs, as well as secondary benefits. These include a decline in anticipatory anxiety, improved mood and sleep, increased productivity, and an overall improvement in quality of life.

Injection Sites and Technique

The FDA-approved dose for chronic migraine is 155 units injected into 31 sites (Figure 43-1). The treatment protocol was standardized for the clinical trials that led to FDA approval. It is important to use this protocol in the initial training. In practice, many providers add injections into the masseter

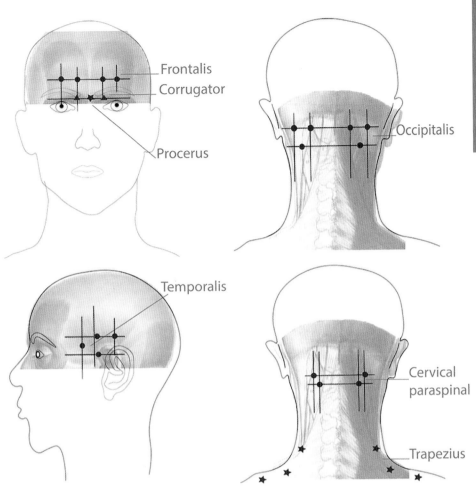

Figure 43-1. These muscle groups correlate with the peripheral innervation of the trigeminal, occipital, and cervical sensory nerves—all implicated in migraine pain. Doses below 155 units did not provide statistically significant benefit. Some evidence supports use of higher doses of an additional 5 units into each temporalis and occipitalis and another 10 units on each side of the trapezius in what is termed a follow-the-pain pattern. (Reproduced with permission from Krel R, Mathew PG. Procedural Treatments for Headache Disorders. *Practical Neurology (US).* 2019;18(4):76-79.)

muscles, and may add injection sites based on patient's unique anatomy or pain distribution. A 30-gauge ½-inch needle is commonly used for all injections.

Adverse Events

The most common side effects seen in registration trials, ironically, were headache, migraine, and neck pain.[4] About 9% of patients developed a headache or migraine and 9% developed neck pain. These side effects occurred soon after the injections. This indicates that they were due to the needle sticks rather than the action of onabotulinumtoxinA. About 4% developed ptosis. This is usually eyebrow ptosis. It tends to occur in older patients and can be avoided most of the time by injecting the frontalis muscle at its uppermost end.

Summary

- OnabotulinumtoxinA is a highly effective and safe treatment for chronic migraine.
- Off-label, onabotulinumtoxinA is used for managing other headaches and facial pain, including episodic migraine, tension-type headache, hemicrania continua, trigeminal neuralgia, and cluster headaches.
- The mechanism of action of onabotulinumtoxinA in preventing chronic migraine involves inhibiting vesicle trafficking and exocytosis of proinflammatory and excitatory neurotransmitters from sensory nerve endings.
- The usual dose of onabotulinumtoxinA for chronic migraine is 155 units injected into 31 sites in the head and neck regions.
- Common side effects of onabotulinumtoxinA included headache, migraine, and neck pain soon after injections, likely due to needle sticks, and about 4% experience ptosis.

REFERENCES

1. Padda IS, Tadi P. Botulinum Toxin. StatPearls. Treasure Island (FL) ineligible companies. Disclosure: Prasanna Tadi declares no relevant financial relationships with ineligible companies. StatPearls Publishing Copyright © 2023, StatPearls Publishing LLC; 2023.

2. Dodick DW, Turkel CC, DeGryse RE, et al. OnabotulinumtoxinA for treatment of chronic migraine: pooled results from the double-blind, randomized, placebo-controlled phases of the PREEMPT clinical program. *Headache.* 2010;50(6):921-936.

3. Burstein R, Blumenfeld AM, Silberstein SD, Manack Adams A, Brin MF. Mechanism of action of OnabotulinumtoxinA in chronic migraine: a narrative review. *Headache.* 2020;60(7):1259-1272.

4. BOTOX® (onabotulinumtoxinA) FDA Label: Available at:https://www.accessdata.fda.gov/drugsatfda_docs/label/2011/103000s5232lbl.pdf

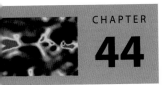

CHAPTER **44**

Nerve Blocks and Trigger Point Injections for Headache Disorders

Paul G. Mathew, Caitlin Hussey, and Sait Ashina

Peripheral nerve blocks (PNBs), sphenopalatine nerve blocks, and trigger point injections (TPIs) in pericranial/pericervical musculature muscles are commonly used in headache management.[1-4]

Peripheral Nerve Blocks

The pain associated with headache and facial pain disorders is primarily mediated through the trigeminal and cervical ganglia (Chapter 4). PNBs target the peripheral nerve branches of the trigeminal and cervical sensory systems. These blocks can be used to address acute pain including termination of a refractory headache cycle or can be used preventatively. PNBs can at times result in pain remission lasting for weeks, months, years, or even indefinitely. The anesthetic agents most frequently used in PNBs are lidocaine and bupivacaine, either with or without steroids. Commonly targeted sites for PNBs include the occipital (greater, lesser, and third), supraorbital, supratrochlear, infraorbital, and auriculotemporal nerves, as well as the sphenopalatine ganglia (SPG).

Indications

Indications for PNBs include several primary and secondary headache disorders.[2] PNBs are often performed in combination depending on the diagnosis and location of pain at the time of presentation. Migraine is the most common headache disorder for which patients present for further evaluation, and PNBs can be used to treat an acute migraine and for the treatment of status migrainosus. This can be a particularly effective strategy for patients who cannot tolerate oral steroids or find them ineffective. In such situations, PNBs may prevent patients from seeking care in emergency departments and urgent care facilities. Similar to the use with status migrainosus, occipital nerve blocks can be effective for the treatment of cluster headache, and at times can help terminate a cluster headache cycle. Although the evidence for steroid use in PNBs is scant for migraine and most other headache disorders, the evidence for using steroids in occipital nerve blocks for the treatment of cluster headache is strong. In clinical practice, serial PNBs are at times performed as a bridge therapy for the treatment of medication overuse headache, post-traumatic headache, and new daily persistent headache. Response to occipital nerve blocks is part of the diagnostic criteria for occipital neuralgia, and thus can have a diagnostic and therapeutic role (Chapter 41). Similarly, PNBs can be effective for the treatment of other neuralgias and primary stabbing headache in clinical practice.

Mechanism of Action

There are multiple potential mechanisms of action of nerve blocks in the management of primary and secondary headache disorders.[4] In addition to the anesthetic effects via sodium channel blockade on peripheral nerves, PNBs may also transiently modulate central pain structures.

For acute pain relief, the mechanism likely bases on a decrease in afferent input, reducing activity in both the trigeminal nucleus caudalis and the cervical dorsal horn.[4] Due to the organization of primary and secondary neurons receiving input from head and neck regions, this diminished activity could influence a wider area than just where the nerve is blocked, especially as the cervical and trigeminal systems are known to converge at brain stem level (trigeminocervical complex).[4] After receiving PNBs, patients often report relief of pain and allodynia in areas outside of the nerve distribution that was infiltrated.[5] In addition, elements of central sensitization including photophobia, phonophobia, and nausea can improve after a PNB. For sustained improvement, temporarily blocking neural activity in a sensitized system might allow for the "winding-down" of central sensitization of nociceptive pathways.[4] Persistent pain, rooted in peripheral sensitization, might also be alleviated in a similar manner, as blocking one set of sensitized nociceptors could elevate the pain threshold in another interconnected set.[3]

Another mechanism of action of PNBs may be volume-dependent decompression of the nerves via hydro-dissection of the connective tissue, muscle, and other adjacent structures that may be causing nerve compression.[6] There is growing evidence suggesting that large volume nerve blocks tend to be more effective, particularly for the treatment of occipital neuralgia and other focal cranial neuralgias where nerve compression may be playing a role.

Injection Sites and Technique

The Procedural Headache Medicine Section of the American Headache Society (IPS-AHS) published expert consensus recommendations in an attempt to provide guidelines for performing PNB and establish some uniformity.[2]

Occipital Nerve Blocks

To perform on occipital nerve blocks, the occiput is palpated, and the inion and mastoid process are identified (Figure 44-1).[2,3] The skin is then prepped with alcohol and volumes between 1.5 and 3 mL per nerve can be injected. If both greater and lesser occipital nerves are being blocked, a total of 6 mL per side could be considered. Care should be taken to confirm that the needle is not advanced intravascularly by obtaining a negative aspiration before injecting. This is particularly important when injecting particulate steroids, which have the potential to embolize. Some patients may have difficulty tolerating bilateral large volume occipital nerve blocks (dizziness, syncope), so it may be prudent to perform unilateral blocks over 2 appointments rather than bilateral blocks during a single appointment.

Supraorbital/Supratrochlear Nerve Blocks

To perform supraorbital and supratrochlear nerve blocks, the supraorbital ridge is palpated, and the supraorbital (superior, mid-pupillary) and supratrochlear (superior, medial) notches are identified (Figure 44-2).[2,3] The skin is then prepped with alcohol and volumes between 0.25 and 1 mL can be injected in the regions of notches, infiltrating the proximal areas of the desired nerve. Care should be taken not to inject steroids in cosmetic areas like the forehead, as steroids can cause atrophy and disfigurement.

Auriculotemporal Nerve Blocks

To perform on auriculotemporal nerve blocks, the temporal artery is located at the level of the tragus; the nerve is typically 1 and 2 cm anterior to the artery (Figure 44-3).[2,3] The skin is then prepped with alcohol, and volumes between 0.5 and 3 mL can be injected above the posterior part of the zygoma

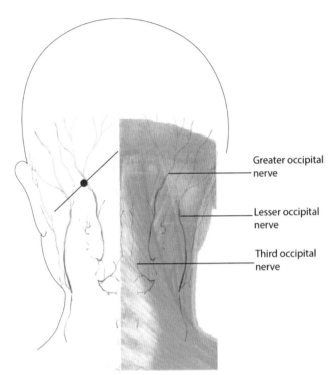

Greater occipital
nerve

Lesser occipital
nerve

Third occipital
nerve

Figure 44-1. Needle enters the skin at red dot and is inserted along the red line toward the inion and then pulled back to ensure there is no blood return. Medication (1.5-3 mL) is then delivered along the red line as the needle is withdrawn. The needle is removed, and the process is repeated along the red line in the opposite direction toward the mastoid, delivering another 1.5 to 3 mL of medication. (Reproduced with permission from Krehl R, Mathew PG. Procedural treatments for headache disorders. *Practical Neurology (US)*. 2019;18(4):76-79.)

infiltrating in the area of the auriculotemporal nerve. Care should be taken not to inject steroids in cosmetic areas like the temples, as steroids can cause atrophy and disfigurement.

Sphenopalatine Ganglion Nerve Blocks

The SPG, also known as the pterygopalatine ganglion, is a sophisticated cluster of cell bodies and fibers, including sympathetic, parasympatehtic, and sensory fibers that contribute to the maxillary branch of the trigeminal nerve.[4,7] Evidence supports the efficacy of SPG blocks for various headache disorders, notably cluster headache, migraine, and trigeminal neuralgia.[7] The mechanism of action of SPG blocks in headache and facial pain disorders is not well understood. There are multiple techniques for performing SPG nerve blocks.[4,7] Due to ease of use, two of the most commonly utilized techniques involve the use of commercially available intranasal catheters that deliver local anesthetic transnasally to the SPG. Alternatively, a Q-tip can be soaked with local anesthetic, and inserted into the nasal cavity. SPG blockade can also be self-administered by the patient using an anesthetic nasal spray that is delivered in the supine position, which affords the patient the convenience of in-home treatment.[7]

Trigger Point Injections

TPI are commonly used for the management of neurological and musculoskeletal disorders. Muscle pain especially involving the neck is a common complaint in patients with migraine, tension-type

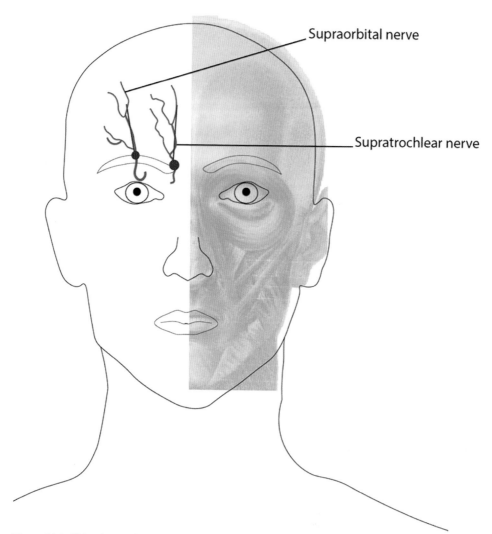

Figure 44-2. Using direct palpation, the supraorbital foramen is identified and the needle is inserted into the red dots (superomedial corner of the orbit for supratrochlear nerve and the mid-pupillary line for the supraorbital nerve), infiltrating the areas of supraorbital and supratrochlear nerves (0.5=1mL per injection site) and being careful to remain superficial throughout the entire process. (Reproduced with permission from Krehl R, Mathew PG. Procedural treatments for headache disorders. *Practical Neurology (US).* 2019;18(4):76-79.)

headache (TTH), cervicogenic, and post-traumatic headaches. Myofascial pain is also common in patients with temporomandibular joint disorders.[8] The pathophysiology of trigger points has not been fully clarified, but it has been suggested that trigger points may be due to abnormal endplate potentials, which result in excessive acetylcholine release at the neuromuscular junction (NMJ), which is a highly specialized synapse between a motor neuron nerve terminal and its muscle fiber. The diagnostic criteria for myofascial trigger points include: (1) a taut band (muscle fibers bundle) in the muscle; (2) pressure-sensitive area with a taut band; (3) referred pain from a trigger point; (4) a local twitch response of the trigger point or taut band and response to mechanical stimulation of the

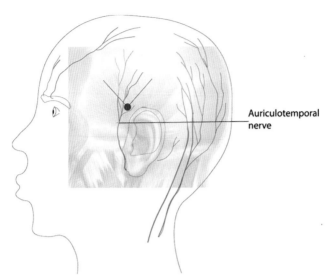

Auriculotemporal
nerve

Figure 44-3. Using direct palpation, the temporal artery pulse is located, and the skin is prepared with alcohol. Next, the needle is inserted into the red dot (anterior to the temporal artery above the posterior part of the zygoma) infiltrating the area of the auriculotemporal nerve and again being careful to remain superficial throughout the entire process. (Reproduced with permission from Krehl R, Mathew PG. Procedural treatments for headache disorders. *Practical Neurology (US)*. 2019;18(4):76-79.)

trigger point. As part of the examination, it is important to identify areas in the head and neck region that can reproduce the patient's headache/head pain.

Indications

Indications for TPIs include several primary and secondary headache disorders, especially when there is associated myalgia/cervicalgia.[1,2] The most common headache diagnoses for which TPIs can be recommended are chronic TTH (CTTH) and chronic migraine (CM). TPIs have been shown to reduce the frequency and intensity of TTH, and may reduce attack frequency in patients with CM. Other indications of TPIs include new daily persistent headache, status migrainosus, episodic TTH, cluster headache, and hemicrania continua. TPIs can also be used in combination with pericranial nerve blocks for the management of migraine.

Mechanism of Action

The mechanism of action of TPIs in the management of primary and secondary headaches is not fully clarified.[1] It is possible that decreased spontaneous electrical activity in the muscles and prevention of local ischemia and hypoxia in the muscles may contribute to the analgesic effect of trigger point injections.[1] Blocking of muscular nociceptors may lead to suppression of pain transmission from first-order to second-order neurons. Finally, the insertion of needle in trigger points may activate diffusion of noxious inhibitory control mechanism leading to pain relief.

Injection Sites and Technique

The most common muscles injected during TPI procedure are trapezius, cervical paraspinal, occipitalis, temporalis, sternocleidomastoid, and levator scapulae muscles.[1] For TPIs, the patient should be seated or recument. Vasovagal reactions can occur, and should be taken into consideration when positioning patients. The injection sites should be cleaned with alcohol if there are no contraindications. Areas that appear inflamed, injured, or edematous should be avoided. A 22-, 25-, or 27-gauge, 1- to 1.5-inch needle is usually used for superficial injections.[1] A 21- or 22-gauge, 2- or 2.5-inch needle is usually used for deeper injections.[1] When the palpable taut band is found, it can be stabilized by holding the overlying skin between the thumb and index finger on the non-injecting hand. It has been recommended to insert the needle approximately 1 to 1.5 cm away from the taut band and then to move it slowly at the 30-degree angle into the trigger point.[1] It is important to aspirate the needle to confirm that a blood vessel has not been penetrated. Approximately, 0.1 to 0.5 mL of local anesthetic can be injected.[1] For injections, 1% lidocaine or 0.25% to 0.5% of bupivacaine can be used.[1] After the injection, the pressure should be applied to the puncture sites.

Procedural Considerations

Precautions and Contraindications

Contraindications for PNBs and TPIs include infections (systemic and local), open skull injury/defect close to the injection areas, active rash, and allergic reaction to local anesthetics.[1,2] Anticoagulation, antiplatelet, and a history of bleeding disorders are not contraindications and generally no special considerations are required from a procedural standpoint, but patients should be informed about the risk of hematoma and increased bleeding. Relative contraindications include history of vasovagal syncope. Steroids should be avoided in the face and all other cosmetic areas given the potential for atrophy and disfigurement. For any procedure, particularly larger volume blocks, it would be reasonable to have the patient be accompanied by someone, and that the patient does not drive immediately after the procedure.

Adverse Events

The adverse events associated with PNBs and TPIs should be discussed with the patient as part of the informed consent process. Adverse events may include nerve or muscle injury, syncope, dizziness/lightheadedness, rapid heart rate, breathing problems, anaphylaxis, hemorrhage, infection, pneumothorax, allergic reaction to anesthetic, worsening of pain or headache, seizure and paralysis. Intramuscular injection with local anesthetics (mostly with bupivacaine) can potentially cause reversible myonecrosis, which is more common in patients receiving serial and high-dose injections. For procedures involving large volumes with the intent of nerve decompression, patients should be advised that after the anesthetic effect of the injection(s) has resolved, there may be some soreness resulting from expansion of tissue planes, which resolves with time. With SPG blocks, the most common side effect was bad taste if anesthetic was swallowed, which can result in oral numbness and lacrimation.

Treatment Outcome

While assessing the acute effect of PNBs and TPIs, pain relief and pain-freedom for 2 hours and sustaining pain-freedom for 24 hours are recommended outcomes. When assessing for a preventative effect, number of headache days, headache attacks, disability, and use of acute headache medications can be assessed. In cases of focal neuralgias, assessing the presence of lancinating pain, paresthesias, and allodynia can be useful, as the patient may have remission of these symptoms, but continue to have symptoms associated with a comorbid headache disorder, which most commonly is CM in patients with occipital neuralgia.

Summary

- PNBs and TPIs can be used for the treatment of primary and secondary headache disorders including migraine, cluster headache, TTH, post-traumatic headache, medication overuse headache, cervicogenic headaches, occipital neuralgia, and other focal cranial neuralgias.

- PNBs that utilize larger injection volumes may exert larger amounts of tissue dissecting pressure resulting in nerve decompression and long-lasting benefit in the case of focal cranial neuralgias.
- Steroids should be avoided in cosmetic areas where disfigurement can result.
- A trigger point is a hyperirritable, palpable, taut band of muscle that can be identified on physical examination.
- Most common muscles injected during the TPI procedure are trapezius, cervical paraspinal, occipitalis, temporalis, sternocleidomastoid, and levator scapulae muscles.
- TPIs can result in improvement of muscle pain and reduction in headache frequency and intensity.

REFERENCES

1. Robbins MS, Kuruvilla D, Blumenfeld A, et al. Trigger point injections for headache disorders: expert consensus methodology and narrative review. *Headache*. 2014;54(9):1441-1459.
2. Blumenfeld A, Ashkenazi A, Grosberg B, et al. Patterns of use of peripheral nerve blocks and trigger point injections among headache practitioners in the USA: results of the American Headache Society Interventional Procedure Survey (AHS-IPS). *Headache*. 2010;50(6):937-942.
3. Krel R, Mathew PG. Procedural treatments for headache disorders. *Pract Neurol*. 2019:76-79.
4. Levin M. Nerve blocks in the treatment of headache. *Neurotherapeutics*. 2010;7(2):197-203.
5. Young W, Cook B, Malik S, Shaw J, Oshinsky M. The first 5 minutes after greater omlipital nerve block. *Headache*. 2008;48(7):1126-1128.
6. Mathew PG, Cooper W. The diagnosis and management of posttraumatic headache with associated painful cranial neuralgias: a review and case series. *Curr Pain Headache Rep*. 2021;25(8):54.
7. Maizels M. Sphenopalatine ganglion block without catheter. *Pract Neurol*. 2021 May:39-42.
8. Simons DG, Travell JG, Simons LS. *Myofascial Pain and Dysfunction: The Trigger Point Manual*. Vol. 1. 2nd ed. Upper Half of Body. Baltimore, MD: Lippincott Williams & Wilkins; 1999.

CHAPTER
45

Infusion Therapy

Michael Marmura

The outpatient headache treatment is not always effective. When established treatment strategies fail to provide adequate headache control, parenteral treatments may be necessary. Clinical trials of acute medication for migraines typically focus on subjects with episodic migraines, treating within a few hours of attack onset, with the goal of achieving pain freedom and relieving the most bothersome symptoms. However, managing status migrainosus or prolonged migraine, particularly in the Emergency Department (ED), requires a different approach (Chapter 9). Highly effective treatments for acute migraines, such as subcutaneous sumatriptan, may be equally or less effective than parenteral treatments, including prochlorperazine, in the ED setting.

Indications for Infusion Therapy

Recommendations for specific therapies are based on placebo-controlled trials in ED or infusion settings, comparison studies of different medications, retrospective analysis of infusion or inpatient outcomes, and expert opinions. Most studies primarily focus on pain relief as the primary endpoint, while the impact on other headache symptoms or the risk of recurrence is often not assessed. When assessing patients with headaches, several important factors indicate the need for parenteral therapy. Some of the most important indications are listed in Box 45-1.

Infusion therapies for headaches are administered in three different settings: ED, infusion centers, and inpatient treatment in a hospital. The ED is the most common setting for patients to receive infusion treatment for migraines, but the environment may pose challenges for individuals with photophobia or phonophobia. The treatment for headache may vary depending on the location, and ED providers do not always follow specific migraine protocols. Outpatient infusion centers may be a preferable option when available, although prior arrangements and scheduling during office hours may be necessary in most cases.

Box 45-1. Common Indications for Infusion Headache Therapy

- Intractable headache
- Refractory migraine
- Moderate-to-severe impact and disability due to headache
- Status migrainosus
- Inadequate response to previous therapies
- Significant nausea, vomiting, or dehydration
- Overuse of acute headache medication
- Medical comorbidities requiring observation

Infusion Therapies for Migraine

Migraine is the most common indication for parenteral headache treatment. The following therapies have shown clinical effectiveness supported by placebo-controlled, prospective, or retrospective studies.

Dihydroergotamine

Dihydroergotamine (DHE), a semi-synthetic formulation of an ergot alkaloid, is a mainstay of parenteral migraine therapy, commonly utilized in both infusion and inpatient settings.[1,2] It acts as a vasoconstrictive agent in veins and arteries, interacting with neurotransmitter receptors such as norepinephrine, epinephrine, dopamine, and serotonin receptors. DHE's therapeutic effects in migraine are attributed to its agonist activity on serotonin receptors, particularly the 5-HT1D receptor subtype. This activity is believed to constrict specific intracranial blood vessels and potentially inhibit the release of proinflammatory neuropeptides from sensory nerve endings in the trigeminovascular system.

The efficacy of intravenous (IV) DHE for intractable migraines was first described by Raskin in 1986.[1] In an initial study, Raskin administered IV DHE to 55 patients suffering from continuous headaches, many of whom had overused acute headache medications. The doses ranged from 0.3 to 1 mg every 8 hours for 2 days. Remarkably, 89% of the patients experienced headache freedom within 2 days, with most reporting sustained relief. Subsequent studies have demonstrated that IV DHE treatment in patients with chronic headaches, including chronic migraine, led to headache freedom within 3 days, along with improvements in headache symptoms. Moreover, DHE is also effective in the prevention of medication overuse relapse, especially in patients who overuse triptans.

In both inpatient and outpatient settings, DHE is typically administered intravenously over a period of 30 to 60 minutes.[2] In the inpatient setting, IV DHE is given every 8 hours until the maximum daily dose of 2 mg is reached, with a maximum weekly dosage of 6 mg. In the emergency department or outpatient environment, the initial dose of IV DHE can be 0.25 to 1 mg, followed by an additional 0.5 to 1 mg, 1 to 4 hours later. To prevent adverse events including nausea, DHE is commonly coadministered with antiemetics. For instance, metoclopramide 10 mg IV approximately 30 minutes prior to the DHE infusion is an effective pretreatment for nausea due to DHE. Before administering IV DHE, it is important to obtain blood pressure readings and an electrocardiogram (EKG) to ensure safety.

Common adverse events of DHE include nausea, diarrhea, abdominal cramps, chest tightness, leg cramps, and acute hypertension. It is worth noting that while headaches may temporarily worsen immediately after DHE administration, this does not necessarily indicate a poor response, as long as nausea can be effectively controlled.[3] Although DHE is commonly given intermittently, continuous infusion of DHE has also been reported to be effective and associated with fewer adverse events.[4] Significant coronary or peripheral artery disease is a contraindication for DHE. Serious or permanent adverse events, such as vasospasm, ischemia, or uncontrolled hypertension, can occur. Patients with uncontrolled hypertension, coronary artery disease, pregnancy, hemiplegic migraine or migraine with brain stem aura, recent use of sumatriptan within the past 24 hours, or current use of macrolide antibiotics or retroviral therapy should not receive DHE.

Antiemetics

Antiemetic dopamine antagonists play a crucial role in the infusion therapy of migraine, serving as effective measures for both prevention of medication-induced nausea, such as with DHE, and treatment of migraine itself (Table 45-1).[2,5] These medications, including metoclopramide, droperidol, and phenothiazines like chlorpromazine and prochlorperazine, are first-line treatments for acute migraine in the ED, as well as in inpatient settings and outpatient infusion clinics. The exact

Table 45-1. Intravenous Antiemetics for Migraine Treatment

Medication	Common Adverse Events	Dose (mg)
Metoclopramide	Akathisia, dystonia, parkinsonism (long-term use), somnolence, serotonin syndrome (rare)	5-20
Prochlorperazine	Dizziness, akathisia, dystonia, parkinsonism (long-term use), somnolence, hypotension	5-10
Promethazine	Dizziness, sedation, akathisia, dystonia (less common than other neuroleptics)	12.5-25
Droperidol	Drowsiness, akathisia, hypotension, tachycardia, chills, higher potential for QT prolongation	0.625-2.5
Chlorpromazine	Dizziness, akathisia, sedation (common), orthostatic hypotension, tachycardia, urinary retention	12.5-50
Haloperidol	Drowsiness, akathisia, hypotension, tachycardia, constipation; rare neuroleptic malignant syndrome or parkinsonism	2-5

mechanism of action of these antiemetic dopamine antagonists in migraine remains unknown. Their benefits in alleviating headache are likely related to their effects on central dopamine receptors, as central dopaminergic pathways are significantly involved in migraine. Furthermore, the antiemetic effect of these drugs may contribute to faster recovery from the migraine attack, particularly in patients experiencing severe nausea and vomiting.

Prochlorperazine IV 10 mg is effective for acute migraine compared to placebo, sumatriptan subcutaneous injection, IV hydromorphone 1 mg, and IV sodium valproate 500 mg. Droperidol doses of 2.75, 5.5, and 8.25 mg/dose are significantly more effective than placebo for acute migraine and repetitive IV droperidol appears effective for refractory migraine as an inpatient treatment.[9] Haloperidol IV 5 mg is also effective for migraine than placebo and is more widely available. Metoclopramide 10 mg IV is effective for migraine as monotherapy and in combination with IV DHE. Chlorpromazine is effective but relatively more sedating than other neuroleptics. Promethazine has a lower risk of akathisia than other neuroleptics, but is likely less effective than other therapies.[5]

Treatment with these medications can be associated with bothersome adverse effects that limit their use, including sedation, hypotension, or akathisia. While significant QT prolongation is rare with lower doses, close monitoring of EKGs is necessary due to the potential for this complication.[5] Prolonged QT interval (QTc) greater than 500 ms increases the risk of torsades de pointes, a potentially life-threatening cardiac arrhythmia. QTc values above 450 to 470 may warrant dose reduction or discontinuation of the neuroleptic. Electrolyte levels, particularly potassium and magnesium, should be monitored as hypokalemia and hypomagnesemia are risk factors for developing torsades. For patients who cannot tolerate neuroleptics due to adverse events, non-neuroleptic antiemetics like ondansetron provide an effective and safe alternative for treating migraine or medication-related nausea.[10] To minimize the risk of extrapyramidal effects associated with dopamine antagonists, the administration of 25 mg IV or IM of diphenhydramine, prior to the infusion of the dopamine antagonist can be useful. Chlorpromazine has been known to induce postural hypotension. This adverse event may be prevented by administering a bolus of 250 to 500 mL of normal saline before initiating the treatment.

Magnesium

Studies on the efficacy of IV magnesium infusion for acute migraine have shown mixed results.[2] Some studies indicate its benefit for migraines with aura, while others report increased pain-free rates.

However, another study found it to be no different from a placebo.[6] When compared, IV magnesium was less effective than metoclopramide but on par with prochlorperazine in migraine treatment.[7,8] Thus, efficacy of IV magnesium in the management of migraine remains uncertain. Nevertheless, it is often utilized due to its favorable tolerability. The recommended dosages for migraine treatment typically range from 500, 1000 to 2000 mg, depending on renal function. While serious side effects are rare, especially when administered over a 30- to 60-minute infusion, potential adverse reactions may include muscular weakness progressing to flaccid paralysis, ataxia, drowsiness, confusion, flushing, sweating, hypotension, hypothermia, and bradycardia. IV magnesium treatment is contraindicated in individuals with a history of heart block or myocardial damage.[11]

Nonsteroidal Anti-inflammatory Drugs

Aspirin and other nonsteroidal anti-inflammatory drugs (NSAIDs) are widely used and well-established treatments for migraine.[2] Frequent NSAID use does not appear to trigger migraine progression, unlike triptans. Intravenous lysine acetylsalicylate (aspirin) at a dosage of 1000 mg has shown moderate improvement in 62% of subjects and a good response in 27% during inpatient treatment of migraine, with good tolerability and minimal adverse events.[12] In the emergency department, ketorolac 30 mg was found to be as effective as 10 mg metoclopramide and more effective than 1000 mg sodium valproate, while dexketoprofen 50 mg IV demonstrated superior and faster action compared to IV ibuprofen 800 mg and metoclopramide 10 mg.

Antiepileptics

Valproic acid and its derivatives have demonstrated efficacy in migraine prophylaxis and may be considered as an intravenous treatment option.[2] An improvement in 80% of chronic migraine patients after they received intravenous valproate sodium, using a loading dose of 15 mg/kg followed by 5 mg/kg every 8 hours, has been reported.[13] A study involving patients with chronic or "transformed" migraine reported a 57.5% response rate to intravenous valproate infusions ranging from 300 to 1200 mg.[14] Limited evidence exists for the use of intravenous levetiracetam in acute migraine treatment.

Corticosteroids

Corticosteroids are commonly used as an alternative to NSAIDs, such as ketorolac, to minimize gastrointestinal side effects.[2] They have shown effectiveness in reducing headache recurrence. Dexamethasone 10 mg has been shown to reduce migraine recurrence compared to metoclopramide alone. Another option for inpatient treatment is methylprednisolone 125 mg every 12 hours for 3 days.[15]

Antihistamines

Antihistamines have shown potential in the treatment of acute migraine. Histamine desensitization has been successful in managing intractable migraine and cluster headache. A study by Swidan et al[16] compared the effects of intravenous diphenhydramine (administered in doses of 25 to 75 mg, three times daily) with IV DHE (administered in doses of 0.25 to 1.0 mg every 8 hours) for severe and refractory migraine headache. While immediate pain relief was better with intravenous diphenhydramine, overall reduction in head pain level after the 3-day protocol was greater with DHE.

Lidocaine

Continuous IV lidocaine infusion is a promising approach for inpatient treatment of migraine and other headaches, especially for patients with acute medication overuse.[17] Studies have shown positive outcomes with lidocaine infusion, including significant improvement and headache freedom in a majority of patients. Common adverse events associated with IV lidocaine include mild nausea, hypotension or hypertension, and arrhythmia, while higher doses may lead to more bothersome neuropsychiatric adverse events such as hallucinations. The usual practice is to initiate treatment at a rate of 1 mg/min, increasing to 2 mg/min after a few hours if tolerated.[17]

Propofol

IV propofol, administered as a subanesthetic or sedating infusion, shows potential effectiveness for refractory migraine. Studies have primarily focused on its use in outpatient or emergency department settings. The doses used in various studies vary significantly from 10 to 1 mg/kg. However, there is no evidence supporting improved long-term outcomes with inpatient treatment using IV propofol for migraine.[18]

Ketamine

Ketamine, a selective N-methyl-D-aspartate (NMDA) receptor antagonist, has potential applications in the treatment of pain and depression with a lower risk of respiratory depression. Studies have shown promising results in the use of IV ketamine for intractable migraine, with patients experiencing improvement in symptoms and reporting significant benefits in both the short and long term. Although neuropsychiatric adverse events were common, they were manageable and often resolved with lower doses or slower titration. In many cases, clinicians use adjunctive medications such as clonidine and benzodiazepines to reduce adverse events. However, the efficacy of low-dose IV ketamine for migraine in the emergency department did not show superiority over placebo. The doses in ketamine studies vary considerably from 0.1 to 1 mg/kg/h, which may explain the differences in effectiveness and adverse events. Further research should explore the role of ketamine in migraine treatment, particularly in less refractory populations.[19]

Infusion Therapy for Migraine: A Practical Approach

Before initiating treatment for migraine, clinicians should conduct a thorough review of the patient's history and overall disease burden, and discuss potential adverse events. Ensuring adequate IV access is crucial, particularly considering the impact of DHE on veins. Most often, patients receive a combination of acute parenteral therapies, which typically includes an NSAID, antiemetic, and DHE. Additional therapies, such as magnesium, anticonvulsants such as valproate, or corticosteroids, can be added. Adding antihistamines, like diphenhydramine, may help reduce the risk of akathisia in susceptible patients. If breakthrough nausea occurs after DHE administration, the use of an additional antiemetic may be necessary. Benzodiazepines or benztropine are commonly used to manage anxiety or dystonic reactions, respectively.[20] It is common for patients to require at least two rounds of treatment to achieve improvement, particularly for those with longstanding migraines or who have not previously received DHE. If feasible, repeating infusions for another 1 to 2 days can enhance treatment outcomes.[21]

Inpatient Treatment of Migraine

While outpatient or ED settings are commonly used for infusion therapy in migraine, inpatient treatment offers a controlled environment and more intensive care for refractory patients. Indications for inpatient treatment include severe disability, unsuccessful infusion therapies, nausea and vomiting, significant medical or psychiatric comorbidities, and acute headache medication overuse involving opioids or barbiturates. Inpatient management often involves therapies that require close monitoring for potential serious adverse effects. Repetitive administration of DHE for up to 7 days is a cornerstone of inpatient treatment, supported by strong evidence for improved long-term outcomes.[1,22] Other commonly utilized therapies include lidocaine, ketamine, chlorperazine, droperidol, and valproate. For patients with intractable symptoms, additional treatments such as magnesium, NSAIDs, corticosteroids, or anticonvulsants may provide added benefits. Inpatient care can enhance the effectiveness of long-term preventive treatments, improve quality of life, and reduce the overuse of acute medications.[13]

Infusion Therapy for Nonmigraine Headache and Trigeminal Neuralgia

Patients experiencing refractory cluster headache often require infusion therapies when other treatments have proven ineffective. Common indications for infusion therapy include poor response to transitional or preventive therapies, severe pain, and functional impairment. Repetitive sodium valproate, high-dose corticosteroids, DHE, IV ketamine, and magnesium are among the parenteral treatments which have been used in severe cluster headache.[23] For patients with short-lasting severe attacks of short-lasting unilateral neuralgiform headache with conjunctival injection and tearing (SUNCT), short-lasting unilateral headache with cranial autonomic symptoms (SUNA), and trigeminal neuralgia, IV treatment is indicated in cases of intractable pain or when there is impairment in essential functions such as eating or drinking. Case reports have reported successful treatment of SUNCT with IV lidocaine, and IV phenytoin, fosphenytoin, and lacosemide may treat acute exacerbations of trigeminal neuralgia (Chapter 39).[24]

Summary

- Infusion therapies in the ED and outpatient setting can provide relief for patients with refractory headache when established acute therapies are ineffective.
- DHE is a mainstay of infusion therapy for headache, but requires prescreening to avoid contraindications and blood pressure monitoring.
- Antiemetics, including dopamine antagonists, effectively treat migraine and associated nausea or vomiting.
- Clinicians often use adjunctive medications such as NSAIDs, corticosteroids, magnesium, and valproate to improve outcomes.
- A few studies have proposed alternative treatments such as lidocaine, propofol, or ketamine for the treatment of severe headache in ED or inpatient settings.
- Infusion therapies are also an option for patients with refractory cluster headache or trigeminal neuralgia.

REFERENCES

1. Raskin NH. Repetitive intravenous dihydroergotamine as therapy for intractable migraine. *Neurology*. 1986;36:995-997.

2. Ashina S, Portenoy RK. Intravenous treatment of migraine. *Tech Reg Anesth Pain Manag*. 2012;16:25-29.

3. Eller M, Gelfand AA, Riggins NY, Shiboski S, Schankin C, Goadsby PJ. Exacerbation of headache during dihydroergotamine for chronic migraine does not alter outcome. *Neurology*. 2016;86:856-859.

4. Ford RG, Ford KT. Continuous intravenous dihydroergotamine in the treatment of intractable headache. *Headache*. 1997;37:129-136.

5. Marmura MJ. Use of dopamine antagonists in treatment of migraine. *Curr Treat Options Neurol*. 2012;14:27-35.

6. Frank LR, Olson CM, Shuler KB, Gharib SF. Intravenous magnesium for acute benign headache in the emergency department: a randomized double-blind placebo-controlled trial. *CJEM*. 2004;6(5):327-332.

7. Cete Y, Dora B, Ertan C, Ozdemir C, Oktay C. A randomized prospective placebo-controlled study of intravenous magnesium sulphate vs. metoclopramide in the management of acute migraine attacks in the Emergency Department. *Cephalalgia*. 2005;25(3):199-204.

8. Ginder S, Oatman B, Pollack M. A prospective study of i.v. magnesium and i.v. prochlorperazine in the treatment of headaches. *J Emerg Med.* 2000;18(3):311-315.

9. Wang SJ, Silberstein SD, Young WB. Droperidol treatment of status migrainosus and refractory migraine. *Headache.* 1997;37:377-382.

10. Gruppo LQ Jr. Intravenous zofran for headache. *J Emerg Med.* 2006;31:228-229.

11. Choi H, Parmar N. The use of intravenous magnesium sulphate for acute migraine: meta-analysis of randomized controlled trials. *Eur J Emerg Med.* 2014;21:2-9.

12. Weatherall M, Telzerow A, Cittadini E, Kaube H, Goadsby PJN. Intravenous aspirin (lysine acetylsalicylate) in the inpatient management of headache. *Neurology.* 2010;75:1098-1103.

13. Marmura MJ, Hou A. Inpatient management of migraine. *Neurol Clin.* 2019;37:771-788.

14. Stillman MJ, Zajac D, Rybicki LA. Treatment of primary headache disorders with intravenous valproate: initial outpatient experience. *Headache.* 2004;44:65-69.

15. Colman I, Friedman BW, Brown MD, et al. Parenteral dexamethasone for acute severe migraine headache: meta-analysis of randomised controlled trials for preventing recurrence. *BMJ.* 2008;336:1359-1361.

16. Swidan SZ, Lake AE III, Saper JR. Efficacy of intravenous diphenhydramine versus intravenous DHE-45 in the treatment of severe migraine headache. *Curr Pain Headache Rep.* 2005;9:65-70.

17. Berk T, Silberstein SD. The use and method of action of intravenous lidocaine and its metabolite in headache disorders. *Headache.* 2018;58:783-789.

18. Piatka C, Beckett RD. Propofol for treatment of acute migraine in the emergency department: a systematic review. *Acad Emerg Med.* 2020;27:148-160.

19. Chah N, Jones M, Milord S, Al-Eryani K, Enciso R. Efficacy of ketamine in the treatment of migraines and other unspecified primary headache disorders compared to placebo and other interventions: a systematic review. *J Dent Anesth Pain Med.* 2021;21:413.

20. Wijemanne S, Jankovic J, Evans RW. Movement disorders from the use of metoclopramide and other antiemetics in the treatment of migraine. *Headache.* 2016;56:153-161.

21. Shafqat R, Flores-Montanez Y, Delbono V, Nahas SJ. Updated evaluation of IV dihydroergotamine (DHE) for refractory migraine: patient selection and special considerations. *J Pain Res.* 2020;13:859-864.

22. Nagy AJ, Gandhi S, Bhola R, Goadsby PJ. Intravenous dihydroergotamine for inpatient management of refractory primary headaches. *Neurology.* 2011;77:1827-1832.

23. Prasad S, Mehadi A, Kaka N, et al. Diagnostic protocols and newer treatment modalities for cluster headache. *Dis Mon.* 2022;68:101316.

24. Muñoz-Vendrell A, Teixidor S, Sala-Padró J, Campoy S, Huerta-Villanueva MJC. Intravenous lacosamide and phenytoin for the treatment of acute exacerbations of trigeminal neuralgia: a retrospective analysis of 144 cases. *Cephalalgia.* 2022;42(10):1031-1038.

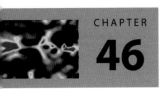

CHAPTER

46

Neuromodulation

Natalia Murinova, Christopher L. Robinson, and Roni Sharon

Often, individuals presenting with headache and migraine disorders have trialed and failed conservative medical management due to either the lack of efficacy or the side effect profile, but there remains another category of noninvasive treatment such as neuromodulation. Neuromodulation, defined as either medication but more often as an electrical stimulation device that alters the transmission of neuronal signaling, has emerged as an alternative noninvasive avenue for addressing headache and migraine disorders. Though the exact mechanism remains to be fully determined, neuromodulation employs electrical currents that modulate neural circuits, historically only accessible through implantable devices. Presently, numerous noninvasive neurostimulation devices are available (discussed here) and are better tolerated since they have a higher safety and lower side-effect profile. These devices offer home-based treatments with remote control and some with paired mobile and web applications, catering to those who have failed or are averse to pharmacotherapy. It suits both headache and migraine sufferers and potentially can extend relief to breast-feeding and pregnant patients, adolescents, and the elderly who may be more sensitive to or where pharmacotherapy may be contraindicated. Trials, including sham-controlled ones, continue to emerge, adding further support to their efficacy and safety profiles. General exclusions to most neuromodulation devices include patients with cranial/body implants, recent trauma, or skin abrasions/breakdown.[1-3]

Remote Electrical Neuromodulation/Nerivio™

Indications

Nerivio™, a product of Theranica Bio-Electronics, is a wireless, wearable, battery-powered neuromodulation device that is noninvasive and can be conveniently controlled via a smartphone app. Nerivio™ is FDA-cleared for the acute management of episodic and chronic migraine with and without aura in patients ≥12 of age.[4]

Contraindications

Individuals with uncontrolled epilepsy or those utilizing active implantable medical devices, such as pacemakers, hearing aid implants, or other implanted electronic devices, should refrain from using Nerivio™. This precaution ensures their safety and prevents any potential complications.[4]

Mechanism of Action

Nerivio™ involves a proprietary electrical stimulation pattern on the upper arm activating specific sensory fibers—mainly small A-delta fibers—above depolarization thresholds, yet under the pain perception threshold. This nonpainful activation of peripheral sensory nerves sends signals to the brainstem's pain control centers, the periaqueductal gray, rostral ventromedial medulla, and subnucleus reticularis dorsalis, triggering descending inhibition

291

pathways. Serotonin and noradrenaline release inhibit pain signaling, particularly in the trigeminal cervical complex (TCC), providing migraine pain relief.[4]

Use of Device

Nerivio™ is a self-administered device designed for home use, providing relief during the onset of a migraine attack or aura. Nerivio™ is placed on the lateral upper arm, specifically between the bellies of the lateral deltoid triceps for a duration of 45 minutes. To maximize efficacy, treatment should commence promptly, ideally within an hour of migraine headache or aura onset. This program features a symmetrical, biphasic, square pulse with a modulated frequency ranging from 100 to 120 Hz. It also includes a pulse width of 400 μs and an output current of up to 40 mA, which can be adjusted in real time by the patient.[4]

Efficacy

In a double-blind randomized controlled trial (252 participants), Nerivio™ use at 2 hours demonstrated 66.7% pain relief versus 38.8% (sham), 37.4% pain freedom versus 18.4%, and the most bothersome symptom relief was 46.3% versus 22.2%.[5] In another randomized, double-blind, placebo-controlled study, REN, administered every other day, demonstrated effectiveness for migraine prevention, showing superiority over placebo by reducing the mean number of migraine days per month.[6]

Safety and Adverse Effects

Adverse events predominantly involved paresthesias around the device site, encompassing warmth, temporary numbness in the arm/hand, redness, itching, tingling, and muscle spasms. Pain in the arm, shoulders, or neck was also reported, and tolerability was high.[4]

Transcutaneous Supraorbital Nerve Stimulation/CEFALY®

Indications

CEFALY® is an FDA-cleared device for acute migraine with or without aura in patients ≥18 years of age and preventive treatment for episodic migraine in patients ≥18 years of age.[2]

Contraindications

CEFALY® is contraindicated in patients with implanted electrical devices, facial trauma, or skin breakdown at the sites of application.[2]

Mechanism of Action

Neuromodulation devices share similar mechanisms of action as the aforementioned. A potential additional mechanism of supraorbital stimulation is that it is thought to modulate the TCC. Research does suggest a functional link between the trigeminal nucleus and cervical nerves, particularly the upper three cervical dorsal horns, forming the TCC. This complex serves as a convergence point for nociceptive afferents from both systems.[2]

Use of Device

Positioned at the forehead's center, CEFALY® administers transcutaneous electrical stimulation to the supraorbital and supratrochlear nerves. For acute migraine management, press the button once, and the 60-minute acute program initiates (max intensity: 16 mA, pulse width: 250 msec, frequency: 100 Hz). For episodic migraine prevention, press the button twice, and the 20-minute prevention program starts (16 mA, 250 msec, 60 Hz).[2]

Efficacy

CEFALY® has led to a reduction of up to 30% in monthly migraine days, accompanied by a notable decrease of up to 37% in the usage of acute migraine medications among users.[2]

Safety and Adverse Effects

Side effects are infrequent and encompass mild sedation, postsession headache, forehead redness, occasional nausea, and a very rare occurrence (0.1%) of an allergy to the electrode adhesive gel.[2]

Single-Pulse Transcranial Magnetic Stimulation

Indications

The single-pulse transcranial magnetic stimulation (sTMS) device is FDA-cleared for acute and preventive management of migraine in patients ≥12 of age.[2]

Contraindications

The sTMS device is contraindicated in patients with implantable devices or history of epilepsy.[3]

Mechanism of Action

The sTMS device curtails cortical hyperexcitability by modulating glutamate and dopamine levels in the hippocampus and caudate, adjusting neuronal excitability, curbing central sensitization, and decreasing headache frequency.[3]

Use of Device

The sTMS is positioned at the back of the head for use. The preventive approach involves two daily sessions of four pulses each (two consecutive pulses, wait 15 minutes, then repeat two consecutive pulses). For acute treatment, if required, administer three sequential pulses at migraine onset, and if necessary, follow up with more pulses at 15-minute intervals.[3]

Efficacy

The sTMS device has demonstrated a decrease of 2.75 migraine days, a 46% rate of achieving a 50% reduction, and reductions in total headache days and headache-related disability.[7]

Safety and Adverse Effects

Adverse events of sTMS include sensations of lightheadedness, tingling, and tinnitus.[2,7]

External Noninvasive Vagal Nerve Stimulation/gammaCore Sapphire™

Indications

The gammaCore Sapphire™ is FDA-cleared for acute pain relief in adults with episodic cluster headache and for acute and preventive pain treatment in migraine patients ≥12 years of age.[2]

Contraindications

The gammaCore Sapphire™ is unsuitable for those with active implants such as pacemakers, defibrillators, or cochlear implants near the treatment site. Caution is urged for carotid atherosclerosis, cervical vagotomy history, vasovagal syncope, and skin irritation near the site.[3]

Mechanism of Action

Continuous vagal nerve stimulation suppresses key components of cluster headache and migraine pain, including the limbic system, thalamus, nucleus tractus solitarius, dorsal pons, and locus coeruleus, potentially by reducing glutamate levels in the trigeminal nucleus caudalis and reversing central sensitization in chronic headache sufferers.[3]

Use of Device

For migraine prevention, patients should apply the device on each side of the neck, giving two treatments daily (morning and night), each comprising two consecutive 2-minute stimulations within an hour of waking and at night. For cluster headache and migraine pain treatment, utilize at the initial sign of migraine pain by administering two stimulations of 2-minute duration each.[8]

Efficacy

Though studies are limited in demonstrating statistical significance for its use and were interrupted by the COVID-19 pandemic, the randomized PRESTO study suggests that gammaCore Sapphire™ may have clinical efficacy for abortive treatment in episodic migraine if used within 30 to 60 minutes postinitiation of attack.[9]

Safety and Adverse Effects

The gammaCore Sapphire™ is well-tolerated, with adverse events including facial pain, gastrointestinal symptoms, and upper respiratory tract infection being the most common side effects.[2]

External Combined Occipital and Trigeminal Nerve Stimulation/Relivion®

Indications

Relivion® is FDA-cleared for the acute management of migraine with and without aura in patients ≥18 years of age.[10]

Contraindications

Contraindications include implant devices or metallic objects, recent facial trauma, or skin breakdown in the area of application.[11]

Mechanism of Action

Relivion® is a self-administered stimulator that delivers electric pulses to 6 branches of the occipital and trigeminal nerves, targeting simultaneously the frontal and occipital pathways of the TCC.[2]

Use of Device

Relivion® is positioned on the head at migraine onset and worn for 20 to 60 minutes. While unlimited treatments are possible, a daily usage limit of 80 minutes is advised, ensuring a comfortable yet effective sensation to relieve pain.[12]

Efficacy

Relivion® users experienced significant pain freedom at 2 hours (46% vs. 12% with sham), achieving resolution of pain and bothersome symptoms (nausea, vomiting, photophobia, or phonophobia) at 47% compared to 14% with sham. Additionally, 36% of Relivion users enjoyed sustained pain freedom at both 2- and 24-hours post-treatment, contrasting with 8% in the sham group.[10]

Safety and Adverse Effects

Side effects were minor and included unpleasant sensations during treatment, pain, skin redness, tingling, and twitching.[10]

Investigational Uses for Neuromodulation

Transcranial Direct Current Stimulation

Transcranial direct current stimulation (tDCS) involves using low current (1-2 mA) and various electrode placements on the head for its use in headache disorders. The quality of available data is limited and requires further studies to better understand if there can be any use in headache disorders as no standardized protocols exist. As with most neuromodulation techniques, the exact mechanism of action remains to be fully elucidated, but it may involve alteration of the central nervous system connectivity and modulation of network-level coding without affecting membrane potential.[2]

Occipital Nerve Stimulation

Only indicated for use in peripheral chronic pain, occipital nerve stimulation (ONS) remains an investigational device treatment for use in headache disorders. Believed to target and modulate the occipital aspect of the TCC, ONS use remains limited due to a higher level of adverse events given its location on the occiput. With further development of the leads and studies (mainly open-label studies), the role of ONS for the management of migraine and other headaches may continue to unfold.[2]

Spinal Cord Stimulation

Spinal cord stimulation (SCS) is currently indicated for failed back surgery syndrome, complex regional pain syndrome, and peripheral diabetic neuropathy. Increasing studies suggest a potential role for SCS in other chronic pain disorders, including refractory chronic migraine, where electrodes induce paresthesia in the epidural space to alleviate pain. Patients start with a trial using temporary SCS leads that are externally powered. If successful, a permanent subcutaneous internal pulse generator (IPG) with leads is implanted for long-term relief. Due to the high-placebo effect in migraine studies, further well-designed, sufficiently powered studies with proper appropriate controls are needed to fully appreciate the effects.[2,13]

Summary

- Noninvasive, neuromodulation devices have become an attractive alternative to traditional pharmacotherapy for migraine and cluster headache, especially for patients who are intolerant to medications or who prefer non-pharmacological options.
- REN with Nerivio™ is a wireless, wearable device controlled by a smartphone app for the acute and preventive treatment of migraine.
- t-SNS with CEFALY® is a device indicated for both acute and preventive migraine treatment in adults, using supraorbital nerve stimulation.
- sTMS provides a portable, non-invasive solution for both acute and preventive migraine management, by delivering magnetic pulses to the occipital cortex.
- External VNS with GammaCore Sapphire™ is indicated for the acute and preventive treatment of migraine and episodic cluster headache, employing non-invasive vagus nerve stimulation.
- eCOTS with Relivion® represents another approach for acute migraine treatment, stimulating both the occipital and trigeminal nerves simultaneously.

REFERENCES

1. Moisset X, Pereira B, Ciampi de Andrade D, Fontaine D, Lantéri-Minet M, Mawet J. Neuromodulation techniques for acute and preventive migraine treatment: a systematic review and meta-analysis of randomized controlled trials. *J Headache Pain.* 2020;21:1-14.

2. Yuan H, Chuang TY. Update of neuromodulation in chronic migraine. *Curr Pain Headache Rep.* 2021;25:3.

3. Tiwari V, Agrawal S. Migraine and neuromodulation: a literature review. *Cureus.* 2022;14:e31223.

4. Nierenburg H, Stark-Inbar A. Nerivio® remote electrical neuromodulation for acute treatment of chronic migraine. *Pain Manag.* 2022;12:267-281.

5. Yarnitsky D, Dodick DW, Grosberg BM, et al. Remote electrical neuromodulation (REN) relieves acute migraine: a randomized, double-blind, placebo-controlled, multicenter trial. *Headache.* 2019;59:1240-1252.

6. Tepper SJ, Rabany L, Cowan RP, et al. Remote electrical neuromodulation for migraine prevention: A double-blind, randomized, placebo-controlled clinical trial. *Headache.* 2023;63(3):377-389.

7. Starling AJ, Tepper SJ, Marmura MJ, et al. A multicenter, prospective, single arm, open label, observational study of sTMS for migraine prevention (ESPOUSE Study). *Cephalalgia.* 2018:38: 1038-1048.

8. Migraine Dosing - gammacore. Available at: https://www.gammacore.com/for-migraine/migraine-dosing/

9. Tassorelli C, Grazzi L, de Tommaso M, et al. Noninvasive vagus nerve stimulation as acute therapy for migraine. *Neurology.* 2018;91:e364-e373.

10. Tepper SJ, Grosberg B, Daniel O, et al. Migraine treatment with external concurrent occipital and trigeminal neurostimulation: a randomized controlled trial. *Headache.* 2022;62(8):989-1001.

11. Important Safety Information - Relivion MG. Available at: https://www.relivion.com/important-safety-information/.

12. Relivion® MG: A New Migraine Device Using "Electricity" to Rewire the Migraine Brain. Available at: https://www.migrainedisorders.org/relivion-migraine-neuromodulation-device/

13. Al-Kaisy A, Palmisani S, Carganillo R, et al. Safety and efficacy of 10 kHz spinal cord stimulation for the treatment of refractory chronic migraine: a prospective long-term open-label study. *Neuromodulation: Technology at the Neural Interface.* 2022;25:103-113.

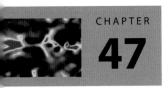

CHAPTER

47

Integrative and Behavioral Treatment of Headache

Deena E. Kuruvilla and Brooklyn A. Bradley

Patients who have less successful responses to mainstream medical therapy may consider other approaches or therapies that are considered outside of typical conventional healthcare. Complementary and integrative medicine (CIM) is a comprehensive realm of treatment approaches which include nutraceuticals, body-based therapies, and mind-body medicine.[1] CIM is increasingly popular in the world of healthcare, especially in the setting of headache disorders.[1] Cognitive behavior therapy (CBT) is also being incorporated into the patient's overall plan of care for their headache disorder. The origin of behavioral treatments is based on the representation of headache as a disorder of psychophysiological origin. CIM and behavioral treatments including biofeedback and CBT may be a new method of effective care for headache disorders in all populations.[2]

Nutraceutical and Herbal Medicine

Riboflavin

Riboflavin (B_2) is a water-soluble B vitamin, and is vital to human health. It is the precursor of the essential coenzymes, which include flavin mononucleotide and flavin adenine dinucleotide.[3] Absorbed in the small intestine, riboflavin is used for metabolic energy production and is naturally present in many different foods. Riboflavin is considered an efficacious treatment in the prophylaxis of migraine as it has a limited side effect profile. The effect of riboflavin 400 mg daily for migraine prevention has been shown in two clinical trials.[3] High-dose riboflavin treatment in comparison with other prophylactic agents has a low number of adverse events.[3] Thus, a high-dose riboflavin treatment of 400 mg/day may alleviate symptoms and reduce the number of migraine days in patients with migraine.[3] An oral route of riboflavin may cause the urine to have a more yellow color than normal, depending on the dosage. The adverse drug events reported in the riboflavin randomized controlled trials (RCTs) were of gastrointestinal origin, including vomiting and diarrhea. However, further research into the side effects of riboflavin is warranted.[3]

Magnesium

Magnesium is an abundant intracellular divalent cation that is involved in numerous cellular functions. It is mostly known for its role as a cofactor of many enzymes central to both glucose metabolism and adenosine triphosphate function.[4] Magnesium is absorbed in the gastrointestinal tract and is largely excreted through the urine. The pathway of magnesium metabolism may play a role in migraine pathogenesis.[4] A case-control study performed in patients with migraine discovered that serum magnesium levels during the migraine attacks and between the attacks are reduced in patients with migraine compared to the healthy group.[5] As a result, daily supplementation of magnesium in patients with migraine may be recommended by the provider.

A double-blind placebo-controlled study where 24 women with menstrual-related migraine were given 360 mg of magnesium pyrrolidine carboxylic acid revealed reductions in the number of days of headache and total pain index.[4] The dosage of magnesium may be recommended depending on the patient's medical history and their degree of migraine headache attacks.[4] Magnesium has a safe side-effect profile, which is why it is being increasingly recommended to migraine patients. Some of the side effects observed in trials included diarrhea and gastric irritation.[4]

Coenzyme Q10

Coenzyme Q10 (CoQ10) is known to improve abnormalities in mitochondrial function, especially in the setting of migraine.[4] In addition, it has demonstrated anti-inflammatory effects.[4]

Past research has shown a relationship between pediatric migraine and CoQ10 deficiency, which led to an open-label, add-on, controlled trial measuring the effectiveness of CoQ10 in prophylactic treatment of migraine headache.[4] A dosage of 100 mg CoQ10 daily reduced the number of attacks in addition to a reduction in severity of headaches (2.3-fold decrease), suggesting that this dose taken three times per day may lessen the frequency of migraine attacks.[4]

Determination of deficiency in patients with migraine may reveal the amount of CoQ10 dosage necessary for clinical improvement. Thus, clinicians can evaluate exact supplementation for each patient.[4]

Butterbur

Butterbur is an herbal supplement derived from the leaves of *Petasites japonicus*, and has been identified as an effective treatment in adult migraine patients.[3] The mechanism of action of butterbur is to decrease vasoconstriction of vessels and excitation of neurons by inhibiting the opening of L-type voltage-gated calcium channels. The active components of butterbur have been discovered to have anti-inflammatory effects as well.[3]

A randomized trial comparing butterbur extract 75 mg BID to placebo in 245 patients with migraine reported that migraine attack frequency was reduced by 48% for *Petasites* extract 75 mg BID.[3] *Petasites* extract 75 mg BID is an effective and well-tolerated preventative treatment for migraine.[3]

Previous randomized controlled trials have not identified any serious adverse effects, and have reported overall tolerance of the drug.[3] Some minor side effects include gastrointestinal manifestations, dyspepsia, headache, itchy eyes, drowsiness, fatigue, and asthma.[3] An area of concern in terms of safety is due to the presence of pyrrolizidine alkaloids (PA) found in the butterbur plant, which are hepatotoxic.[3] According to the National Center for Complementary and Integrative Health, U.S. National Institutes of Health, only butterbur products which have been processed to remove PAs and are labeled or certified as PA-free should be considered for use.

Feverfew

Feverfew, known scientifically as *Tanacetum parthenium L.*, is a medicinal plant typically used for treating fevers, migraine headaches, and insect bites. It is an inhibitor of prostaglandin synthesis and is associated with anti-inflammatory activity.[3,4]

In a double-blind placebo-controlled cross-over trial studying feverfew as a prophylactic treatment for migraine, the results showed that feverfew caused a decrease in pain intensity and symptom severity compared to placebo,[3] while another study reported that feverfew extract decreased migraine frequency.[3]

The adult feverfew dosage for migraine headaches is 100 to 300 mg up to four times daily. Feverfew can be used to prevent or stop a migraine headache. For feverfew supplements that are CO_2 extracted, it is recommended to take 6.24 mg three times daily for up to 16 weeks.[3] Adverse events in previous trials were reported to be generally mild and reversible.

Omega-3

Omega-3 fatty acids are a component of cell membrane phospholipids. Dietary intake of fish oil that is rich in eicosapentaenoic acid (EPA) and docosahexaenoic acid (DHA) allows for increased quantity of long-chain fatty acids in the phospholipids of blood cells membrane. This contributes to the inflammatory properties of omega-3.[3]

In a double-blind RCT measuring omega-3 polyunsaturated fatty acids in the prevention of migraine in chronic migraine patients, it was found that the group receiving omega-3 had a reduction of more than 80% per month in the number of days of headache.[3]

Most studies utilize daily doses of 15 to 20 g of fish oil containing about 30% EPA. Providers may also recommend patients to increase their natural intake of fish oil through two 8 oz fish meals per week. Omega-3 fish oil supplements are generally a safe and effective treatment in headache prevention and treatment. There are not many reports of adverse events in these RCTs due to the overall safe side-effect profile.

Vitamin D

Vitamin D, also called calciferol, is a fat-soluble vitamin that can be obtained through the diet or taken as a dietary supplement. This vitamin can be obtained through sun exposure, foods, and supplements. Vitamin D is necessary for bone growth and bone remodeling, and it also has a role in the reduction of inflammation throughout the body.[3] A case-control study measuring vitamin D deficiency with chronic tension-type headache (TTH) found that decreased serum 25-hydroxy D levels were lower in chronic TTH patients than in controls (14.7 vs. 27.4 ng/mL).[3] A randomized, double-blind, placebo-controlled trial of vitamin D_3 supplementation in adult migraine patients reported that when patients receiving 100 µg/day D_3 demonstrated a decrease in migraine frequency from baseline to week 24 compared to placebo.[3] The recommended dietary allowance of vitamin D for adults is 600 international units a day (IU).[3] Long-term use of vitamin D can damage the patient's bones, tissues, and organs. It is important for the provider to identify the best dosage for the patient.

Melatonin

There is increasing evidence supporting the idea that melatonin secretion is related to headaches.[3] Melatonin is a hormone produced by the pineal gland, and its secretion is increased in darkness. It plays a major role in regulating circadian rhythms and the sleep-wake stages.[3]

A pilot study evaluating the use of melatonin 4 mg as prophylactic therapy for primary headaches found a reduction in headache frequency between baseline and follow-up after 6 months of treatment with melatonin.[3] The melatonin 10 mg given orally, when introduced early in a cluster period, was found to be superior to placebo at decreasing cluster attack frequency.[3] According to the Sleep Foundation, a safe starting dose for adults is between 0.5 and 5 mg of melatonin.[3] To ensure safe usage, it is important that the provider knows the personal medical history of the patient and use this information to recommend the appropriate melatonin dosage. The most commonly reported side effects of melatonin include headache, dizziness, nausea, and drowsiness.[3]

Menthol

Menthol ($C_{10}H_{20}O$) is an ingredient of peppermint that has been used to treat many different pain conditions, most importantly the treatment of headache.[6] Menthol is considered a vasoactive agent that can produce cutaneous vasodilation. When it is applied to the skin, it leaves a cooling effect and can depress cutaneous nociception at low concentrations.[6]

A randomized, triple-blind, placebo-controlled study for the evaluation of efficacy and tolerability of the cutaneous application of menthol 10% as a treatment for migraine without aura revealed that menthol solution was superior to placebo on pain relief. In addition, the menthol solution was able to alleviate nausea and vomiting in the study population.[6] In an interventional uncontrolled study measuring the cutaneous application of menthol 10% solution on the temporal area in acute treatment of common migraine, the menthol solution was well tolerated by patients and was able to relieve the pain and related symptoms.[6] In the trials above, 1 mL of menthol was applied to the forehead and temporal area of the painful side using a piece of sponge. The menthol medication is for the skin only, and the substance can be applied no more than three to four times a day. The most common adverse effect of menthol solution is skin irritation.

Lavender

Lavender, of the genus *Lavandula*, is a flowering plant.[7] The leaves of lavender are recognized for their volatile oil, and can be used in aromatherapy. Lavender is often used in supportive therapy alongside mainstream medical therapy. Lavender essential oil has been used in the treatment of digestion, colds, and loss of appetite. It also is beneficial for patients with stress, anxiety, headaches, and migraines.[7] An RCT investigating the effect of lavender as a prophylactic therapy for migraine reported that after 3 months of lavender therapy, the Migraine Disability Assessment Scores (MIDAS) questionnaire score was reduced in comparison to the baseline and control group.[7] In a placebo-controlled clinical trial, patients with migraine inhaled lavender essential oil for 15 minutes and reported a mean reduction of headache severity.[7] The method of application of lavender essential oil may depend on the patient and their type of headache disorder. Providers should have a conversation about the aromatherapeutic use of lavender essential oils and which route would be optimal for their particular diagnosis. There are no reported major side effects or adverse events with this treatment.

Ginger

Ginger is a spice that is used for medicinal purposes in China and India. It is most commonly used to treat stomach pain, nausea, diarrhea, and respiratory disorders.[3] The analgesic action of ginger may be due to the inhibition of arachidonic acid metabolism via the cyclooxygenase (COX) pathways.[3] A double-blind placebo-controlled RCT of ginger addition to migraine acute management revealed that in adults with episodic migraine who received 400 mg of ginger extract (5% active ingredient), they showed better clinical response after 1, 1.5, and 2 hours.[3] The researchers also reported a reduction in pain and improvement on functional status following treatment with ginger.[3] A double-blind RCT comparing the efficacy of ginger to sumatriptan in the abortive treatment of common migraine found that, 2 hours after administering either drug, the mean headache severity decreased.[3] The effectiveness of ginger powder was statistically comparable to sumatriptan, but the clinical adverse effects of ginger powder were less than that of sumatriptan.[3]

There are various ways to use ginger for the treatment of migraine or headache disorders. Diluted ginger oil can be massaged into the temples, forehead, or back of neck. In addition, powdered ginger in the correct dose can be used in the prevention of migraine.[3] It is important for the provider to discuss with the patient different options for their particular headache diagnosis. Ginger may cause abdominal discomfort, heartburn, and mouth irritation if not taken properly. However, more trials need to be conducted to confirm this.

Mind-Body Medicine

Biofeedback

Biofeedback, also called biological feedback, is a well-known approach to lessen symptoms in patients with recurrent headache. It is an established nonpharmacological technique in the migraine community, and there are many published studies to support its impact on the frequency and severity of headaches in migraine patients. Two types of biofeedback include electromyography (EMG) and thermal or hand-warming feedback. An additional method includes feedback on sweat gland activity, in order to oppose the sympathetic nervous system arousal that initiates in response to stress.[8] The mechanism of biofeedback in migraine patients may be largely dependent upon its influence on oxidative stress. It has been reported that biofeedback impacts serum nitric oxide (NO) stable metabolites, peroxide activity, and superoxide dismutase (SOD) serum activity.[8] A study identifying the relationship between biofeedback and oxidative stress in patients with chronic migraine found that peroxide levels were higher in patients before biofeedback treatment, and reported that NO serum levels and SOD activity were lower prior to biofeedback treatment.[8] Various types of biofeedback are effective for migraine and TTH. An RCT has shown that there is a reduction in medication use and medical care in people who use both biofeedback and relaxation techniques over a 36-month period.[8]

Cognitive Behavioral Therapy

CBT is used as a behavioral headache treatment that targets the patient's behaviors, emotions, and cognitive responses.[9] It is the combination of two psychological treatment approaches, using cognitive- and behavioral-based techniques. The goal of CBT is to modify behavior by altering thoughts and behavioral patterns of reacting to an event or stressor. For headaches in particular, patients are guided to modify their thought process when responding to a stressor, and learn how to cope with stress, as stress is often a trigger of headaches. CBT is often administered in combination with biofeedback for relaxation training.[9]

An RCT measuring the effects of CBT for migraine headaches found that there was a significant reduction in headache frequency, duration and peak intensity following a minimal-therapist-contact approach and a clinic-based approach in the migraine patients.[9] In a two-factor experiment with repeated measures, CBT for chronic headache allowed for improved coping strategies, less disability, improved mood, increased pain-free days, and better control over pain following CBT.[9] An open/pilot trial of CBT in patients with refractory chronic migraine found that CBT made a statistically significant difference on pain severity, number of migraine attacks, and overall disability in the patients.[9]

Studies have reported that CBT alters pain severity, number of migraine attacks, and degree of disability in migraine patients.[9] As a result, CBT should be recommended by providers to migraine patients and patients suffering from other headache disorders. Overall, CBT may best be used in combination with other behavioral or pharmacological approaches than CBT alone. For example, providers may recommend CBT plus relaxation, CBT plus antidepressants (amitriptyline), or CBT plus biofeedback.[9]

Relaxation Training

Relaxation training is a systematic approach recommended for headache management where the patient learns how to reach a physical and mental state of relaxation within a few minutes of experiencing a stressor.[8] The goal of relaxation training is to slow down the sympathetic nervous system, which is closely connected to the stress response. Once the patient is in deep relaxation, they are able to reverse many of the physical responses that can stimulate a headache. Deep breathing and progressive muscle relaxation (PMR) are two of the techniques of relaxation training.[8]

A randomized trial comparing acupuncture, relaxation training, and physical training in the treatment of chronic TTH revealed that headache-free periods and headache-free days were higher in the relaxation group than the acupuncture group; however, an RCT is necessary to confirm statistical significance.[8] An RCT studying the effects of PMR on migraine frequency and contingent negative variation (CNV) reported that migraine patients randomized to the PMR group experienced a reduction of migraine frequency, illustrating the clinical importance of PMR and other relaxation techniques for migraine prophylaxis.[3]

PMR is a well-researched approach for the prevention and improvement of headache symptoms.[3] PMR is an efficacious nonpharmacological intervention for migraine prophylaxis. Providers should discuss this option with patients and recommend its combination with other integrative or behavioral approaches.

Meditation

Meditation is a mind-based practice that has been used for thousands of years, originating from Eastern tradition.[3] Meditation includes many different techniques, such as mindfulness meditation, mantra meditation, transcendental meditation, and spiritual meditation. The main goal is to integrate the body and mind, and use this connection to improve well-being.[3] Spiritual meditation is commonly used in the setting of migraine and physiological reactivity to stress. Thus, meditation is increasingly being recommended as a nonpharmacological option for patients experiencing disorders that involve chronic pain, such as migraine.

In a study measuring the effects of a month-long meditation protocol on meditation naïve participants with frequent migraines, the frequency of migraine headaches decreased in the spiritual meditation group compared to the other groups.[3] In addition, medication usage for migraine headaches was lower in the spiritual meditation group. The researchers proposed that the decrease in use of medications may be due to increased pain tolerance to migraine headache pain, which was mediated by the meditation intervention.[3] In a study of meditation-based treatment yielding immediate relief for meditation-naïve migraine patients, participants reported a 33% decrease in pain following the meditation intervention.[10] The patients had a single brief exposure to meditation, illustrating that meditation as an immediate intervention for reducing migraine pain is effective and is clinically relevant.[10] Meditation may be used in combination with yoga and other mindfulness practices. Providers should recommend meditation as an option for adults with migraines who have not been successful with mainstream medical therapy. Meditation has the capacity to improve migraine frequency, disability, and quality of life in patients suffering from migraine or other headache disorders.

Manipulative and Body-Based Practices

Acupuncture

Acupuncture is a body-based practice that involves applying small needles or pressure to specific points in the body. It is a nonpharmacological treatment option for various diseases and symptoms. It is often recommended for patients with migraine. However, there are few high-quality RCTs measuring the effectiveness of this treatment. It is known that the application of acupuncture induces a sensation in the patient and is often considered efficacious in the treatment of chronic pain.[3]

In an RCT studying the effectiveness of acupuncture for patients with migraine, the acupuncture group experienced a decrease by 2.2 days in the number of days with headache or moderate-to-severe intensity when compared to baseline.[3] In an RCT evaluating the efficacy of acupuncture for the prophylaxis of migraine, there was a mean reduction of 2.3 migraine days in the verum acupuncture group, which was statistically significant compared to baseline.[3] However, an RCT studying acupuncture for migraine prophylaxis reported that acupuncture only had clinically minor effects on migraine.[3]

Acupuncture is widely used as a preventative treatment for migraine. However, there is a lack of high-quality evidence investigating its effectiveness. It is important for patients to discuss this treatment option with their providers before proceeding with the intervention.

Massage Therapy

Massage therapy is a popular complementary and integrative therapy especially for pain treatment.[3] It involves the manipulation of soft tissue to improve pain and discomfort.[3] Massage therapy also promotes mental relaxation. It is generally viewed as a safe therapeutic intervention with few risks and adverse events.[3] For migraine in particular, massage therapy has the goal of reducing stress and improving symptom.[3]

In an RCT assessing the effects of massage therapy on migraine patients, patients in the massage group had greater improvements in migraine frequency and sleep quality both during the intervention and postintervention.[3] In a study measuring the reduction of current migraine headache pain following neck massage and spinal manipulation, headache pain intensity was reduced following treatment.[11] However, future RCTs should be conducted to evaluate the long-term effects of massage therapy. In addition, it is important that patients discuss the option of massage therapy with their provider to see if it is a viable option for their specific case.

Chiropractic Therapy

Chiropractic medicine has become increasingly popular over the last few decades. It focuses mainly on neuromusculoskeletal system disorders, and the impact they have on overall well-being. Chiropractic treatment procedures use manual techniques, such as joint adjustment and/or manipulation in the treatment of these disorders.[3] However, this therapy needs further assessment of its effectiveness for the management of specific diseases, especially migraine.[3]

In an RCT assessing the efficacy of chiropractic spinal manipulative therapy (SMT) in the treatment of migraine, 2 months of chiropractic SMT at vertebral fixations was established and the treatment group showed a statistically significant improvement in migraine frequency, duration, disability, and medication use in comparison to the control group; however, some patients were unable to complete the trial due to increased migraine frequency.[12] In an RCT studying chiropractic SMT for migraine, the researchers reported that migraine days were reduced in the treatment groups; however, the reduction in migraine days was not statistically different.[3] Some of the adverse events included tenderness, neck pain, and provoked migraine attack.[3]

While some studies report chiropractic therapy as an efficacious route for patients with migraine, it is important to address the history of adverse effects in this area of care. One study in 2017 determined the frequency of patients seen at an institution who were diagnosed with a cervical vessel dissection and symptoms of stroke in relation to a chiropractic neck manipulation.[3] Out of the 141 patients with cervical artery dissection, 12 patients had documented chiropractic neck manipulation prior to the dissection. The 12 patients had a total of 16 cervical artery dissections. In addition, all 12 patients experienced symptoms of acute stroke[3] In addition, there was a case report of a 32-year-old woman who had a chiropractic manipulation and subsequently developed vertebral artery dissection and brainstem infarct. Her condition quickly worsened and she died shortly after.[3]

Some studies show a improvement in migraine following chiropractic therapy. However, it is vital to consider the potential adverse effects of such a treatment. Chiropractic therapy should always be discussed with a provider and the patient be closely monitored following treatment. Thus, patients who are at an increased risk for dissections should avoid chiropractic therapy.

Summary

- Integrative medicine and behavioral approaches are a viable option for patients who do not respond to mainstream pharmacological treatments.
- Nutraceutical products commonly used in migraine include riboflavin, magnesium, coenzyme Q10, butterbur, feverfew, omega-3, vitamin D, and melatonin.
- Herbal medicine is a category of integrative medicine that involves herbs and herbal formulas that can be used for both acute and preventive treatment of headache.
- Mind-body medicine, including biofeedback, CBT, relaxation training, and meditation, can be used for headache management.
- Manipulative and body-based practices for headaches include acupuncture and massage therapy, while chiropractic therapy should be cautiously considered for potential adverse effects, particularly in patients at risk for dissections.

REFERENCES

1. Institute of Medicine (US) Committee on the Use of Complementary and Alternative Medicine by the American Public. Complementary and Alternative Medicine in the United States. Washington, DC: National Academies Press (US); 2005. 1, Introduction. Available at: https://www.ncbi.nlm.nih.gov/books/NBK83804/.

2. Kuruvilla DE, Mehta A, Ravishankar N, Cowan RP. A patient perspective of complementary and integrative medicine (CIM) for migraine treatment: a social media survey. *BMC Complement Med Ther*. 2021;21(1):58.

3. Wells RE, Beuthin J, Granetzke L. Complementary and integrative medicine for episodic migraine: an update of evidence from the last 3 years. *Curr Pain Headache Rep*. 2019;23(2):10.

4. Guilbot A, Bangratz M, Ait Abdellah S, Lucas C. A combination of coenzyme Q10, feverfew and magnesium for migraine prophylaxis: a prospective observational study. *BMC Complement Altern Med*. 2017;17:433.

5. Assarzadegan F, Asgarzadeh S, Hatamabadi HR, Shahrami A, Tabatabaey A, Asgarzadeh M. Serum concentration of magnesium as an independent risk factor in migraine attacks: a matched case-control study and review of the literature. *Int Clin Psychopharmacol*. 2016;31(5):287-292.

6. Borhani Haghighi A, Motazedian S, Rezaii R, et al. Cutaneous application of menthol 10% solution as an abortive treatment of migraine without aura: a randomised, double-blind, placebo-controlled, crossed-over study. *Int J Clin Pract*. 2010;64(4):451-456.

7. Rafie S, Namjoyan F, Golfakhrabadi F, Yousefbeyk F, Hassanzadeh A. Effect of lavender essential oil as a prophylactic therapy for migraine: a randomized controlled clinical trial. *J Herb Med*. 2016;6(1):18-23.

8. Millstine D, Chen CY, Bauer B. Complementary and integrative medicine in the management of headache. *BMJ*. 2017;357:j1805.

9. Onur OS, Ertem DH, Karsidag C, et al. An open/pilot trial of cognitive behavioral therapy in Turkish patients with refractory chronic migraine. *Cogn Neurodyn*. 2019;13(2):183-189.

10. Tonelli ME, Wachholtz AB. Meditation-based treatment yielding immediate relief for meditation-naïve migraineurs. *Pain Manag Nurs*. 2014;15(1):36-40.

11. Noudeh YJ, Vatankhah N, Baradaran HR. Reduction of current migraine headache pain following neck massage and spinal manipulation. *Int J Ther Massage Bodywork*. 2012;5(1):5-13.

12. Tuchin PJ, Pollard H, Bonello R. A randomized controlled trial of chiropractic spinal manipulative therapy for migraine. *J Manipulative Physiol Ther*. 2000;23(2):91-95.

PART VI

Special Populations

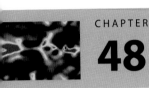

48

Headache During Pregnancy and Lactation

Huma U. Sheikh and Susan Hutchinson

Migraine is very common in the female population, occurring in 18% of all women in the United States (vs. 6% of men) (see Chapter 5). The prevalence of migraine peaks during child-bearing years to 25% to 30%. Given that 50% of pregnancies are unplanned, the choice of migraine medications for women in this population is important to protect against maternal and fetal complications of pregnancy.

Headache and Pregnancy

Reproductive events such as pregnancy influence the course of migraine in females. Fortunately, most women with migraine experience improvement during pregnancy especially if they have migraines without aura.[1] Migraine with aura is less likely to improve with pregnancy. New onset headache or migraine during pregnancy needs to be further investigated with an appropriate workup to rule out a secondary headache condition such as pre-eclampsia, stroke, cerebral venous thrombosis, pituitary tumor, and choriocarcinoma.

Epidemiology

Headache is a common occurrence in pregnant women, with some case reports recording it as high as 35%.[2] These occur most commonly in women who have a prior history of a primary headache disorder, mostly migraine, but many are also of new onset. Up to 75% of women with a prior history of migraine with and without aura will note a significant improvement in their headaches during the pregnancy.[12] However, some women may also have the first onset of a primary headache syndrome like migraine during pregnancy, with some reports of the first onset of migraine in pregnancy in up to 14%.[3]

Pathophysiology

Headaches in pregnancy can be a concerning condition. Most of these will be due to migraine, but there are also secondary conditions to consider. One retrospective study over 5 years showed that in addition to migraine, other diagnosis to be on the lookout for include hypertensive disorders, pre-eclampsia, posterior reversible encephalopathy syndrome (PRES), reversible cerebral vasoconstriction syndrome (RCVS), venous thrombosis in addition to other primary headache disorders including tension-type headache.[4] All of these can cause headache as a symptom of the underlying disease (see Chapter 1). The characteristics of the headache along with other symptoms and signs can help to narrow down the diagnosis. In the postpartum period, in addition to worsening of migraine due to shift in hormones, secondary causes including a low-pressure headache are important to keep in mind, in women who underwent an epidural analgesia.

Diagnosis and Clinical Presentation

It is important to keep in mind that a new headache during pregnancy requires a complete workup (see Chapters 1-3). Given that this is a hypercoagulable state, it is important to rule out secondary causes of headache, including sinus venous thrombosis, stroke, or headache related to pre-eclampsia, in addition to others. Once a secondary cause is ruled out, most women with headache in pregnancy will likely be diagnosed with migraine. The diagnosis of migraine or other primary headache during pregnancy is similar as in other women, guided by the diagnostic criteria of the third edition of *International Classification of Headache Disorders* (ICHD-3). It is based on the characteristics of the headache as well as ruling out secondary causes.

Treatment

The treatment of secondary causes of headache will be based upon etiology. Considerations for effects on the developing fetus need to be taken into account. There have been no randomized controlled trials of migraine preventive medications for efficacy during pregnancy. For the most part, practitioners would prefer to be conservative and rely on lifestyle measures like getting adequate sleep and hydration. Acupuncture, biofeedback, massage and physical therapy, as well as mindfulness and relaxation therapies have been found to be effective and safe for pregnant women.[5,6] For more severe headaches, nerve blocks with either lidocaine or ropivacaine have been found to be generally safe and well tolerated, effective in the acute period as well as a preventive. There is some evidence for using propranolol as a preventive, although there are reports for decreased placental perfusion or bradycardia. Magnesium can be used in oral doses although when given intravenously, there are some reports of skeletal issues in the fetus. When deciding on an acute or a preventive medication, it can be helpful to refer to the manual to see if it is safe in pregnancy (see Tables 48-1 and 48-2).[7]

Prognosis

The prognosis for the majority of women with headache during pregnancy is excellent. Many will experience marked lessening of migraine headaches in particular due to stable levels of estradiol achieved by the second trimester.[8] Recognition of warning signs of a secondary headache is important to keep in mind for this population. The prognosis for headache due to secondary headaches will depend on the specific etiology. Hypertensive disorders such as pre-eclampsia or HELLP (Hemolysis, Elevated Liver enzymes, and Low Platelets) can have detrimental effects on both the mother and child and should be recognized and treated immediately.

Headache and Lactation

Approximately one-third of women will experience headache during the postpartum period.[9] Postpartum is defined as the 6-month period following delivery. Headache is more common in women with a history of migraine prior to delivery. Fortunately, most of the headache medications that were taken prior to pregnancy can be resumed with a few exceptions, depending on whether the mother is deciding to breastfeed.

Table 48-1. Acute Migraine and Headache Treatment Use Considerations During Pregnancy and Breastfeeding

Preferred	Allowed	Possible	Contraindicated	No Information
Acupuncture	Tylenol, caffeine	Neuromodulators	Ergotamine	Ubrogepant
Yoga, mindfulness	Nerve blocks, trigger points		NSAIDs	Lasmiditan
Biofeedback	Metoclopramide			Rimegepant
Adequate sleep and hydration	Ondansetron (not in first trimester)			
	Sumatriptan[a]			

NSAIDs: nonsteroidal anti-inflammatory drugs.

[a]Recommendation based on a registry.

Table 48-2. Preventive Migraine and Headache Treatment Use Considerations During Pregnancy and Breastfeeding

Preferred	Possible	Contraindicated
Acupuncture	Propranolol	Divalproex sodium
Yoga, mindfulness	Neuromodulator	Topiramate
Biofeedback	OnabotulinumtoxinA	ARBs, CGRP inhibitors[a]
Relaxation therapies	SSRI (not paroxetine)	CGRP inhibitors[a]

ARB, angiotensin receptor blockers; CGRP, calcitonin gene-related peptide; SSRI, serotonin reuptake inhibitors.

[a]Insufficient data and so should be avoided.

Clinical Presentation and Diagnosis

The immediate postpartum time frame of 6 to 12 hours following delivery can be referred to as the acute phase of postpartum. This is a common time for several types of headache including a low-pressure headache from leakage of spinal fluid if an epidural was done, blood loss, headache from dehydration, headache from elevated blood pressure often associated with pre-eclampsia, and migraine. The time frame of the first 6 weeks after delivery may be referred to as the puerperium. Recognition of signs of serious secondary headaches during this time is critical. Cerebral venous thrombosis, stroke, arterial dissection, and postpartum angiopathy/RCVS all need to be considered in the evaluation of severe headache in the postpartum patient. Postpartum ends at 6 months after delivery.

Treatment

Triptans, NSAIDs, acetaminophen, and trigger point injections can be used during this postpartum time for acute migraine management.[9,10] If a woman is breastfeeding, there are two medications to avoid. Ergots and ergot alkaloids should be avoided as they can interfere with milk production. In addition, aspirin should be avoided. It peaks in breast milk in 3 hours and has been associated with Reye syndrome in infants. Low-dose "baby" aspirin (75-81 mg daily) can still be used. There is not enough data for the newer oral migraine medications including gepants and ditans to make any statements about their relative safety during breastfeeding. However, a recent study investigated rimegepant concentration in the breast milk of 12 women.[11] This open-label, single-center study enrolled healthy lactating women aged 18 to 40 years with a gestation of 37 to 42 weeks and uncomplicated delivery of a single healthy child ≥2 weeks (14 days) and ≤6 months before study drug administration. Plasma samples were collected 0, 1, 2, 4, and 8 hours postdose; human milk samples were collected at 0, 1, 2, 4, 8, 12, 16, 24, 32, and 36 hours. The milk/plasma drug concentration ratio was estimated as the ratio of the human milk/plasma areas under the curve. The Relative Infant Dose (RID) (%) was calculated as 100 times the quotient of the body weight-normalized infant and maternal doses. The conclusion was that on a weight-adjusted basis, the mean RID of rimegepant was <1% of the maternal dose. However, more studies are needed before advising women to resume an oral gepant for the acute treatment of migraine during lactation, but these results of the above-mentioned study are reassuring.

Breastfeeding can serve as a protective effect but often fades when menses returns.[12] As a result, it may not be necessary to resume a prescription preventive medication during this time. Nonpharmacological treatments should be emphasized. If a preventive medication is felt to be needed, it should be started at a low dose and increased gradually while watching the effect on the infant. OnabotulinumtoxinA may be an option as systemic levels are not seen after intramuscular administration, and it is unlikely there would be any passing into breast milk. Other standard oral migraine preventives can be used but the effect on the breastfeeding infant needs to be considered. For the newer calcitonin gene-related peptide (CGRP) targeting preventive medications, there is no data on safety of use during lactation. When making decisions about medications compatible with breastfeeding, several references can be useful including the National Library of Medicine's Drugs and Lactation database (LactMed). LactMed is a peer-reviewed, fully referenced database and is updated regularly. It can be accessed at https://ncbi.nlm.nih.gov/books/n/lactmed. Other resources include a comprehensive manual *Medications and Mothers Milk* written by Thomas Hale, PhD, and *Drugs in Pregnancy and Lactation* by Briggs et al. Both are updated regularly. An app is available for both Hale's manual and LactMed. In addition, MothertoBaby is a service available from the Organization of Teratology Information Specialists (OTIS) and can be accessed at http://mothertobaby.org/.

Prognosis

Prognosis for headache, especially migraine, is excellent in the lactating female. For many, breastfeeding serves a protective effect until menses returns. Most prepregnancy headache medications can be resumed with the exception of the ergots/ergot alkaloids and aspirin. For those wanting to take a conservative approach, the "pump and dump" method can be adopted by discarding breast milk for a specific number of hours after an acute medication is taken. The number of hours will depend on the specific medication and when it peaks in the breast milk. New clinically relevant information is expected in coming years of the effect of the new CGRP-mediated medications on both pregnancy and breastfeeding. It is important for all clinicians managing headache to stay informed of new recommendations of headache medications for pregnancy and breastfeeding.

Summary

- Headache, most frequently migraine, is a common occurrence in the pregnant female.
- A new headache during pregnancy requires a full workup given the hypercoagulable state during this time.
- Nonpharmacologic treatments, such as acupuncture, biofeedback, and relaxation therapy, are safe and effective in the treatment of headache in pregnancy and lactation, and should be tried prior to medications.
- Breastfeeding can delay the return of migraine by suppressing cyclical hormonal fluctuations.

- Triptans, nonsteroidal anti-inflammatory drugs, and acetaminophen can be used in the management of postpartum headache.
- Ergots, ergot alkaloids, and regular-strength aspirin should be avoided in women who are breastfeeding.

REFERENCES

1. Kvisvik EV, Stovner LJ, Helde G, Bovim G, Linde M. Headache and migraine during pregnancy and puerperium: the MIGRA-study. *J Headache Pain.* 2011;12(4):443-451.

2. Zimmermann JSM, Fousse M, Juhasz-Böss I, Radosa JC, Solomayer EF, Mühl-Benninghaus R. Neurologic Consultations and Headache during Pregnancy and in Puerperium: A Retrospective Chart Review. *J Clin Med.* 2023;12(6):2204.

3. Raffaelli B, Siebert E, Korner J, Liman T, Reuter U, Neeb L. Characteristics and diagnoses of acute headache in pregnant women: a retrospective cross-sectional study. *J Headache Pain.* 2017;18 (1):114.

4. Robbins MS, Farmakidis C, Dayal AK, Lipton RB. Acute headache diagnosis in pregnant women: a hospital-based study. *Neurology.* 2015;85(12): 1024-1030.

5. Holdridge A, Donnelly M, Kuruvilla DE. Integrative, interventional, and non-invasive approaches for the treatment for migraine during pregnancy. *Curr Pain Headache Rep.* 2022;26(4):323-330.

6. Parikh SK, Delbono MV, Silberstein SD. Managing migraine in pregnancy and breastfeeding. *Prog Brain Res.* 2020;255:275-309.

7. Burch R. Headache in pregnancy and the puerperium. *Neurol Clin.* 2019;37(1):31-51.

8. Melhado EM, Maciel JA Jr, Guerreiro CA. Headache during gestation: evaluation of 1101 women. *Can J Neurol Sci.* 2007;34(2):187-192.

9. Negro A, Delaruelle Z, Ivanova TA, et al. Headache and pregnancy: a systematic review. *J Headache Pain.* 2017;18(1):106.

10. Hutchinson S, Marmura MJ, Calhoun A, Lucas S, Silberstein S, Peterlin BL. Use of common migraine treatments in breast-feeding women: a summary of recommendations. *Headache.* 2013;53(4):614-627.

11. Baker TE, Croop R, Kamen L, et al. Human milk and plasma pharmacokinetics of single-dose rimegepant 75 mg in healthy lactating women. *Breastfeed Med.* 2022;17(3):277-282.

12. Sances G, Granella F, Nappi RE, et al. Course of migraine during pregnancy and postpartum: a prospective study. *Cephalalgia.* 2003;23(3):197-205.

Special Populations

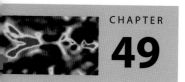

CHAPTER

49

Headache in Children and Adolescents

Lauren Doyle Strauss, Robert Charles Goodrich, and Jaclyn M. Martindale

Headache and migraine are common in children. The evaluation, diagnosis, and treatment in children have special considerations.

Clinical Approach to Diagnosis

In the headache evaluation of children and young adults, it is important to involve them and their caregivers in the history gathering (Table 49-1). Having consensus on symptoms and the episode frequency will be important. Some children may not report all of their milder headaches because they do not want to leave the class and may want to avoid medication. Younger children who are experiencing neurologic symptoms of paresthesias or visual disturbances may not report them to their family because they may not be bothersome to them. Children often are in multiple settings between school, home, sports, and other caregiver's care; so, a headache log or diary may be needed to clarify episode frequency. If more information is needed on pain intensity, quality, and location or associated features, the patient's family is advised to try ask questions during the episodes and record in the log/diary. With the guardian's permission, the treating physician can speak to the school teacher or nurse to understand more about symptoms, frequency, and medication-taking behaviors. A detailed medical history is essential to determine if the condition is a migraine or to identify any concerns indicative of a secondary headache. Although most headaches that occur in childhood are from primary headaches, the treating physician needs to be aware of family's anxiety over possible malignant causes.

Imaging to evaluate for structural causes of headache can be considered when headaches do not meet criteria for a primary headache disorder or are worsening or not responding to treatment.[1] Occipital location alone does not need to warrant imaging as long as there is a reassuring neurologic examination. MRI would be preferred due to the absence of radiation, and younger children require sedation. Incidental findings and anatomical variants can be revealed on imaging such physiologic pituitary enlargement in adolescence, cysts, mega cisterna magna, periventricular leukomalacia, and cortical dysplasia or cysts.[2] Blood tests may include screens for anemia, thyroid disease, diabetes, as well as low levels in ferritin, vitamin B12, and vitamin D. Screening for pregnancy or toxicology/drug exposure may be indicated if applicable.

Primary Headaches

Migraine

The third edition of *International Classification of Headache Disorders* (ICHD-3) has different requirements to meet criteria for migraine in children and adolescents (age <18 years) as compared to adults.[3] There need to be five attacks where the minimum duration of an attack must be 2 hours which is shorter compared to adults where the minimum is 4 hours. It is important to highlight that if a child sleeps during a migraine, the time sleeping is included in duration. Other notable differences include that migrainous-associated

Table 49-1. History Taking in Pediatric Headache in Pediatric Patients

Onset	Time of Year (Consider in Context to Season, Start of School, Start of Menses)
Headache pattern and frequency	Acute vs. chronic; stable or worsening; daily from the start; episodes or continuous; number of headaches/week or month; headaches occurring during the week and weekends
Headache quality	Give examples and try demonstrating or give additional descriptors (e.g., dull "like pushing down," pressure "like a balloon blowing up," sharp "like a knife," throbbing "like your heart is beating," pounding "like a hammer hitting")
	Encourage parents to help translate into words their child would understand
Location of pain	Ask the child to point on their head where pain starts and where it moves to; specifically ask if it involves eyes, ears, or neck
Aura	Timing before/during/after headache or without headache, type, order if multiple neurologic symptoms, how symptoms start/spread/resolve
	Consider using nonmedical terms and descriptions such as:
	Numbness "trouble feeling"
	Paresthesias "tickling or butterfly wings, or the sensation when you fall asleep on your arm/leg"
	Aphasia "trouble speaking or understanding the people around you?"
	In younger children, may need to specifically ask "Do you see or feel anything funny or different?" "Do you see any colors, lights, or sparkles?"
Associated symptoms	Ask about tinnitus "bee buzzing in your ear," dizziness, blurred or double vision, sensitivity to light/sound/smell, fatigue
Alleviating factors	Sleep, cold/warm compress, distraction or fun activity, medications, position (standing vs. supine)
Life impact	Missed days of school/work, urgent care or Emergency Department visits, missed events or family activities, discontinuing or missing sports
Patient-focused concerns	"Do you feel comfortable telling your teacher or coach when you have a headache?"
	"What bothers you the most about the headaches?"
	If needed, you can ask parent/guardian to step out of room to take additional history
Parental-focused concerns	"What do you think is causing these headaches?"
	"What are you concerned about?"
	"What made you ask for this evaluation?"
	"Does the nurse have the needed forms filled out to give medication access?"
	"Have you discussed with the school about creating a migraine action plan or placing a 504 plan for migraine?"

Special Populations

features, photophobia and phonophobia, may be inferred from behaviors such as blocking out the light under a blanket or telling others to be quiet. Bilateral location is often seen in children. Criteria for aura are the same across the age spectrum. Migraine prevalence has a reported range in the pediatric population from 5% to 40%.[4] The prevalence increases with age and varies with 3% for 3 to 7 years, 11% for 7 to 11 years, and 23% in 11 to 15 years. There is an equal prevalence in girls and boys before puberty. After puberty, the prevalence in girls is two to three times more common.

Tension-type Headache

Tension-type headache is considered relatively common in children and adolescents. However, little is known about tension-type headache in children. Tension-type headache classification in the International Classification of Headache Disorders, 3rd edition (ICHD-3) uses the same criteria for children and adolescents as adult-aged patients (Chapter 13). There are high rates of headache transformation between a diagnosis of tension-type headache and migraine which can complicate diagnosis.

Secondary Headaches

Idiopathic Intracranial Hypertension

As discussed in Chapter 23, idiopathic intracranial hypertension (IIH), also called pseudotumor cerebri syndrome, is an increase in intracranial pressure that typically manifests clinically as headache, visual obscurations, and variable degrees of papilledema and visual loss. It is a rare condition in children with an annual incidence of 0.71 per 100,000. Symptoms are similar to those found in adults, although headache is interestingly not as prominent among younger children (1-6 years) and may be absent in as many as 13%.[5] Papilledema is reported in 90% and visual field deficits are present in 70% to 85% at the time of presentation. The diagnostic criteria for IIH are the same in adults and children. In children, the elevated opening pressure in a nonsedated, nonobese child is considered $\geq$28 cm H_2O, compared to $\geq$25 cm H_2O in an adult.[6] There is a female predominance among children IIH. However, obesity becomes a much stronger risk factor after puberty, and many prepubescent patients with IIH have a thin body habitus. Secondary causes in the pediatric population include cerebral venous sinus thrombosis (CVST) secondary to otitis media and mastoiditis, severe iron deficiency anemia from high cow's milk intake, acne treatment use with tetracycline and vitamin A derivative, growth hormone therapy, and Down and Turner syndromes. Acetazolamide from 20 to 30 mg/kg/day in divided doses is the mainstay of treatment, but furosemide 1 to 2 mg/kg/day three times per day can be used as an adjunct or alternative. Topiramate is considered second line and dosing is not well established, but it adds the benefits of headache prophylaxis and weight loss. Surgical interventions such as ventriculoperitoneal shunting, intravenous stenting, and optic nerve fenestration can be considered when there is rapid vision loss, intolerance to medications, or difficulty with medication adherence.

Cerebral Venous Sinus Thrombosis

CVST is a rare cause of headache in children. The incidence in childhood is 0.4 to 0.7 per 100,000, and 40% occur in the neonatal period where headache would be difficult to determine.[7] Risk factors include contraceptive use, prothrombotic disorders, dehydration, anemia, head injury, autoimmune conditions, malignancy, congenital heart disease, renal disease, Down syndrome, and infection (especially otitis media and mastoiditis). The headache associated with CVST is nonspecific, but can include features such as nausea and any of the systemic symptoms caused by the underlying condition leading to the CVST (Chapter 20).

Chiari Malformation

Chiari I malformation, or the downward herniation of the cerebellar tonsils >5 mm through the foramen magnum in a peg-like fashion, is typically asymptomatic (Chapter 25). When symptomatic in children, headache is the most common presenting complaint and is more common in older ages. Although for adults the headache typically fits the ICHD-3 criteria of occipital or suboccipital location, of short duration (less than 5 minutes), and provoked by cough or other Valsalva-like maneuvers, children seldom fit this pattern, with only 6% reporting occipital location and only 4% having worse symptoms with Valsalva according to one cohort study.

Obstructive Sleep Apnea

Obstructive sleep apnea and other sleep disorders such as insomnia, bruxism, and restless leg syndrome are correlated with migraine in children and adults, and sleep apnea can also independently cause its own headache as defined by the ICHD-3, so screening for sleep disorders is an important step in the treatment of headaches. The prevalence of pediatric OSA is estimated to be in the range of 1% to 5%.[8] Importantly, the most common cause of OSA in children is tonsillar and adenoid hypertrophy, so the treatment for this condition is often surgical.[9]

Epilepsy

Patients with epilepsy have an increased risk of migraine and migraine patients have an increased risk of epilepsy (Chapter 21). Importantly, headaches and migraine often co-occur with seizures. It has been reported that 35% of children experience headache at the same time as their seizures,[10] whether it be preictal, interictal, and postictal. The ICHD-3 recognizes headaches related to epileptic seizures as a secondary headache disorder and classifies them as either ictal or postictal (Chapter 21). There are certain childhood epilepsy syndromes that are more highly associated with headache, including benign Rolandic epilepsy, and the childhood occipital epilepsies. The later conditions (Gastaut and Panayiotopoulos syndromes) are often associated with features commonly found in migraine such as visual aura, autonomic disturbance, nausea, and vomiting. An important way to distinguish between seizures and migraine can be through a description of the aura a patient is experiencing. Although exceptions exist, the visual aura associated with epilepsy tends to be more colorful, circular, hemifield in location, and sudden in onset compared with the black and white, linear or zig-zag, centrally located, and more gradually progressive aura of migraine. A thorough history and description of the events in question are essential, but if suspicion for seizure exists, obtaining an electroencephalogram (EEG) may be necessary to investigate epilepsy as a cause or comorbidity of pediatric headache.

Treatment Considerations

The decision to initiate treatment should take into consideration the frequency, severity, duration, and disability of youth with migraine. Pediatric-specific considerations may include school absences, missed activities, time away from friends, or even the parent or caregiver's missed days from work. The goals of treatment—whether it be lifestyle modifications, nutraceutical, behavioral, pharmacologic, or neuromodulation—should aim to improve the patient's function and minimize the degree of headache-related disability. Engaging the patient and their family in shared decision-making and setting appropriate outcome expectations may aid in treatment adherence and effectiveness. Families should discuss with their school strategies for child or adolescent's unique needs for quick successful headache treatment to minimize interference with their school and daily function. Having a migraine action plan and completed medication administration forms at school can help minimize delays to treatment and headache-related disability.

Lifestyle Modifications

Healthy habits are an important and practical way to reduce the likelihood of headaches. Use the mnemonic SMART (sleep, meals, activity, relaxation, triggers) to assess and address healthy habits. The American Academy of Sleep Medicine (AASM) recommends school-aged children get 9 to 12 hours of sleep and adolescents get 8 to 10 hours of sleep per night.[11] Insufficient duration, consistency, or quality of sleep can be a trigger for headache or may be indicative of a primary sleep disorder. A healthy lifestyle should be encouraged to include consistent well-balanced meals, adequate hydration, maintaining healthy weight, and regular exercise. Avoiding caffeinated beverages or specific food triggers can be effective in headache reduction. It is important to evaluate various sources of stressors such as at school, home, or in social relationships. Stressors may be perceived differently depending on the age,

Special Populations

culture, or beliefs of the individual and their caregivers. When discussing with the patient and their caregiver, the normalcy of stressors should be validated. Stress coping or relaxation strategies can be an important aspect of headache prevention. Working toward a consistently healthy lifestyle may help minimize the risk of headache. However, it is important to acknowledge some factors may be out of the child or family's control such as school start times, homework burden, or caregiver work schedule. Special care should be taken to explore food and housing insecurity, barriers to care, financial strains, or other psychosocial stressors. Involving the social work team to create individualized solutions can help address some of these barriers. Accommodations at school such as being able to rest in a cool, dark room, ability to freely hydrate and use the restroom, and icepacks are recommended.

Behavioral Therapy

Behavioral interventions are both safe and effective for youth with headaches. The most commonly used therapy is cognitive behavioral therapy (CBT), which has demonstrated to be efficacious in combination with amitriptyline. Many therapies focus on muscle relaxation that can also help with stress reduction. These therapies are nonpharmacological options that can provide lifelong strategies to effective pain coping. These may include physical therapy, massage therapy, acupuncture, osteopathic manipulation, guided imagery, diaphragmatic breathing, biofeedback, mindfulness, or meditation. Behavioral therapies require motivation by the patient and their caregivers, time commitment, potentially missed time from work/school, and can be challenging to access due to limited resource or cost. Device applications are available for many relaxation techniques and may help overcome access challenges by using technology in the home.

Nutraceuticals

There is limited evidence on the efficacy of nutraceuticals in the prevention of childhood and adolescent headaches. While the Food and Drug Administration (FDA) regulates nutraceuticals, the safety and efficacy regulations are more limited compared to conventional pharmaceutical agents. Riboflavin, coenzyme Q10, magnesium, feverfew, and vitamin D have shown to be possibly effective in adults and are generally well tolerated (Chapter 47).[12] There needs to be careful use of butterbur due to the risk of hepatotoxicity although there are pyrrolizidine alkaloid (PA) free available preparations. Additionally, omega-3 polyunsaturated fatty acids have limited evidence at this time in migraine prevention. It is important to inquire about the use of nutraceuticals and counsel on the limited evidence of efficacy, out-of-pocket costs, potential drug-nutraceutical interactions, and safety concerns.

Pharmacologic Treatment Considerations

With limited research available on pharmacologic treatments in pediatrics, the American Academy of Neurology (AAN) and the American Headache Society (AHS) released practice guideline recommendations for both acute and preventative treatments in children and adolescents with migraine.[13,14] There is a high placebo responder rate in pediatric migraine trials, which hinders demonstration of pediatric-specific evidence for these medications. There are several medications approved by the FDA for use in children and adolescents. In clinical practice providers may use "off-label" medications acknowledging limited pediatric-specific evidence but demonstrated efficacy in adults, balanced with tolerability, side-effect profile, and patient or caregiver preference. Additionally, when choosing medication, it is important to consider these practice guidelines in addition to the individual characteristics of the headache, the individual's age, childbearing potential, route of administration, and co-occurring conditions. Insurance authorization and financial barriers may be another important component in the decision-making process.

Acute Pharmacological Treatments

Adjustments to treatment strategies and dosing of acute and preventative medications need to be made based on age and weight and tolerated route of administration. Children who are unable to swallow pills or who have vomiting may require nontablet routes of administration. Taking medications early in migraine onset is associated with improved effectiveness. The AAN–AHS guidelines recommend initiating acute treatment with ibuprofen and escalating therapy to triptans or combination treatment if not effective. Caution should be used with aspirin-containing medications due to the risk of Reye syndrome in children. Table 49-2 outlines the commonly used acute therapies available. It is important to counsel families that variety of medications may be tried to find the most

Table 49-2. Acute Headache Therapies for Children and Adolescents

Name	Formulations	Dosing	Considerations/Side Effects
Antiemetics[14–16]			
Ondansetron	P, L, D	0.15 mg/kg Max 8 mg/dose	Drowsiness, constipation
Promethazine	P, L, R	0.25-0.5 mg/kg Q6H, Max 25 mg/dose	Anticholinergic side effects, drowsiness, extrapyramidal symptoms
Metoclopramide	P, L, D, R	0.4-0.8 mg/kg/day divided Q6H Max 10 mg/dose	Drowsiness, dystonic reactions, hyperprolactinemia
Prochlorperazine	P, L, R, T	0.1 mg/kg Q6H Max 10 mg/dose	Drowsiness, anticholinergic side effects, extrapyramidal symptoms
Dimenhydrinate	P, L, D, R	12.5-100 mg Q6H-8H	Drowsiness
NSAIDs[14–16]			
Acetaminophen	P, L, D, R	15 mg/kg Q4H Max 4 g/day	
Ibuprofen	P, L, D, R	10 mg/kg Q6H Max 3200 mg/day	Avoid in renal or hepatic dysfunction
Ketorolac	P, L	1 mg/kg Q4-6H Max 10 mg/dose	Duration of therapy should not exceed 5 days
Naproxen sodium	P, L	5-7 mg/kg Q8-12H Max 1 g/day	
Antihistamine[14–16]			
Hydroxyzine	P, L	0.5 mg/kg Q6H	Drowsiness, also used in anxiety
Diphenhydramine	P, L, D	1 mg/kg Q4-6H Max 50 mg/dose	Drowsiness
Cyproheptadine	P, L	0.2-0.5 mg PRN QHS to TID	Drowsiness, increased appetite
Fast-acting triptans[14–16]			
Sumatriptan	P	25-100 mg Max 200 mg/day	Preparation available with naproxen[a]
	Powder	11-22 mg	

(Continued)

Table 49-2. Acute Headache Therapies for Children and Adolescents (*Continued*)

Name	Formulations	Dosing	Considerations/Side Effects
	SC	3-6 mg	
	NS	5-20 mg	
Zolmitriptan	P, D, NS[a]	2.5-5 mg	
Rizatriptan[b]	P, D	5-10 mg	
Almotriptan[a]	P	6.25-12.5 mg Max 25 mg/day	
Eletriptan	P	20-40 mg	Limit grapefruit
Slow-acting triptans[14–16]			
Naratriptan	T	1-2.5 mg	
Frovatriptan	T	2.5 mg	
Ergot derivatives[14–16]			
Dihydroergotamine	NS	0.5 mg	Max 6 sprays/day, 8 sprays/week
Neuromodulation[14–16]			
Single pulse transmagnetic stimulation (sTMS)[a]	Device	3 pulses at onset, may repeat 3 pulses after 15 minutes if needed up to 2 times for total of 9 pulses in 30 minutes	Dizziness, site paresthesias; contraindicated in epilepsy or recent head injury, implantable metal devices, suspected or diagnosed heart condition, family history of epilepsy, or family history of stroke
Noninvasive vagal nerve stimulation (nVNS)[a]	Device	2-minute stimulation, may repeat in 20 minutes for additional 2 minutes if necessary. May repeat a third time after 2 hours for an additional 2 minutes if necessary	Neck discomfort, shoulder or facial pain/twitching, site pain/irritation; caution if history of abnormal blood pressure or heart rate; contraindicated if implantable medal device
Remote Electrical Neuromodulation (REN)[a]	Device	Up to 45 minutes of treatment starting at migraine symptom onset	Site pain, irritation, paresthesia

[a]FDA-approved for children ≥12.

[b]FDA-approved for children ≥6.

D, Chewable or Oral-Disintegrating Tablet; L, Liquid; MAOi, Monoamine Oxidase Inhibitor; Max, Maximum; NSAID, Non-Steroidal Anti-Inflammatory Drug; NS, Nasal Spray; P, Pill; PRN, Pro Re Nata (as needed); Q12H, Every 12 Hours; Q4H, Every 4 Hours; Q6H, Every 6 Hours; Q8H, Every 8 Hours; QHS, Every Night at Bedtime; R, Rectal; SC, Subcutaneous; T, Topical; TID, Ter in Die (three times a day).

effective treatment for the patient. With any acute treatment, it is important to counsel on avoidance of medication overuse (Chapter 28) and risk of medication overuse headache. This occurs with use of analgesics (nonsteroidal anti-inflammatory drugs [NSAIDs], acetaminophen, etc.) more than 14 days per month and triptans or combination analgesics (containing caffeine) for 9 days per month for more than 3 months.

The US Food and Drug Administration (FDA)-approved triptans for adolescents 12 years or older include sumatriptan/naproxen, zolmitriptan nasal spray, and almotriptan. For younger children, rizatriptan is FDA-approved for use in children 6 years or older. Nonoral forms of triptans have quicker absorption and faster onset of action, which are ideal for migraines that rapidly peak in severity or if the child is unable to tolerate oral medications. There are cautions and misconceptions surrounding use of triptans in pediatric migraine. While these cardiovascular and cerebrovascular conditions are less common in the pediatric population, the morbidity and mortality associated with aggravating these conditions are important to consider.

Preventative Pharmacological Treatment

The AAN–AHS guidelines recommend lifestyle modifications as first-line approaches to headache prevention. Many pediatric studies for preventive medications use a minimum of four headache days per month for at least 3 months or a PedMIDAS (disability) score over 30, indicating moderate to severe migraine-related disability. In clinical practice, preventative treatments should be considered based on the degree of headache-related disability, frequency, severity, and risk of medication overuse headache. When considering preventative medications, it is important to engage the patient (and parents) in shared decision-making and set realistic treatment expectations. The CHAMP study was the first large, randomized, double-blinded, placebo-controlled multicenter trial designed to evaluate the effectiveness of topiramate and amitriptyline in pediatric migraine prevention.[17] Unfortunately, there were no significant differences in improvement between the medications or placebo. Individuals who received medications were more likely to report adverse events. Similarly, in many pediatric studies, preventative medications fail to show superiority to placebo. This may be related to high placebo response in pediatric trials, trial design, or other contextual factors. Although topiramate is the only FDA-approved medication for treating migraine in children 12 years or older, there are several classes of therapies used in clinical practice for headache prevention (Table 49-3). The AAN–AHS guidelines recommend amitriptyline in combination with CBT, topiramate, and propranolol to be more likely than placebo to reduce headache frequency or disability. Monoclonal antibodies (mAbs) or small molecule antagonists to calcitonin gene-related peptide (CGRP) are FDA-approved for the treatment of migraine and episodic cluster headache adults. While these do show some promise, pediatric trials will lag, and it will likely be several years to obtain definitive efficacy and safety data for use in the child and adolescent population. The Pediatric and Adolescent Headache special interest group the AHS published an expert consensus statement on the use of CGRP mAbs suggesting indications, contraindications, and necessary monitoring until more data becomes available.[21]

Interventional Treatments

OnabotulinumtoxinA is FDA-approved for preventative treatment of chronic migraine in adults. Clinical trial in adolescence with migraine failed to meet its efficacy endpoints but demonstrated tolerability of onabotulinumtoxinA in the adolescent population.[22] In clinical practice, it is used for prevention when adolescents have failed several therapies. Insurance approval and financial barriers are important to consider.

While limited evidence exists in the pediatric population, peripheral nerve blocks, trigger point injections, or sphenopalatine ganglion blocks are used for both acute and short-term preventative treatment in select youth. As there is no consensus of use in the pediatric population, there is variability of injection sites, medications used, and use of repeat injections in clinical practice.

Neuromodulation

While the neuromodulation devices are not included in the AAN–AHS guidelines, there are three devices with FDA approval for acute and preventative treatment of migraine in adolescents (see also Chapter 46). Single-pulse transcranial magnetic stimulation (sTMS) and noninvasive vagal nerve

Special Populations

Table 49-3. Preventative Headache Therapies for Children and Adolescents

Name	Formulations	Dosing	Considerations/Side Effects
Nutraceuticals[12,13,15,16,18]			
Magnesium	P	Elemental magnesium 9 mg/kg/day with food	Diarrhea
Coenzyme Q10	P, D, L	1-3 mg/kg/day in the morning with food	GI upset, insomnia
Riboflavin	P	50-400 mg/day either daily or divided BID	Urine discoloration, GI upset
Melatonin	P, D, L	2-3 mg QHS	Sleepiness
Ferrous sulfate			Dark stools, GI upset
Vitamin D	P, D, L	Normal Vit D levels: 400 IU/day; Mild Vit D deficiency 800 IU/day; Moderate Vit D Deficiency 5000 IU/day	
Polyunsaturated fatty acids	P	Fish oil compound	
Feverfew			
Antidepressants[13,15,16]			
Amitriptyline	P	0.25-1 mg/kg/day QHS	Max 200 mg/day. Do not use within 14 days of MAOi; side effects: sedation, anticholinergic side effects, prolonged QTC, black box warning: increased suicidality in children
Nortriptyline	P	Dosing not well established; 0.5-1 mg/kg/day QHS	Similar to amitriptyline but less sedation and anticholinergic effects
Venlafaxine	P	Dosing not well established; 12.5-25 mg/day	Black box warning increased suicidality in children
Antihypertensives[13,15,16]			
Propranolol	P, L	0.5-4 mg/kg/day divided BID or TID	Max 120 mg/day; caution in asthma; also used in anxiety, essential tremor and hypertension
Nimodipine		10-20 mg TID	GI upset
Calcium channel blockers[13,15,16]			
Verapamil	P	40-80 mg Q6-8H	Do not use in patients with poor liver function or hear block; avoid grapefruit as can increase serum levels
Antihistamine[13,15,16]			
Cyproheptadine	P, L	0.2-0.5 mg/kg/day either divided BID or given all QHS	Max 16 mg/day; side effects: appetite stimulant, weight gain, sleepiness; Ok to continue other antihistamines

Table 49-3. Preventative Headache Therapies for Children and Adolescents (*Continued*)

Name	Formulations	Dosing	Considerations/Side Effects
Antiepileptics[13,15,16]			
Gabapentin	P, L	300-1200 mg TID	Max 3600 mg/day; can be used for neuropathic pain
Topiramate[a]	P, L	2-3 mg/kg/day divided BID	Max 200 mg/day; can be used for tics or seizures; side effects: weight loss, paresthesia, cognitive impairment, renal stones, angle closure glaucoma, suicidal ideation; teratogenicity; lowers efficacy of oral contraceptives especially at doses >200 mg/day
Valproic acid	P, L	10-30 mg/kg/day divided BID	Max 1000 mg/day or 45 mg/kg/day; caution in females of child-bearing age; side effects: weight gain, somnolence, tremor, alopecia, thrombocytopenia, lymphopenia, hepatotoxicity, hyperammonemia, pancreatitis
Zonisamide	P	4-10 mg/kg/day	Max 200 mg/day; side effects: anorexia, increased suicidal ideation
Lamotrigine			
Levetiracetam	P, L	20-40 mg/kg/day divided BID; Max 3000 mg/day	Irritability, behavior changes, worsening depression
Neurotoxins[15,16]			
OnabotulinumtoxinA		74 units or 155 units injected per PREEMPT protocol every 12 weeks	
Neuromodulation[16,19,20]			
Single pulse transmagnetic stimulation (sTMS)[a]	Device	4 pulses in morning and 4 pulses at night	Dizziness, site paresthesia; contraindicated in epilepsy or recent head injury, implantable metal devices, suspected or diagnosed heart condition, family history of epilepsy, or family history of stroke
Noninvasive vagal nerve stimulation (nVNS)[a]	Device	2-minute stimulation TID	Neck discomfort, shoulder or facial pain/twitching, site pain/irritation; caution if history of abnormal blood pressure or heart rate; contraindicated if implantable medal device

[a]FDA-approved for children ≥12.
See Chapter 43 for PREEMPT protocol details. BID, Twice Daily; D, Chewable or Oral-Disintegrating Tablet; GI, Gastrointestinal; IU, International Units; L, Liquid; MAOi, Monoamine Oxidase Inhibitor; Max, Maximum; NS, Nasal Spray; P, Pill; PRN, Pro Re Nata (as needed); Q6H, Every 6 Hours; Q8H, Every 8 Hours; QHS, Every Night at Bedtime; R, Rectal; SC, Subcutaneous; T, Topical; TID, Ter in Die (three times a day).

stimulation (nVNS) are FDA-approved for both acute and preventative treatment for adolescents 12 years and older.[19,23] Both these devices are contraindicated in patients with implantable metal or electronic devices. A third option, the smartphone-controlled remote electrical neuromodulation (REN) device, is also FDA-approved for acute treatment in adolescents. All three devices require prescriptions from the clinician and have been relatively well tolerated. Practical disadvantages include device size, storage, necessity to charge, time commitment, and noise. Out-of-pocket cost and insurance approval may also be financial barriers.

Treatment of Headache in Emergency or Urgent Care Setting

When the headache persists or leads to prolonged debilitation, an escalation of therapy may be required. In addition to SMART healthy habits, behavioral modifications, and acute therapies, patients may need a bridge or transitional therapy, such as oral steroids, scheduled NSAIDs, or triptans for a few days. When patients fail to respond to acute therapies or are unable to tolerate oral therapies, they may require nonoral medications in the infusion center, urgent care, or emergency room. Headache is a frequent cause of pediatric emergency room visits. When presenting to the emergency room, many patients will receive a combination of medications. While many clinicians still refer to this as a "migraine cocktail," this terminology is outdated, stigmatizing, and poorly accepted by both patients and providers. Additionally, it is vague and does not clearly define the combination of medications administered, which can be confusing for patients and other healthcare providers.

Evidence is limited and consensus on emergency room treatment guidelines is lacking. Despite this, common medications used in these settings are included in Table 49-4. These are given in combination with intravenous fluids or each other. Symptom improvement and anticipatory guidance can set the patient up for successful discharge to home. Despite these therapies if symptoms persist, admission for dihydroergotamine (DHE) has the most evidence; however, it does not guarantee rapid resolution of symptoms. Additionally, the necessity of admission does have pitfalls such as disruption of sleep patterns, loud noises, lights, and added stressors. When possible, facilitating a peaceful, dark, and quiet environment can help the recovery process.

Prognosis

Pediatric migraine has many similar diagnostic and treatment considerations with adult migraine. There is limited literature on the lifelong prognosis in children looking at the natural history of disease. It has been reported that only 27% of pediatric patients with headache were headache free 20 years later.

Summary

- Although most headaches in childhood are from primary headache disorders, it is important to screen for secondary causes with a detailed history from both the patient and their caregivers.

- There are important differences in the ICDH-3 criteria for migraine in children compared to adults: the minimum duration of an attack is 2 hours instead of 4, and the headache is more often bilateral than unilateral.

- Tension-type headache is relatively common with similar diagnostic criteria to adults, but not much is known about this primary headache in the pediatric population.

- Secondary causes of headache in children include IIH, CVST, obstructive sleep apnea, Chiari malformations, importantly, seizures, as they can often co-occur and/or mimic migraine.

- Headache-related disability should be considered when planning treatment and can be measured using the PedMIDAS.

Table 49-4. Emergency Headache Treatments[24]

Name	Formulations	Dosing	Considerations/Side Effects
NSAIDs			
Ketorolac	IV, IM	0.5 mg/kg Q6-8H, Max 30 mg	
Diclofenac	IM	75 mg	
Antiemetics			
Chlorpromazine	IV, IM	0.1 mg/kg, Max 25 mg	Drowsiness, hypotension can be reduced with pretreatment of fluids
Prochlorperazine	IV, IM	0.15 mg/kg, Max 25 mg	Drowsiness, anticholinergic side effects, extrapyramidal symptoms
Promethazine	IV, IM	25 mg	IM preferred; caution with IV administration due to extravasation risk; anticholinergic side effects, drowsiness, extrapyramidal symptoms
Metoclopramide	IV, IM	0.15 mg/kg, Max 10 mg	Drowsiness, dystonic reactions
Ondansetron	IV, IM	0.15 mg/kg, Max 8 mg	Drowsiness, constipation
Antihistamines			
Diphenhydramine	IV, IM	1 mg/kg Q4-6H, Max 50 mg	Drowsiness
Nutraceuticals			
Magnesium	IV	30 mg/kg, Max 2000 mg	Limited evidence, well tolerated
Antiepileptics			
Valproic acid	IV	8-20 mg/kg; Max 2000 mg loading dose; limited evidence for continuous infusion 1 mg/kg/hr	Caution in child bearing potential
Steroids			
Decadron	IV		Lacks supporting evidence
Ergot Derivatives			
Dihydroergotamine	IV, IM	0.5-1 mg	>6 years; may require premedication to reduce nausea/vomiting; contraindicated in pregnancy, history of cerebrovascular disease or hypertension

ᵃFDA-approved for children ≥ 12.

IM, Intramuscular; IV, Intravenous; Max, Maximum; Q4H, Every 4 Hours; Q6H, Every 6 Hours; Q8H, Every 8 Hours.

Special Populations

• First-line treatment for pediatric headache should include lifestyle modifications, certain triptans, topiramate, and some neuromodulation devices; practice guidelines and patient-specific considerations should also be used in treatment decisions.

REFERENCES

1. Conicella E, Raucci U, Vanacore N, et al. The child with headache in a pediatric emergency department. *Headache*. 2008;48:1005-1011.

2. Strauss LD, Cavanaugh BA, Yun ES, Evans RW. Incidental findings and normal anatomical variants on brain MRI in children for primary headaches. *Headache*. 2017;57:1601-1609.

3. Headache Classification Committee of the International Headache Society (IHS). *The International Classification of Headache Disorders*, 3rd edition. *Cephalalgia*. 2018;38:1-211.

4. Barnes N, Millman G, James E. Migraine headache in children. *Clin Evid*. 2006(15):469-475.

5. Cleves-Bayon C. Idiopathic intracranial hypertension in children and adolescents: an update. *Headache*. 2018;58:485-493.

6. Avery RA, Shah SS, Licht DJ, et al. Reference range for cerebrospinal fluid opening pressure in children. *N Engl J Med*. 2010;363:891-893.

7. Dlamini N, Billinghurst L, Kirkham FJ. Cerebral venous sinus (sinovenous) thrombosis in children. *Neurosurg Clin N Am*. 2010;21:511-527.

8. Marcus CL, Brooks LJ, Draper KA, et al. Diagnosis and management of childhood obstructive sleep apnea syndrome. *Pediatrics*. 2012;130:576-584.

9. Lin SY, Su YX, Wu YC, Chang JZ, Tu YK. Management of paediatric obstructive sleep apnoea: a systematic review and network meta-analysis. *Int J Paediatr Dent*. 2020;30:156-170.

10. Kanemura H, Sano F, Ishii S, Ohyama T, Sugita K, Aihara M. Characteristics of headache in children with epilepsy. *Seizure-European Journal of Epilepsy*. 2013;22:647-650.

11. Paruthi S, Brooks LJ, D'Ambrosio C, et al. Recommended amount of sleep for pediatric populations: a consensus statement of the American Academy of Sleep Medicine. *J Clin Sleep Med*. 2016;12:785-786.

12. Orr SL, Venkateswaran S. Nutraceuticals in the prophylaxis of pediatric migraine: evidence-based review and recommendations. *Cephalalgia*. 2014;34:568-583.

13. Oskoui M, Pringsheim T, Billinghurst L, et al. Practice guideline update summary: pharmacologic treatment for pediatric migraine prevention. Report of the Guideline Development, Dissemination, and Implementation Subcommittee of the American Academy of Neurology and the American Headache Society. *Neurology*. 2019;93:500-509.

14. Oskoui M, Pringsheim T, Holler-Managan Y, et al. Practice guideline update summary: acute treatment of migraine in children and adolescents. Report of the Guideline Development, Dissemination, and Implementation Subcommittee of the American Academy of Neurology and the American Headache Society. *Neurology*. 2019;93:487-499.

15. Szperka C. Headache in children and adolescents. *Continuum (Minneap Minn)*. 2021;27:703-731.

16. Gladstein J, Szperka CL, Gelfand AA. *Pediatric Headache*. Amsterdam, the Netherlands: Elsevier; 2021.

17. Powers SW, Coffey CS, Chamberlin LA, et al. Trial of amitriptyline, topiramate, and placebo for pediatric migraine. *N Engl J Med*. 2016;376:115-124.

18. Gelfand AA, Goadsby PJ. The role of melatonin in the treatment of primary headache disorders. *Headache*. 2016;56:1257-1266.

19. Irwin SL, Qubty W, Allen IE, Patniyot I, Goadsby PJ, Gelfand AA. Transcranial magnetic stimulation for migraine prevention in adolescents: a pilot open-label study. *Headache: The Journal of Head and Face Pain*. 2018;58:724-731.

20. Dodick DW, Turkel CC, DeGryse RE, et al. OnabotulinumtoxinA for treatment of chronic migraine: pooled results from the double-blind, randomized, placebo-controlled phases of the PREEMPT clinical program. *Headache: The Journal of Head and Face Pain*. 2010;50:921-936.

21. Szperka CL, VanderPluym J, Orr SL, et al. Recommendations on the use of anti-CGRP monoclonal antibodies in children and adolescents. *Headache*. 2018;58:1658-1669.

22. Winner PK, Kabbouche M, Yonker M, Wangsadipura V, Lum A, Brin MF. A randomized trial to evaluate onabotulinumtoxinA for prevention of headaches in adolescents with chronic migraine. *Headache*. 2020;60:564-575.

23. Grazzi L, Egeo G, Liebler E, Padovan AM, Barbanti P. Non-invasive vagus nerve stimulation (nVNS) as symptomatic treatment of migraine in young patients: a preliminary safety study. *Neurol Sci*. 2017;38:197-199.

24. Gelfand AA, Goadsby PJ. A neurologist's guide to acute migraine therapy in the emergency room. *Neurohospitalist*. 2012;2:51-59.

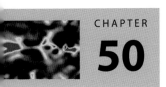

Headache in the Elderly

50

Brinder Vij

Primary headache syndromes are more commonly seen in younger adults and the overall prevalence remains very high. The incidence of secondary headache though increases with older age but 52% to 81% of the headaches in geriatric population are still primary.[1] Changing population demographics with increasing proportion of older adults in the United States and globally makes it further important for clinicians to be skilled with geriatric headache management. According to U.S. census bureau projections nearly one in four American is going to be an older adult by year 2060.

Primary Headache Disorders in Elderly

Headache disorders in older adults are essentially diagnosed in a similar way as in young adults using third edition of the *International Classification of Headache Disorders* (ICHD-3). Most common primary headache in elderly is tension-type headache (TTH), followed by migraine and trigeminal autonomic cephalalgias (TACs). Short-lasting unilateral neuralgiform headache attacks with conjunctival injection and tearing (SUNCT) and short-lasting unilateral neuralgiform headache with autonomic features (SUNA) are also more often seen in older adults with mean age of onset above 50 for both. The diagnosis and treatment of these headaches is similar in both young and older adults.[2] Table 50-1 describes specific features and general recommendations for managing common primary headaches in older adults.

Secondary Headache Disorders in Elderly

It is well known that incidence of secondary headaches increases with age (Chapter 1). It has been estimated that approximately 15% of geriatric headaches can be due to serious and potentially life-threatening underlying cause. It is important to be educated about the existence of secondary headaches because inability to recognize them can lead to significant morbidity and mortality in seniors and impact their families. Table 50-2 describes specific features and general recommendations for managing common secondary headaches in older adults.[3,4] Trigeminal neuralgia, a face pain syndrome common in the elderly population, is described in detail in Chapter 39.

Specific Geriatric Headache Syndromes

Hypnic Headache

This is a classic geriatric headache syndrome and is seen almost exclusively in adults above the age of 50 years (see Chapter 17 for details). Headache develops only during sleep and awakens the patient. It can have both migraine and TTH features. It is more common in women. The typical time for hypnic headache occurrence is 2 to 4 AM (alarm clock headache). The headache lasts from 15 minutes to 4 hours. The headache is not accompanied

Table 50-1. Specific Features and General Recommendations for Managing Common Primary Headaches in Older Adults

Headache Type	Clinical Features	Specific Treatment Recommendations
Tension-type headache	• Most common headache disorder in older adults. • Headache intensity is generally low in elderly.	• Nonpharmacological options like biofeedback and relaxation techniques should be first to all. • Consider low starting dose of tricyclic antidepressants like amitriptyline because of higher incidence of anticholinergic side effects.
Migraine	• Incidence of new onset migraine decrease with age. One-year prevalence of migraine remains 3-6% in older adults. • Migraine is a more commonly seen in elderly women but the incidence/prevalence gap between men and women decreases with aging. • Older adults can present with aura only symptoms without any headache. These symptoms are usually visual, sensory, and speech and can be confused with stroke symptoms. Unlike cerebrovascular events, the aura symptoms are reversible. Also, progression of symptoms is more abrupt in stroke compared to aura.	• All the traditional treatments like antiseizure, antidepressant, and anti-hypertensive medications can be used as in younger adults but consider comorbidities and use lower possible doses to avoid adverse reactions. • Anti-CGRP treatments (CGRP monoclonal antibodies and gepants) can be used in elderly because of minimal side effects. Cost of these medications sometimes could be hindrance. • OnabotulinumtoxinA and different FDA-approved devices are another safe option for elderly and have advantage of avoiding polypharmacy and may have better adherence. • Involving neurovascular/stroke team is recommended when treading a fine line between aura-like symptoms versus TIA/stroke.

Trigeminal autonomic cephalalgias	• Cluster headache is typically seen in middle-aged men but has been reported in up to ninth and tenth decades of life.
	• Peak incidence for men is 40-49 years and 60-69 years for women.
	• Secondary cluster should be suspected:
	  o If pain attack lasts more than 4 hours.
	  o Absence of circadian or circannual rhythm.
	  o Interictal pain.
	  o Inadequate response to treatment.
		• MRI and MRA is recommended for a new onset cluster headache in older adults.
		• Can use oxygen for acute treatment but caution is advised in case of comorbid primary lung conditions like COPD in older adults.
		• While using steroids be mindful of unique side effects like psychosis, osteoporosis, avascular necrosis, and uncontrolled BP and diabetes in elderly.

BP, blood pressure; CGRP, calcitonin gene-related peptide; COPD, chronic obstructive pulmonary disease; MRA, magnetic resonance angiography; MRI, magnetic resonance imaging; TIA, transient ischemic attack.

Table 50-2. Specific Features and General Recommendations for Managing Common Secondary Headaches in Older Adults

Headache Type	Clinical Features	Diagnosis	Treatment
Headache related to vascular etiologies	• Older age is a risk factor for stroke. Headache is common in cases of sinus venous thrombosis (50%), hemorrhage (21.3%), and ischemic (8.4%). Among ischemic strokes posterior circulation strokes are more likely to have headache. In TIA headache is reported in 28% of cases, possibly because aura symptoms might be counted as TIA. • Post cerebral angiography and carotid enterectomy headaches are clearly defined by ICHD-3 and are possible in older adults as they are more likely to undergo these procedures.	• Neuroimaging with MRI, MRA, MRV, or CT as appropriate. At times carotid doppler, echocardiogram, and cardiac arrythmia work up. • No specific testing required for post-procedure headaches, and they can be subclassified using ICHD-3 criteria.	• Generally, symptomatic but be aware of the hemorrhage risk even in ischemic stroke and avoid NSAIDs during acute phase of management. • Most of the time headache treatment is for short duration but if long-term treatment is needed then empirical treatments based on the phenotype of the chronic headache could be used.
Medication-related headache	• Headache can be a side effect of medication use (8%). • MOH is more common (30.1% of headache patients) in older adults because they may be using analgesic for other pain issues. • Triptans and combination analgesics are likely culprits for MOH.	• Careful history of headache in context of starting or stopping a medication is critical diagnosis and ICHD-3 provides guidance for this. • For MOH clear documentation of number of acute medication use is critical.	• Treatment usually will involve stopping the offending medication. • Every MOH should be considered for migraine preventive treatment.

(Continued)

Table 50-2. Specific Features and General Recommendations for Managing Common Secondary Headaches in Older Adults (*Continued*)

Headache Type	Clinical Features	Diagnosis	Treatment
Cervicogenic headache	• The estimated prevalence of cervicogenic headache varies from 1% to 4%. Neck pain incidence peaks in middle age but can be seen in older adults also. • Pain typically starts in the neck and radiates anteriorly to occipital and to the top of head and at times to the forehead on ipsilateral side. Neck movement often triggers headache.	• Could use ICHD-3 criteria or Cervicogenic Headache International Study Group criteria.	• Fluoroscopy-guided blocks like intra-articular atlantoaxial blocks, third occipital nerve block, and medical branch blocks in upper cervical (C1-4) region could be both diagnostic and therapeutic. • Neck muscle strengthening exercises may be beneficial to relieve pain. • Acupuncture and medical massage can also be used for temporary symptom management.
Sleep apnea–related Headache	• Aging is a risk factor for sleep apnea and morning headache is about four times more often in patients with snoring and OSA compared to normal population. • Headache is typically bilateral upon waking up and usually resolve within 4 hours and does not have migraine features (nausea, photo/phonophobia).	• Screen patients suspected of having sleep apnea–related headache with STOP-Bang questionnaire. • Use ICHD-3 criteria for diagnosing sleep apnea–related headache.	• Treatment should be focused on primary sleep disorder and headache usually would improve in conjunction with it. • Symptomatic treatment with simple analgesics could also be used.

CT, computer tomography; ICHD-3, third edition of International Classification of Headache Disorders; MOH, medication overuse headache; MRA, magnetic resonance angiography; MRI, magnetic resonance imaging; MRV, magnetic resonance venography; TIA, transient ischemic attack.

by restlessness or associated autonomic features. Generally, it is a persistent headache disorder happening almost daily but episodic hypnic headache (<15 days/month) has also been reported. Because it follows a circadian rhythm, hypothalamus is considered to be involved in the pathophysiology as evidenced by decreased gray matter volume in some patients. Treatment includes use of caffeine before bed or lithium. Other less effective treatment options are topiramate and indomethacin. In older adults, the differential to hypnic headache includes nocturnal hypertension, hypoglycemia, sleep apnea, medication overuse headache, and secondary intracranial pathology.[2,4,5]

Cardiac Cephalalgia

This headache happens in context of acute myocardial infarction as a referred head pain from stimulation of trigeminovascular nervous system via vagal nerve afferents or somatic afferents from chest pain. According to ICHD-3 criteria, cardiac cephalgia improves with improvement in cardiac ischemia and responds to nitroglycerin. This headache is very important to recognize because of the associated high morbidity.[6,7]

Primary Cough Headache

This headache is also known as Valsalva maneuver headache. It occurs only with cough or straining and is relatively short-lived, lasting few seconds to 2 hours. Headache is usually bilateral and typically involves occipital region. It has a very rare incidence of <1% in specialty headache clinics. Patients with this headache may present to a pulmonary clinic first. Nausea, vertigo, and sleep disturbance are common features in patients with cough headache. Indomethacin 50 to 200 mg/day may be effective in treating this headache. Acetazolamide, metoclopramide, and melatonin can also be used. Rarely CSF removal can also provide relief.[4] If cough remains persistent in older adults, it may need full evaluation for any lung pathology.

Exploding Head Syndrome

This is a unique and rare headache syndrome mostly seen in older adults. Patients typically wake up and describe a sense of loud painless explosive noise that occurs suddenly in the head. It is different from the thunderclap headache due to subarachnoid hemorrhage which is also abrupt but presents with severe pain without reported explosive noise. The feeling of this syndrome could be very frightening but the patient needs to be assured about its benign nature. The polysomnography may be ordered to rule out sleep disorders. Treatment with clomipramine and topiramate has been used for recurrent cases.[8,9]

Chronic Subdural Hematoma

Headache associated with chronic subdural hematoma (CSDH) needs a special mention because this is more common in elderly especially after age 70 years. It is characterized by a very slow abnormal collection of blood in subdural space. Older adults are considered more prone because of cerebral atrophy and subclinical brain injury causing bridging vein trauma leading to leakage of blood and starting a neuroinflammatory cascade leading to formation of hematoma. Initial symptoms may include subacute to chronic headaches but would eventually develop some more ominous features like nausea, ataxia, seizures, mental status changes, weakness, or coma. Treatment generally would need a neurosurgical evaluation and intervention. With recent advances in understanding pathophysiology, some anti-inflammatory treatments like steroids or antifibrinolytic therapies like tranexamic acid have potential to modulate growth of CSDH.[10,11]

Temporal Arteritis

The headache due to temporal arteritis is common in elderly populations and more so in those with age above 70. Temporal arteritis is discussed in detail in Chapter 22.

Treatment

It is generally recommended that when titrating medications in elderly, start low, go slow, and aim for the lowest effective dose. It is important to pay attention to age-related pharmacokinetic and pharmacodynamic changes while choosing a starting dose of acute or preventative medication.

For TTH, first-choice treatment is nonpharmacological intervention (such as biofeedback or relaxation techniques) whenever accessible and accepted by patients (Chapter 13). Acetaminophen is the drug of first choice for acute treatment (nonsteroidal anti-inflammatory drugs should be avoided) and amitriptyline for prevention of TTH, followed by venlafaxine and mirtazapine. Close monitoring is required owing to the risk of adverse effects.

In the elderly, certain medication-specific considerations are helpful for migraine management. Triptans are not contraindicated in elderly just because of age. Topiramate has challenges of complicating cognition and acute angle glaucoma in older adults. Tricyclic antidepressants (TCAs) are prone to give significant anticholinergic side effects in older adults like dry mouth, urinary retention, and cardiac arrhythmias. Vitamin B2 (riboflavin), magnesium, coenzyme Q10, anti-CGRP treatments, and onabotulinumtoxinA seem to be effective and safe options. They are particularly attractive because of low risk for adverse effects (Chapters 7, 8, 43, 47).

Noninvasive neuromodulator devices like Cefaly, Nerivio, and Gammacore also come with minimal side effects and can be suitable options for many elderly (Chapter 46). At times offering multidisciplinary approach involving physical therapy, acupuncture, psychological interventions, and optimal medical care can be considered for long-term headache management in senior adults.

When administering oxygen therapy for cluster headaches in elderly patients, caution must be exercised regarding the potential for acute and chronic toxicity, particularly in the presence of concomitant lung pathology such as chronic obstructive pulmonary disease. It is also important to remain vigilant for acute and chronic side effects of steroids in older adults. Sleep disorders are common in older adults and there is a potential interplay between cluster headache and sleep pathophysiology.[12] Recognizing and addressing sleep issues in older adults may decrease their cluster headache burden also.[13]

Summary

- Headache disorders in elderly should be classified using ICHD criteria.

- Differentiate late-life accompaniments of migraine with persistent aura from aura without headache and transient ischemic attack/stroke with comprehensive history and examination.

- Secondary causes of headache should always be considered in the differential diagnosis of headaches in elderly individuals, even if the headache phenotype appears similar to that of a primary headache.

- Older adults, being susceptible to falls, are at risk for tears of intracerebral veins, leading to subdural hemorrhage, which can manifest as subacute headache.

- When titrating medications in elderly, it is recommended to start with a low dose, go slow, and aim for the lowest effective dose.

- Attention should be paid to age-related pharmacokinetic and pharmacodynamic changes when choosing a starting dose.

REFERENCES

1. van Oosterhout WPJ, Cheung C, Haan J. Primary headache syndromes in the elderly: epidemiology, diagnosis and treatment. *J Clin Transl Res.* 2016; 2(2):45-51.

2. Berk T, Ashina S, Martin V, Newman L, Vij B. Diagnosis and treatment of primary headache disorders in older adults. *J Am Geriatr Soc.* 2018; 66(12):2408-2416.

3. Robblee J, Singh RH. Headache in the older population: causes, diagnoses, and treatments. *Curr Pain Headache Rep.* 2020;24(7):34-38.

4. Bamford CC, Mays M, Tepper SJ. Unusual headaches in the elderly. *Curr Pain Headache Rep.* 2011;15(4): 295-301.

5. Evers S, Goadsby PJ. Hypnic headache: clinical features, pathophysiology, and treatment. *Neurology.* 2003;60(6):905-909.

6. Navarro-Pérez MP, Bellosta-Diago E, Olesen J, Santos-Lasaosa S. Cardiac cephalalgia: a narrative review and ICHD-3 criteria evaluation. *J Headache Pain.* 2022;23(1):136.

7. Sun L, Zhang Q, Li N, Bao S, Wang D, Li X. Cardiac cephalalgia closely associated with acute myocardial infarction. *Am J Emerg Med.* 2021;47:350.e1-350.e3.

8. Pearce JM. Clinical features of the exploding head syndrome. *J Neurol Neurosurg Psychiatry.* 1989;52(7): 907-910.

9. Palikh GM, Vaughn BV. Topiramate responsive exploding head syndrome. *J Clin Sleep Med.* 2010; 6(4):382-383.

10. Edlmann E, Giorgi-Coll S, Whitfield PC, Carpenter KLH, Hutchinson PJ. Pathophysiology of chronic subdural haematoma: inflammation, angiogenesis and implications for pharmacotherapy. *J Neuroinflammation.* 2017;14(1):108.

11. Feghali J, Yang W, Huang J. Updates in chronic subdural hematoma: epidemiology, etiology, pathogenesis, treatment, and outcome. *World Neurosurg.* 2020;141:339-345.

12. Tatineny P, Shafi F, Gohar A, Bhat A. Sleep in the elderly. *Mo Med.* 2020;117(5):490-495.

13. Barloese M, Lund N, Petersen A, Rasmussen M, Jennum P, Jensen R. Sleep and chronobiology in cluster headache. *Cephalalgia.* 2015;35(11): 969-978.

Special Populations

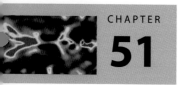

51

Headache in Sexual and Gender Minority Individuals

Patrick Ebbert, Anna Pace, and Eric A. Kaiser

Managing headache disorders in sexual and gender minority individuals poses several questions. Are individuals who are using gender-affirming hormone therapy (GAHT) at higher risk for certain secondary headache disorders? What effects may GAHTs have on primary headache disorders? What drug-drug interactions should be considered for individuals using GAHTs when prescribing acute and preventive headache medications? How does sexual and gender minority stress influence headache prevalence and severity? How can you as a neurologist provide welcoming, affirming clinical care for sexual and gender minorities? Unfortunately, there is a large scientific gap in how best to provide care for this underserved, stigmatized population. The following will outline some key considerations when providing headache care for individuals who identify as lesbian, gay, bisexual, transgender, and gender diverse (Table 51-1).

Epidemiology

Data from the 2013–2018 National Health Interview Survey demonstrated prevalence of headache/migraine was higher in bisexual women (36.8%) and lesbians (24.7%) as compared to heterosexual women (19.7%), and higher in bisexual men (22.8%) and gay men (14.8%) as compared to heterosexual men (9.8%).[1] The precise prevalence of primary headache disorders in the transgender and gender-diverse population is not known, and there have been no large population-based studies assessing this question. In a small sample study, the rate of migraine among transgender women who had received GAHT was reported to be similar to that of cisgender women in the general population, at about 25%.[2] Even the estimated proportion of transgender individuals itself has been difficult to specify given a wide range of heterogenous studies over decades, although a recent survey by the U.S. Census Bureau indicates that approximately 0.6% of U.S. adults identify as transgender.[3] With 2020 U.S. census data of 258.3 million adults, all else being equal, this would estimate adult transgender individuals with migraine at more than 246,000 in the United States alone.

Pathophysiology

Sex hormones play a role in migraine pathophysiology, both influencing migraine prevalence as well as directly correlating with migraine attacks. It is well known that migraine is more common in cisgender women than cisgender men overall (see Chapter 5). Links between estrogens, androgens, and hormonal supplementation and migraine have been shown. It stands to reason then that differences in hormonal profiles, whether endogenous or exogenous, could play a role in shaping migraine pathogenesis. Estrogens have a complex relationship with migraine and have been shown to have both analgesic and hyperalgesic

Table 51-1. Glossary of Terminology and Nomenclature

Gender identity	Describes one's personal sense of their own gender, which may or may not align with one's sex assigned at birth; e.g., man, woman, no gender, or something else
Sex assigned at birth	Based on an infant's external genitalia, can be male or female
Assigned male at birth (AMAB)	Term used to refer to being assigned "male" at birth
Assigned female at birth (AFAB)	Term used to refer to being assigned "female" at birth
Cisgender	Describes a person whose gender identity is congruent with their sex assigned at birth
Transgender	Describes a person whose gender identity is different than the person's sex assigned at birth
Trans-masculine	Describes a person who was assigned female sex at birth and identifies with masculinity more than femininity
Trans-feminine	Describes a person who was assigned male sex at birth and identifies with femininity more than masculinity
Gender nonbinary	Describes a person whose gender identity falls outside of the traditional gender binary structure
Gender queer	An umbrella term that describes a person whose gender identity falls outside the traditional gender binary of male and female; some people use the term *gender expansive*
Gender fluid	Describes a person whose gender identity is not fixed, a person may feel more aligned with a certain gender some of the time, another gender at other times, a mix of both genders sometimes, and sometimes no gender at all
Intersex	Describes a group of congenital conditions in which the reproductive organs, genitals, and/or other sexual anatomy do not develop according to traditional expectations for females or males; intersex can also be used as an identity term for someone with one of these conditions
Sexual orientation	Describes a person's sexual, romantic, or emotional attraction to another person and is unrelated to one's gender identity
Lesbian	Describes a woman who is primarily emotionally and physically attracted to other women
Gay	Describes people who are physically attracted to people of the same sex and/or gender as themselves
Bisexual	Describes a person who is physically attracted to women and men
Asexual	Describes a person who experiences little or no sexual attraction to others
Heterosexual/ straight	Describes women who are primarily physically attracted to men, and men who are physically attracted to women

Special Populations

Source: Adapted with permission from Pace A, Barber M, Ziplow J, Hranilovich JA, Kaiser EA. Gender Minority Stress, Psychiatric Comorbidities, and the Experience of Migraine in Transgender and Gender-Diverse Individuals: a Narrative Review. *Current Pain and Headache Repo.* 2021;25(12):82.

properties in different contexts. Relative estradiol withdrawal has been linked to menstrual-related migraine. Stable estrogen supplementation during states of relative estrogen withdrawal such as during the menstrual cycle or menopause has been shown to have a relative analgesic effect.[4] Estrogen receptors are highly expressed in the thalamus and trigeminal nucleus of humans,[5] which may explain the underlying mechanism of estrogen's relationship to migraine.

There is very limited data on the effect of hormonal therapy on migraine in transgender individuals. These limited data suggest that estrogen-based GAHT in transwomen may cause a worsening of headache, while testosterone-based GAHT in transmen may cause an improvement. A 2007 study reported that 2/47 (4.3%) of transwomen pre-GAHT had headaches, while 5/47 (10.6%) reported headaches post-GAHT; the two participants in this study with preexisting headaches developed worsened symptoms post-GAHT.[6] In transmen, 10/26 (38.5%) participants reported preexisting headache, with three developing new headaches post-treatment. Of the 10 participants who experienced headaches prior to GAHT, testosterone improved pain in six, increased severity in one, and had no change in three participants. Another study in 2021 assessing headache prevalence in transmen found an overall prevalence of 32 out of 88 (36.4%) transmen with symptoms diagnostic of migraine according to ICHD-3 criteria.[7] Of those with migraine headache, half (16/32) were on GAHT; of these, eight participants noted an improvement in their headaches post-GAHT, seven participants noted no change, and one participant noticed worsening.

Clinical Presentation

For gender minority individuals, the presentation of primary headache disorders is unlikely to be altered significantly by GAHT. GAHT may have ill-described effects on headache frequency or increase certain features (i.e., aura with estrogen therapy). However, it is important to consider potential secondary headache disorders that present in transgender and gender-diverse individuals receiving GAHT. Cerebral venous sinus thrombosis (CVST), reversible cerebral-vasoconstriction syndrome (RCVS), and idiopathic intracranial hypertension (IIH) have been described in individuals receiving GAHT,[8] but there is a lack of clinical studies to determine whether there is an actual increase in risk. Large cohort studies have found an increased risk of venous thromboembolism in transgender women, which is thought to be at least in part due to estrogen-containing GAHT, suggesting that there may be an increased risk of CVST.[8] Nevertheless, it is recommended to avoid unilaterally discontinuing estrogen-containing GAHT, which can lead to increased gender dysphoria and risk of suicide. Instead, carefully discuss risks and benefits of estrogen therapy, and consider lowering the dose and/or switching formulations.

Treatment Considerations

For individuals using GAHT, take caution in prescribing new medication to avoid potential drug-drug interactions. Antiepileptic drugs (AEDs) for prevention pose the greatest risk as they are often inducers (and occasionally inhibitors) of the CYP 3A4 pathway, which metabolizes endogenous and exogenous sex hormones.[9] For transgender women receiving GAHT, avoid topiramate (especially doses >200 mg/day), carbamazepine, and oxcarbazepine, which are CYP 3A4 inducers and may reduce estrogen levels.[9] Valproate, zonisamide, and gabapentin have no significant impact on estrogen levels, thus are relatively safe to use.[9] Monitor lamotrigine levels for patients using estrogen-containing GAHT.[9] For transgender men, avoid zonisamide, carbamazepine, and oxcarbazepine, which may reduce testosterone levels.[9] Valproate may increase testosterone levels.[9] Topiramate and gabapentin have no significant impact on testosterone levels.[9] If considering AEDs that may alter hormone levels, discuss potential interactions with the patient and coordinate hormone level monitoring with their GAHT prescriber. OnabotulinumtoxinA and anti-CGRP monoclonal therapies may be a safe and effective alternative that avoids these potential drug-drug interactions.

Prognosis

Recent studies suggest that transgender and gender-diverse individuals with migraine may experience a significant burden of disease, as they report higher pain scores and a lower quality of life compared to cisgender counterparts.[10] There is a high prevalence of anxiety, depression, and other psychiatric conditions in sexual and gender minority individuals, along with a prior history of trauma, which may affect migraine incidence and severity, though this has not been explicitly studied.[11] Sexual and gender minority stress may also play a role in worsening health outcomes, as many sexual and gender minority individuals experience stigma, discrimination, and microaggressions in healthcare as well as in other life circumstances.[12] It is crucial to screen for psychiatric comorbidities when patients are seen in clinic for headache, to allow for appropriate behavioral health referrals and collaborative multidisciplinary care.

Summary

- Sexual minorities report higher rates of migraine than heterosexual individuals, but the prevalence of headaches in gender minority individuals remains poorly characterized.
- Estrogen-based hormone therapy has been associated with an increased risk of CVST, but this risk can potentially be reduced by lowering the estrogen dosage and considering transdermal administration methods.
- GAHTs may exacerbate or improve underlying primary headache disorders.
- For patients receiving GAHT, be cautious of potential drug-drug interactions when prescribing acute and preventive headache medications.
- It is important to screen for psychiatric comorbidities in sexual and gender minority patients and refer for behavioral health management when needed to reduce headache burden.

REFERENCES

1. Heslin KC. Explaining disparities in severe headache and migraine among sexual minority adults in the United States, 2013–2018. *J Nerv Ment Dis.* 2020;208(11):876-883.
2. Pringsheim T, Gooren L. Migraine prevalence in male to female transsexuals on hormone therapy. *Neurology.* 2004;63(3):593-594.
3. US Census Bureau. New Household Pulse Survey Data Reveal Differences between LGBT and Non-LGBT Respondents During COVID-19 Pandemic [Internet]. Census.gov. 2021. Available at: https://www.census.gov/library/stories/2021/11/census-bureau-survey-explores-sexual-orientation-and-gender-identity.html.
4. Brandes JL. The influence of estrogen on migraine: a systematic review. *JAMA.* 2006;295(15):1824-1830.
5. Cseh A, Farkas KM, Derzbach L, et al. Lymphocyte subsets in pediatric migraine. *Neurol Sci.* 2012;34(7):1151-1155.
6. Aloisi AM, Bachiocco V, Costantino A, et al. Cross-sex hormone administration changes pain in transsexual women and men. *Pain.* 2007;132 (Supplement 1):S60-S67.
7. Yalinay Dikmen P, Ertas M, Kosak S, et al. Primary headaches among gender dysphoric female-to-male individuals: a cross-sectional survey on gender transition experience. *Headache: The Journal of Head and Face Pain.* 2021;61(8):1194-1206.
8. Hranilovich JA, Kaiser EA, Pace A, Barber M, Ziplow J. Headache in transgender and gender-diverse patients: a narrative review. *Headache: The Journal of Head and Face Pain.* 2021;61(7):1040-1050.
9. Johnson EL, Kaplan PW. Caring for transgender patients with epilepsy. *Epilepsia.* 2017;58(10):1667-1672.
10. Nagata JM, Ganson KT, Tabler J, Blashill AJ, Murray SB. Disparities across sexual orientation in migraine among US adults. *JAMA Neurol.* 2020;78(1):117-118.
11. Freitas LD, Léda-Rêgo G, Bezerra-Filho S, Miranda-Scippa Â. Psychiatric disorders in individuals diagnosed with gender dysphoria: a systematic review. *Psychiatry Clin Neurosci.* 2019;74(2):99-104.
12. Pace A, Barber M, Ziplow J, Hranilovich JA, Kaiser EA. Gender minority stress, psychiatric comorbidities, and the experience of migraine in transgender and gender-diverse individuals: a narrative review. *Curr Pain Headache Rep.* 2021;25(12):82.

Special Populations

PART VII

Special Topics

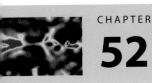

CHAPTER

52

Practical Professional Ethics in Headache Medicine

Morris Levin and Robert E. Shapiro

Medical ethics is concerned with principles that are intended to guide behavior by members of the medical community. Medical professionalism might be defined as the behavior that is expected of members of our profession. The two are different but obviously overlap. This chapter focuses on common and important professional ethical issues which are particularly likely to arise in research, practice, and teaching in Headache Medicine, and provides some practical ways of approaching them.

Ethical Principles

Basic tenets of modern medical ethics consist of four principles outlined by Thomas Beauchamp and James Childress in their authoritative text *Principles of Biomedical Ethics* (see Reference list): (1) Respect for our patients' *Autonomy* (their rights to informed choices in therapy), (2) *Beneficence* (that we act in the best interest of the patient), (3) *Nonmaleficence* (to not be the cause of harm), and (4) *Justice* (general fairness and equity).[1] A case could be made to add two more: *Honesty* and *Confidentiality*. Most ethical questions that arise involve one of these major areas but often, multiple principles may be at play and, not uncommonly, principles may collide. And, in many common medical ethical controversies, clear answers are not available, and practical compromises are often necessary. Guidance is available, such as the American Medical Association (AMA) Codes of Conduct (found at www.ama-assn.org) and guidelines of the Ethics Committee of the American Headache Society, as well as other published resources.[2,5] Why is it important for clinicians to adopt a strict code of behavior? One reason is that ethical standards often mirror the law—and naturally clinicians want to avoid legal problems. But another reason is that we want our patients to be able to trust us, so they will come to see us, follow our recommendations, and pay us for the services; and for that to happen we need to present ourselves as having a strong professional code of ethics. Sadly, trust in the medical profession has declined. Attention to professionalism can hopefully begin to reverse that trend.

Conflict of Interest

Conflict of interest (COI) in medicine, the clash between one's self-interest and one's professional obligations (especially patients' interests) is almost unavoidable. The obvious example is the tension between achieving the net income to support a practice or department and the imperative to providing service to patients who might be struggling to afford to pay for care. But the existence of the COI is not the problem—it is the way in which it is managed. For example, if a physician has been paid to promote a migraine prophylactic medication and later gives a lecture at a medical conference about headache prevention, but makes their relationship with the pharmaceutical company clear, and also specifically points out to the audience all areas of potential bias—many would consider this to be adequate COI management. Of course, some COI cannot be managed and needs to be eliminated—the simple example being the nearly universal prohibition on selling treatments that one prescribes.[4]

The *appearance* of COI, even when there is a good case to be made for there not being *actual* COI, is also to be avoided for the simple reason that it reduces trust. An example might be a researcher whose published study results are authored by an employee of the company that produces the therapeutic agent studied in the trial. Prudent management would be for the investigator to either write or thoroughly review all published material.

It has been argued that the problem of unaddressed COI has been exaggerated, and that small payments or gifts from industry are inconsequential. However, it has been shown that our prescribing behavior can be influenced by even modest drug company inducements, and that patients believe pharmaceutical companies do influence our practices.

Issues of Justice: Equity in Headache Medicine Care

Discrimination against patients for any reason, including race, gender, religion, lack of religion, appearance, age, and medical diagnoses, obviously violates ethical principles. And in the United States, it is against the law (Federal Civil Rights Act of 1964 and the Age Discrimination Act of 1975). Yet there is good evidence that some groups are cared for differently than others (see also Chapter 53). A notable example involves the racial disparities in receiving appropriate testing and treatment of pain conditions. To overcome discrimination, it is imperative that we educate ourselves about our biases, especially unconscious ones (implicit bias).

Health equity, the ability of everyone to have the same opportunity to have good healthcare, is an ethical imperative. But health inequity is widespread, exemplified by the existence of medically underserved populations and areas (MUPs, MUAs). These have traditionally referred to groups or areas with sparse primary care resources, but the concepts should also pertain to all important medical services, including headache care. At the time of writing, there are around 700 board-certified headache specialists in the United States where there are arguably many millions of people with headache disorders who warrant specialty care. This dramatic undersupply of important specialists requires governmental attention but also would seem to require those already established in the field to support training in Headache Medicine in any way we can.

Another equity issue involves access to effective treatments. New powerful tools like calcitonin gene-related peptide antagonist medications and neuromodulatory devices are unaffordable for many. In the United States, where drug prices are high and rising, we do need to talk to patients about therapies in a balanced way, including cost-benefit analyses. And we probably do need to advocate for fairly priced treatments from pharmaceutical manufacturers and reasonable coverage from health insurance companies.

Analgesic Use: Overprescribing Versus Withholding

Our prime mission is to relieve the suffering caused by headache disorders, both preventively and, when that fails, acutely. But knowing the risks of tolerance, toxicity, and withdrawal with some of the most potent (opioid) analgesics produces conflict between our mission to relieve suffering and the principle of nonmaleficence. And in Headache Medicine we have the additional proviso to avoid medication overuse headache. Careful prescribing, vigilance, and the use of state pharmaceutical monitoring systems can allow prudent prescribing in selected patients. Further, for headache patients that are already receiving chronic opioid maintenance therapies, it is important to respect that physician-forced tapering of these medications, no matter how well-intended, may potentially lead to more harm than benefit.

Identifying and Learning from Medical Errors

Kohn and colleagues, in their 1999 groundbreaking study "To Err Is Human,"[3] found that between 44,000 and 98,000 hospital deaths each year resulted from medical errors. Subsequent studies have found significantly higher numbers. Naturally, some degree of medical error occurrence is inevitable, despite our best efforts to minimize it, whether outpatient or inpatient. However, examining medical errors tends to lead to systemic improvements, which improve patient outcomes. Establishing an effective reporting system that focuses not on blame but on identification of errors for the purpose of system improvement is the best way to manage medical errors, and individual physicians must become comfortable using whichever reporting system is in place in their institutions.

A challenging question in the medical error area is that of "disclosure," i.e., letting the patient know about an error involved in their care. To withhold information from patients and families in these situations seems unethical, yet full disclosure has traditionally not occurred, for reasons including embarrassment, legal liability, and lack of experience in disclosing unpleasant information. Surprisingly, patients are actually less likely to file malpractice suits when physicians apologize and fully disclose errors. It has been shown that patients are keenly interested in (1) how the error happened, (2) how the effects on them will be mitigated, and (3) what is being done to prevent it from happening to someone in the future. It is becoming clear that clinicians and institutions who practice this type of transparency benefit both financially and more importantly, in their relationships and reputations in their communities.

Research Design and Participation

There are several general ethical guidelines that one should follow when becoming involved in clinical research. One is the importance of designing and conducting drug or device trials that could be made available to and actually help a great number of patients (rather than, for example, helping to market products or extend patents for existing drugs). Informed consent should always be truly informed. One should be completely comfortable with the methods of analyzing and subdividing data. And one should remember to maintain independence from clinical trial sponsors for any trials we participate in, including the right to publish negative outcomes.

Physician Responsibilities and Burnout

Burnout has been defined as the state of emotional, physical, and mental exhaustion caused by excessive and prolonged stress. It occurs when one feels overwhelmed, emotionally drained, and unable to meet constant demands. Burnout in medicine is an ethical concern as it can lead to reduced health resources and has been shown to lead to increased harm to patients. And it just makes sense to preserve the health of those who help to maintain our health. It has been recently noted that neurologists and, in particular, headache specialists have a high burnout rate—nearly 60%—arising from dissatisfaction with work schedules, insurance company policies, malpractice concerns, patient telephone calls, compensation, frustrations with the electronic health record (EHR), the assignment of previously nonphysician tasks like coding and billing, time limits on patient visits, and productivity benchmarks. Unfortunately, health systems often try to address physician burnout with programs to improve individual efficiency and resilience, whereas successfully addressing this problem requires system-wide solutions. Negotiating for minimum time standards for outpatient visits, limits on active caseloads, and flexible schedules will help. Encouraging and providing time and resources for maintaining balanced personal and social connections, good sleep hygiene, eating, and exercise routines are all essential ingredients—aka, self-care.

And finally, a timely question: what are our responsibilities in times of crisis like the COVID-19 pandemic? Does self-care direct us to be cautiously self-protective in risky situations? This has been explored in the past with the conclusion being that in times of crisis, we do need to incur some risk and "step up" when called. This had included headache specialists deployed to inpatient neurological services, caring for contagious patients. In addition, many of us had continued to provide necessary procedures like botulinum injections, nerve blocks, and myofascial trigger point injections. The rationale behind this service is that we are uniquely trained to do it, and the time to balk at selfless patient care would have been prior to entering the field. However, we can and should demand the best possible safety precautions, a schedule that does not promote sleep deprivation, and mental health services when needed for stressed clinicians. And in academic settings, temporary emphasis on direct clinical care during times of crisis should not become permanent, to the detriment of research and education missions that are essential to ensuring the best possible care for future patients.

Summary

- Maintaining high standards of professional behavior is essential for all physicians for a number of reasons.

- In Headache Medicine, patients are often in very vulnerable and sometimes desperate positions, and rely on specialists for unbiased, patient-centered advice; therefore, managing COI properly is essential.

- Disparities in healthcare continue to exist and it is imperative for practitioners to think about and attempt to rectify inequities they encounter.

- Disclosing medical errors in both inpatient and outpatient settings is considered an ethical imperative.

- In times of pandemic, it is expected that practitioners will continue to provide in-person services as long as they are provided protective equipment and processes.

- At the same time practitioners should practice appropriate self-care in order to avoid burnout.

REFERENCES

1. Beauchamp T, Childress J. *Principles of Biomedical Ethics.* 8th ed. New York, NY: Oxford University Press; 2019.
2. Bernat JL. *Ethical Issues in Neurology.* Philadelphia, PA: Lippincott Williams & Wilkins; 2008.
3. Kohn LT, Corrigan JM, Donaldson M. *To Err Is Human: Building a Safer Health System.* Washington, DC: Institute of Medicine; 1999.
4. Levin, M. Practical professional ethics in headache medicine. *Headache.* 2020;60:2053-2058.
5. Russel JA, Hutchins JC, Epstein LG; on behalf of the AAN Ethics Law and Humanities Committee. American Academy of Neurology Code of Professional Conduct. *Neurology.* 2021;97:489-495.

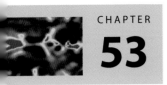

CHAPTER

53

Headache Medicine and Racial/Ethnic Disparities

Larry Charleston, IV

According to the Center for Disease Control and HealthyPeople.gov 2030, health disparities are defined as differences in the prevalence and severity of disease and/or disease treatment that are rooted in social inequalities and adversely affect groups of people who have systematically experienced greater obstacles to health based on the following factors: racial or ethnic group; religion; socioeconomic status; gender; age; mental health; cognitive, sensory, or physical disability; sexual orientation or gender identity; geographic location; or other characteristics historically linked to discrimination or exclusion. Health disparities are also considered the measure of health equity. Health equity strives to improve the standard of health of all people and reducing health disparities by improving the health of marginalized, vulnerable, and socially disadvantaged individuals and not by worsening the health of advantaged groups.[1] Headache Medicine disparities exist but may not be fully known. Headache Medicine disparities are likely due to multifactorial processes and effect several areas of headache healthcare. This chapter focuses on racial/ethnic disparities in Headache Medicine.

Factors Associated with Healthcare Disparities

Racism

Race is not inherently biological but rather a social construct.[2] This is important to understand as both laypeople and medical professionals can hold false beliefs with regard to race based on skin color or self-identified country of origin. A "race"-conscious society lends itself to racial biases and, importantly, racism. Racism is a social determinate of health marked by discrimination of particularly groups deemed be "inferior" or "minority." People are not minorities, rather, certain populations have been minoritized. For example, for over 80% of the U.S. history, Blacks or African-Americans (AA) were subject to slavery or laws that institutionalized discriminatory practices against them. These discriminatory practices led to suboptimization of housing, health, wealth, education, environments, social interactions, and affluency for many AA. Moreover, AA have faced health inequities for 100% of the U.S. history. Other groups of color have also faced discriminatory practices. AA were "legally" enslaved for approximately 60% of American history. Thus, it is important to have cultural sensitivity or humility when engaging with patients from different backgrounds and cultures, and acknowledge a sense of individuality while avoiding stereotypes.[3]

Bias

Bias is the evaluation of something or someone that can be positive or negative. Unchecked biases can result in untoward behaviors done with awareness, conscious or explicit bias (e.g., prejudice) or without awareness, unconscious or implicit bias (e.g., unintended discrimination).[4] Implicit and explicit biases toward people of color have been pervasive throughout the U.S. history, including in medicine. Negative biases toward people of color have been documented in clinical settings.[5] These biases untowardly impact treatment recommendations, health outcomes, patient-provider relations, patient adherence, and trust. Racial bias in pain perception is positively associated with racial bias in treatment recommendations. Weak racial bias in pain can be seen in children as early as of age 7 years old and strong reliable racial bias in pain at age 10.[6] Specific racial bias in Headache Medicine needs further elucidation.

Other Factors

A social determinant of health is the social factors that drive health outcomes. The social determinants of health thought to play a role in headache disparities include:

- Historical injustices, discrimination (e.g., redlining), and its implications
  ○ Unconscious (implicit) biases
    ■ Microaggressions
  ○ Conscious (explicit biases)
    ■ Macroaggressions
  ○ Institutional or systemic racism
- Socioeconomic status
- Social environment
  ○ Adverse childhood events (ACEs)
- Insurance status
- Lack of specialists
- Lack of diverse representation in research
- Provider biases
- Decreased "race" and social concordance with headache providers
- Low headache literacy (patient and providers)
- Miscommunication and/or misperceptions about the presence and/or severity of pain
- Healthcare, medication, and therapy costs
- Limited access to healthcare and the appropriate treatments
- Mistrust
- Attitudes, beliefs, and behaviors that influence the acceptance of appropriate analgesics and analgesic doses

While it is important to have variables and comparators to understand differences, for centuries, there has often been a comparison of ethnic groups to white Americans in studies, as such, may be presented in the data shared in this chapter. Nevertheless, we have to be careful to avoid the subtle inference that white Americans are the "standard" group. While currently this may help us make sense of data and disparities, as we look to make positive changes in equity diversity inclusion and belonging, a comparison of expected and observed may provide another approach to obtain feasible data.

Examples of Disparities in Headache Care in U.S. Populations

There is a research framework to examine racial/ethnic disparities in healthcare. Nevertheless, very few studies have investigated racial/ethnic disparities in Headache Medicine.[7] The data are limited with some derived from epidemiological studies. AA have received less accurate diagnosis and have a decreased quality of life compared to Non-Hispanic White (NHW) Americans.[8] AA report the second highest ictal cutaneous allodynia, second to American Indian Alaskan Natives (AIAN). There is increased associated depressive symptoms, severity, chronicity, and frequency with migraine. AA have a higher mistrust of the healthcare system and may be less likely to visit ambulatory care settings for the treatment of migraine disorders. Nearly half of AA patients who do visit ambulatory care do not receive any abortive medication for migraine. It is possible AA patients are more likely to visit the emergency department (ED) for headache care. Although studies have been mixed, AA may also receive lower-value care for migraine. Pediatric populations are affected as well.[7] Children of color were less likely to receive neuroimaging in and, less likely to receive any acute medications compared to NHW pediatric populations. AA children are less likely to have ED visits for sports-related head injuries and less likely to receive a concussion diagnosis than NHW.

AIAN population has the highest prevalence of migraine and severe headache in the United States. Compared to all Americans, AIAN population has ~39% more reports of migraine and severe headache.[8] AIAN populations report the highest ictal cutaneous allodynia. The annual incidence of traumatic brain injury (TBI) and concussion among AIAN is ~104% higher than all population groups in the United States.

Hispanic/Latinx (H/L) populations are 50% less likely to receive a migraine diagnosis than NHW.[8] H/L children who presented to the ED with mild TBI had a higher likelihood of decline in social, academic, and/or physical functioning at 3 months than NHW children. H/L ethnicity is a predictor of decreased access to medical care for chronic pain.

Box 53-1 presents ten strategies to mitigate racial and ethnic disparities in the clinical practice of Headache Medicine.

Box 53-1. Ten Suggestions to Address and Ameliorate Racial/Ethnic Disparities in Headache Medicine Clinical Practice

1. Understand that racial/ethnic disparities in Headache Medicine are likely due to multifactorial processes and affect several areas of headache healthcare
2. Increase self-awareness and bystander training
3. Bias and cultural sensitivity assessments and training
4. Make significant and enduring changes in organizational leadership to enhance inclusion in key decision-making processes
5. Incorporation of education of Headache Medicine disparities in curricula, grand rounds, etc.
6. Continued education regarding racism (especially as social determinants of health and unconscious bias), health and headache disparities
7. Increasing means of headache care access by engaging underrepresented communities in clinical care and research
8. Work to earn trust with marginalized communities (build social concordance)
9. In organizations: enhance their focus on disparities and equity in meetings, symposia, and continuing medical education offerings for members
10. Implement the "Golden Rule" principle with clinical, education, and professional encounters ("Do unto others as you will have them do unto you")

Special Topics

Summary

- Racial/ethnic disparities in Headache Medicine exist but may not be fully known.
- Headache Medicine disparities are likely due to multifactorial processes and affect several areas of headache healthcare.
- Social determinants of health including discriminatory practices may play a significant role in disparities.
- Headache Medicine data and inclusion of diverse populations are lacking.
- Implicit biases in pain perception may be culturally relevant, more apparent with time pressures, and contribute to disparities in pain/headache management; racial/ethnic biases in pain perception may begin as early as 7 years old.
- Populations underrepresented in medicine are needed in the Headache Medicine pipeline and headache research.

REFERENCES

1. Centers for Disease Control and Prevention. *What is Health Equity?* Retrieved on July 11, 2023. Available at: https://www.cdc.gov/nchhstp/healthequity/

2. Bailey ZD, Feldman JM, Bassett MT. How structural racism works: racist policies as a root cause of U.S. racial health inequities. *N Engl J Med.* 2021;384(8): 768-773.

3. Charleston L 4th. Cross-cultural headache care within the United States: speaking the unspoken. *Headache.* 2020;60(8):1832-1836.

4. Charleston L 4th, Spears RC, Flippen C 2nd. Equity of African American men in headache in the United States: a perspective from African American headache medicine specialists (Part 1). *Headache.* 2020;60(10):2473-2485.

5. Hall WJ, Chapman MV, Lee KM, et al. Implicit racial/ethnic bias among health care professionals and its influence on health care outcomes: a systematic review. *Am J Public Health.* 2015;105(12):e60-e76.

6. Dore RA, Hoffman KM, Lillard AS, Trawalter S. Children's racial bias in perceptions of others' pain. *Br J Dev Psychol.* 2014;32(2):218-231.

7. Charleston L 4th. Headache disparities in African-Americans in the United States: a narrative review. *J Natl Med Assoc.* 2021;113(2):223-229.

8. Kiarashi J, VanderPluym J, Szperka CL, et al. Factors associated with, and mitigation strategies for, health care disparities faced by patients with headache disorders. *Neurology.* 2021;97(6):280-289.

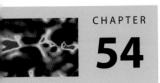

CHAPTER

54 Telemedicine in Headache Medicine

Nina Riggins and Raissa Villanueva

Due to the public health emergency with the COVID-19 pandemic in March 2020, the removal of legislative barriers, historically faced by clinicians, allowed for the timely adoption of telehealth as a mode of healthcare delivery. With major regulatory and health policy changes, telemedicine visits allowed for the safe management of patients while protecting both patients and the healthcare workforce in a time of rapid spread of the COVID-19 disease.[1] The authors believe that telemedicine is here to stay for a variety of applications in the field of headache medicine.

According to a survey of members of the American Headache Society (AHS), responders were comfortable treating persons living with migraine via telehealth.[2]

New advancements in technology, including the use of artificial intelligence, may pose greater benefits along with substantial ethical considerations.[3] Other advances in technology such as remote patient monitoring and wearable devices are also important in the future care of patients. With these advances, there will always be a need to recognize when a face-to-face visit is necessary.

Telehealth

The American Academy of Neurology defines telehealth as various electronic and telecommunication technologies for the delivery of virtual medical services. Telehealth allows clinicians to provide care when participants (members of the healthcare team and patients with their families) are separated by distance or time. Telehealth includes synchronous (such as audio and video two-way interactive communication) or asynchronous communication (such as patient portal messages or images sent through secure email). The term "telemedicine" often refers to synchronous two-way, real-time interactive audio (such as phone appointments if audio only) and video exchange (telemedicine appointments). Telehealth allows providers to remotely perform a neurologic assessment and gather a history, including review of headache diaries and medications, thereby optimizing patient care.[4]

Telemedicine

Patients with headache disorders and other neurologic diseases can be complex and chronic; they may require more frequent follow-up appointments. Telemedicine visits can enhance patients' access to medical care in headache medicine. For patients with known diagnosed primary headache disorders, without new neurologic symptoms, telemedicine can be the preferred method of delivering care because there is less reliance on performing a neurologic exam and clinicians can rely on obtaining the history virtually to make medical management decisions. Telemedicine can decrease the financial cost, time burden, and potential stress of traveling to appointments, and minimizes disruption of daily routines for patients such as time away from work and family. For patients with headache disorders, in particular, these telemedicine visits can also decrease exposure to possible triggers for migraine attacks such as light, noise, and smells. Telemedicine visits can be a powerful tool for counseling and patient education. Social determinants of health may also be reviewed during remote visits.

However, there is a role for face-to-face appointments, especially for new patient visits when "red flags" in history may suggest a secondary headache disorder (see Chapter 1). When medical history suggests reliance on the neurologic exam to help in diagnosis, a face-to-face visit may be more appropriate for evaluating the patient. Patients may also not have access to proper technology such as wireless internet or video cameras to allow for a telemedicine visit. Patients may not have the privacy to discuss medical issues around family members at home. The hybrid model combining in-person and remote visits has a promise in the future of headache medicine.

Preparation for Telemedicine Visit

Prior to the virtual visit, the clinician should do the following:

- Make sure that glare and distracting noises are minimized.
- For image quality, ensure lighting is positioned in front of the person on video. Blue-blocking screens and glasses can be suggested for use by patients in order to prevent triggering a migraine attack from looking at the screen.
- Position your image in the middle of the video frame and optimize eye contact with the patient by looking at the camera directly. Try to have the camera at the level of your face so you do not have to look from upside down.
- Minimize distracting noises. Turn any sound notifications off for email and other applications on the computer. Silence any office phone or cell phone notifications as well.
- Background should be professional and nondistracting.
- Dress professionally.
- It is recommended making sure that you have patient's phone number handy. This way, if wireless connection fails, you might be able to conduct a phone appointment.
- Be prepared to arrange a face-to-face visit when appropriate.

Beginning the Telemedicine Visit

Upon entering the visit, the clinician should do the following:

1. Introduce yourself and any others accompanying the visit from the clinical side.
2. Use two patient identifiers at the start of the visit.
3. Patient should be consented to perform the visit by video.
4. Discuss with the patient that a Health Insurance Portability and Accountability Act (HIPAA)-compliant technology is utilized during the visit.
5. You should inform the patient of the limitations of the remote visit, such as conducting a limited neurologic exam.
6. You need to confirm the location of the patient. It includes making sure that the patient is in the state/region where you are allowed by law to perform this telemedicine visit.
7. If the patient connects to video visit from a situation, when you do not feel comfortable to continue telemedicine visit (e.g., if you see that patient is driving during telemedicine appointment), you should immediately communicate the reason that you will need to discontinue and offer to reschedule an appointment or reconnect by video or phone after they stop driving.
8. You should ask the patient to introduce other people in the same room with them.

History Taking in Telemedicine Visit

Taking a history for a telemedicine visit for a patient with headache should be similar to an in-person visit. The headache diary should be reviewed with the patient, including frequency, intensity of symptoms, and use of acute pain medications. See Chapter 1 for further details on history taking.

Physical and Neurological Examination in Telemedicine Visit

If the patient has home-monitoring devices such as blood pressure machine and weight scale, this data can be very useful and should be collected as part of the telemedicine visit. Evaluation of mental status and general appearance usually mirrors the one conducted in the medical office.

If you suspect a secondary headache during a telemedicine appointment and need a fundoscopic exam, in-person tests, or imaging to make a diagnosis, you should immediately arrange for an in-person evaluation and the necessary tests. For example, if patient has reports visual changes and pulsatile tinnitus, you should consider timely face-to-face evaluation for intracranial hypertension. Clinician may ask the patient to remove the glasses if needed for part of the neurologic exam.

Head and Neck Examination

Observe if the head is normocephalic and atraumatic, and note any changes in the range of motion in the neck.

Mental Status

Mental status can be assessed by the patient's ability to give a history and recall events in the history. This also allows you to assess language, dysphasia, mood and affect. If chief complaint warrants assessing language in more depth, you can ask the patient to name, read, and repeat phrases. Recall of words can be tested during the visit if there are cognitive complaints are in the history.

Cranial Nerves

Make a note of any cranial autonomic symptoms such as redness of the eyes, ptosis, and runny nose. A detailed cranial nerve examination during a video telemedicine visit is described below.

Cranial Nerve I (Olfactory)

Always ask the patient about their sensation of smell.

Cranial Nerve II (Optic)

Changes in pupils might be observed when the video quality is good. You may need to ask the patient to move closer to the camera when possible, for an optimal look at their pupils. Flashlights can be used to evaluate pupillary constriction. Visual fields can be assessed by asking the patient to count fingers in the four quadrants of the screen.

Cranial Nerves III, IV, and VI (Oculomotor, Trochlear, and Abducens)

You can ask the patient to look up, down, and side to side, and then have them follow your finger with their gaze. In addition, you may be able to identify nystagmus and ptosis when present when the patient is close enough to the camera.

Special Topics

Cranial Nerve V (Trigeminal)

You can ask the patient to check sensation to touch in all three branches of trigeminal nerve by using their finger or a tissue.

Cranial Nerve VII (Facial)

Similar to a face-to-face visit, you can ask the patient to move their facial muscles (e.g., smile, raise their eyebrows, etc.). Asymmetry of the face at rest and during facial movement should be noted.

Cranial Nerve VIII (Vestibulocochlear)

Patient can perform finger rub test on themselves and report if they have a difference in hearing between left and right sides.

Cranial Nerves IX and X (Glossopharyngeal and Vagus)

It might be challenging to check for palate elevation but this can be attempted. Changes in voice and dysarthria should be noted.

Cranial Nerve XI (Accessory)

Shoulder shrug and neck rotation can be assessed visually.

Cranial Nerve XII (Hypoglossal)

Observe tongue protrusion, ask to move their tongue side to side, and evaluate for changes, such as asymmetry, atrophy, and fasciculations.

Motor Examination

Muscle strength can be tested against gravity only. Toe walking and heel walking could be observed when there are no concerns about unsteadiness and risk of falls. Severe muscle tone changes can be visible, such as spastic gait, but subtle changes in tone cannot be assessed in a telemedicine visit. If you believe that examination of reflexes is necessary, you will need to arrange for a face-to-face visit. Pronator drift or bicycling of arms can be performed to assess for subtle arm weakness.

Sensory Examination

The patient can be asked to use a tissue to check sensation to touch. Be careful when asking them to perform a Romberg test and stay on the safe side: if you have any concerns about any risk of falls, please document that as a reason for the Romberg test not being performed.

Coordination

Finger-to-nose, finger tapping, and heel-to-sheen maneuvers are used similar to in-person visits.

Gait

The patient can be asked to show you how they are walking, when possible and appropriate.

Overall, the neurologic exam in a telemedicine visit can be informative, but an in-person examination may be necessary to perform the fundoscopic exam, confrontational muscle strength testing, and reflex testing to assess muscle tone.[5]

Webside Manner: Addressing Patients Professionally

Physicians must approach telemedicine visits with enhanced listening skills and empathy. Since some subtleties in communication can be more difficult to pick up during audio-video communication, clinicians must be conscious of this difference and come prepared for this type of interaction on video.

Summary

- Telehealth allows the relaying of digital information to provide care, and may include two-way interactive conferencing, mobile health applications, virtual check-ins, electronic consultations, telephone services, or remote patient monitoring.

- History taking and physical examination during a telemedicine visit allow the clinician to remotely assess the patient and evaluate the necessity for a timely in-person visit.

- Telemedicine provides value in the evaluation of chronic medical conditions such as in headache medicine, where there is more reliance on the clinical history and less reliance on the neurologic exam for known primary headache disorders.

- Telemedicine serves as a tool for optimizing resource utilization.

- Telemedicine supports patient-centered care and can enrich in-person care.

- More research studies are needed to assess the best telehealth techniques and overcome limitations and concerns about cybersecurity.

REFERENCES

1 Grinberg AS, Fenton BT, Wang K, et al. Telehealth perceptions and utilization for the delivery of headache care before and during the COVID-19 pandemic: a mixed-methods study. *Headache.* 2022;62(5):613-623.

2. Minen MT, Szperka CL, Kaplan K, et al. Telehealth as a new care delivery model: the headache provider experience. *Headache.* 2021;61(7):1123-1131.

3. Dave T, Athaluri SA, Singh S. ChatGPT in medicine: an overview of its applications, advantages, limitations, future prospects, and ethical considerations. *Front Artif Intell.* 2023;6:1169595.

4. Hatcher-Martin JM, Busis NA, Cohen BH, et al. American Academy of Neurology telehealth position statement. *Neurology.* 2021;97(7):334-339.

5. Robblee J, Starling AJ, Halker Singh RB, Riggins N. Teleneurology for primary headache disorders. *Pract Neurol.* 2020:31-39.

Index

Note: Page numbers followed by *b*, *f*, and *t* indicate boxes, figures, tables, respectively